T0263105

Neonatal and Perinatal Nutrition

Editors

AKHIL MAHESHWARI
JONATHAN R. SWANSON

CLINICS IN PERINATOLOGY

www.perinatology.theclinics.com

Consulting Editor
LUCKY JAIN

June 2022 • Volume 49 • Number 2

ELSEVIER

1600 John F. Kennedy Boulevard • Suite 1800 • Philadelphia, Pennsylvania, 19103-2899

http://www.theclinics.com

CLINICS IN PERINATOLOGY Volume 49, Number 2
June 2022 ISSN 0095-5108, ISBN-13: 978-0-323-89766-2

Editor: Kerry Holland
Developmental Editor: Karen Solomon

Clinics in Perinatology (ISSN 0095-5108) is published quarterly by Elsevier Inc., 360 Park Avenue South, New York, NY 10010-1710. Months of issue are March, June, September, and December. Business and Editorial Offices: 1600 John F. Kennedy Blvd., Ste. 1800, Philadelphia, PA 19103-2899. Customer Service Office: 3251 Riverport Lane, Maryland Heights, MO 63043. Periodicals postage paid at New York, NY and additional mailing offices. Subscription prices are $331.00 per year (US individuals), $823.00 per year (US institutions), $376.00 per year (Canadian individuals), $860.00 per year (Canadian institutions), $448.00 per year (international individuals), $860.00 per year (international institutions), $100.00 per year (US and Canadian students), and $195.00 per year (International students). International air speed delivery is included in all Clinics subscription prices. All prices are subject to change without notice. **POSTMASTER:** Send address changes to *Clinics in Perinatology*, Elsevier Health Sciences Division, Subscription Customer Service, 3251 Riverport Lane, Maryland Heights, MO 63043. **Customer Service: Telephone: 1-800-654-2452** (U.S. and Canada); **1-314-447-8871** (outside U.S. and Canada). **Fax: 1-314-447-8029. E-mail: journalscustomerservice-usa@elsevier.com** (for print support); **journalsonlinesupport-usa@elsevier.com** (for online support).

Reprints. For copies of 100 or more, of articles in this publication, please contact the Commercial Reprints Department, Elsevier Inc., 360 Park Avenue South, New York, NY 10010-1710. Tel. 212-633-3874; Fax: 212-633-3820; E-mail: reprints@elsevier.com.

Clinics in Perinatology is also published in Spanish by McGraw-Hill Interamericana Editores S.A., P.O. Box 5-237, 06500 Mexico D.F., Mexico.

Clinics in Perinatology is covered in *MEDLINE/PubMed (Index Medicus) Current Contents, Excepta Medica, BIOSIS and ISI/BIOMED.*

Contributors

CONSULTING EDITOR

LUCKY JAIN, MD, MBA
George W. Brumley Jr Professor and Chairman, Department of Pediatrics, Emory University School of Medicine, Chief Academic Officer, Children's Healthcare of Atlanta, Executive Director, Emory + Children's Pediatric Institute, Atlanta, Georgia, USA

EDITORS

AKHIL MAHESHWARI, MD
Neonatologist and Vice-President for Academic Affairs, Millennium Medical Group, Jackson Heights, New York; Chair, Global Newborn Society, Clarksville, Maryland, USA

JONATHAN R. SWANSON, MD, MSc
Professor of Pediatrics, Division of Neonatology, University of Virginia, Chief Quality Officer for Children's Services, Medical Director for the Neonatal Intensive Care Unit, University of Virginia Children's Hospital, Charlottesville, Virginia, USA

AUTHORS

BELAL ALSHAIKH, MD, MSc
Neonatologist, Community Health Sciences, O'Brien Institute of Public Health, Alberta Children's Hospital Research Institute, Pediatrics, Cumming School of Medicine, University of Calgary, Calgary, Alberta, Canada

NITASHA BAGGA, MBBS, DNB
Department of Neonatology, Rainbow Children's Hospital, Hyderabad, India

STEPHANIE MERLINO BARR, MS, RDN
Neonatal Dietitian, Department of Pediatrics, MetroHealth Medical Center, Cleveland, Ohio, USA

ERYNN M. BERGNER, MD
Section of Neonatal-Perinatal Medicine, Assistant Professor, Department of Pediatrics, University of Oklahoma Health Sciences Center, Oklahoma City, Oklahoma, USA

CYNTHIA L. BLANCO, MD
Professor, Pediatrics, UT Health San Antonio, Division Director, Neonatology Services, University Health System, San Antonio, Texas, USA

CATHERINE O. BUCK, MD
Assistant Professor, Department of Pediatrics, Yale School of Medicine, New Haven, Connecticut, USA

SUSAN DAI, MSc, RD
Clinical Dietitian, Nutrition Services, Alberta Children's Hospital, Neonatal Follow-Up Clinic, Alberta Health Services, Calgary, Alberta, Canada

KEYUR DONDA, MD
Department of Pediatrics, University of South Florida Health Morsani College of Medicine, Tampa, Florida, USA

TANIS R. FENTON, PhD, RD
Professor, Community Health Sciences, O'Brien Institute of Public Health, Alberta Children's Hospital Research Institute, Cumming School of Medicine, University of Calgary, Nutrition Services, Alberta Health Services, Calgary, Alberta, Canada

LAURA A. GOLLINS, MBA, RD, LD, CNSC
Clinical Program Coordinator, Neonatal Nutrition Program, Neonatology, Texas Children's Hospital, Houston, Texas, USA

SHARON GROH-WARGO, PhD, RDN
Professor, Nutrition and Pediatrics, Case Western Reserve University, MetroHealth Medical Center, Cleveland, Ohio, USA

AMY B. HAIR, MD
Associate Professor, Section of Neonatology, Assistant Professor, Department of Pediatrics, Baylor College of Medicine, Texas Children's Hospital, Houston, Texas, USA

KATHRYN A. HASENSTAB, BS BME
Innovative Infant Feeding Disorders Research Program, Center for Perinatal Research, Abigail Wexner Research Institute, Nationwide Children's Hospital, Columbus, Ohio, USA

SUDARSHAN R. JADCHERLA, MD, FRCPI, DCH, AGAF
Nationwide Foundation Endowed Chair in Neonatology, Professor of Pediatrics and Associate Division Chief, Innovative Infant Feeding Disorders Research Program, Center for Perinatal Research, Abigail Wexner Research Institute, Division of Neonatology, Division Pediatric Gastroenterology, Hepatology and Nutrition, Department of Pediatrics, Nationwide Children's Hospital, Department of Pediatrics, College of Medicine, The Ohio State University College of Medicine, Columbus, Ohio, USA

SANGEETA JAIN, MD
Associate Professor, Division of Maternal-Fetal Medicine, University of Texas Medical Branch, Galveston, Texas, USA

SUNIL K. JAIN, MD
Professor of Pediatrics and Obstetrics, Medical Director, Premature Infant Follow-Up Clinic, Division of Neonatology, Department of Pediatrics, University of Texas Medical Branch, Galveston, Texas, USA

AAMIR JAVAID, BS
Department of Medicine, University of Virginia School of Medicine, Charlottesville, Virginia, USA

JONATHAN MEDERNACH, DO
Fellow of Pediatric Gastroenterology, Hepatology, and Nutrition, Department of Pediatrics, University of Virginia Children's Hospital, University of Virginia, Charlottesville, Virginia, USA

JENNIFER KIM, MD
Department of Pediatrics, Division of Neonatology, University Hospital, San Antonio, Texas, USA

VIKKI LALARI, MSc, RD
Clinical Dietitian, Neonatal Intensive Care Unit, Vancouver, British Columbia, Canada

AKHIL MAHESHWARI, MD
Chair, Global Newborn Society, Clarksville, Maryland, USA

CAMILIA R. MARTIN, MD, MS
Associate Director, NICU, Department of Neonatology, Beth Israel Deaconess Medical Center, Associate Professor of Pediatrics, Harvard Medical School, Boston, Massachusetts, USA

L. ADRIANA MASSIEU, RD, LD, CNSC
Department of Clinical Nutrition Services, Texas Children's Hospital, Houston, Texas, USA

JEREMY P. MIDDLETON, MD
Associate Professor, Department of Pediatrics, University of Virginia Children's Hospital, University of Virginia, Charlottesville, Virginia, USA

ANGELA M. MONTGOMERY, MD, MSEd
Assistant Professor, Department of Pediatrics, Yale School of Medicine, New Haven, Connecticut, USA

MOHAN PAMMI, MD, PhD, MRCPCH
Professor, Section of Neonatology, Department of Pediatrics, Baylor College of Medicine, Texas Children's Hospital, Houston, Texas, USA

RAVI M. PATEL, MD, MSc
Associate Professor Division of Neonatal-Perinatal Medicine, Department of Pediatrics, Emory University School of Medicine and Children's Healthcare of Atlanta, Georgia, USA

MEGAN E. PAULSEN, MD
Assistant Professor, Department of Pediatrics, University of Minnesota Medical School, Minneapolis, Minnesota, USA

PATTI H. PERKS, MS, RDN, CNSC
Neonatal Intensive Care Unit, University of Virginia Children's Hospital, Charlottesville, Virginia, USA

MURALIDHAR H. PREMKUMAR, MBBS, DCH, DNB, MRCPCH, MS
Division of Neonatology, Department of Pediatrics, Baylor College of Medicine, Texas Children's Hospital, Houston, Texas, USA

RAGHAVENDRA B. RAO, MD
Professor, Department of Pediatrics, University of Minnesota Medical School, Minneapolis, Minnesota, USA

KRISTIN SANTORO, MD
Neonatal-Perinatal Medicine Clinical Fellow, Division of Newborn Medicine, Department of Pediatrics, Boston Children's Hospital, Boston, Massachusetts, USA

AMUCHOU SORAISHAM, MBBS, MD, DNB, DM, FRCPC
Department of Pediatrics, Cumming School of Medicine, University of Calgary, Calgary, Alberta, Canada

JONATHAN R. SWANSON, MD, MSc
Professor of Pediatrics, Division of Neonatology, University of Virginia, Chief Quality
Officer for Children's Services, Medical Director for the Neonatal Intensive Care Unit,
University of Virginia Children's Hospital, Charlottesville, Virginia, USA

SANA SYED, MD, MSCR, MSDS
Division of Pediatric Gastroenterology and Hepatology, Department of Pediatrics,
University of Virginia School of Medicine, Charlottesville, Virginia, USA

SARAH N. TAYLOR, MD, MSCR
Section of Neonatology, Associate Professor, Department of Pediatrics, Yale School of
Medicine, New Haven, Connecticut, USA

RACHAEL TROTMAN, RD, CNSC
Neonatal Intensive Care Unit, University of Virginia Children's Hospital, Charlottesville,
Virginia, USA

JACLYN B. WIGGINS, MD
Division of Neonatology, Department of Pediatrics, University of Virginia, Charlottesville,
Virginia, USA

Contents

> Prematurity and other complications at birth are nutritional emergencies. Parenteral nutrition is a bridge to enteral nutrition for a few days or months, and sometimes the sole source of nutrition for life. Parenteral nutrition regimens are constructed to provide adequate and balanced energy, macronutrients, and micronutrients to support growth and prevent deficiencies. Neonatal parenteral nutrition regimens are complicated by periodic shortages of essential products, compatibility challenges, and contaminants. Newborns benefit from serial growth assessments, monitoring of biochemical status, nutrition-focused physical examinations, and management by a multidisciplinary team to ensure adequacy of parenteral nutrition and promote best outcomes.

> Fatty acids are critical bioactives for fetal and neonatal development. Premature delivery and current nutritional strategies pose several challenges in restoring fatty acid balance in the preterm infant. The impact on fatty acid balance and outcomes using lipid emulsions, enteral nutrition, and enteral supplements are reviewed, including a summary of the most recent large clinical trials of enteral fatty acid supplementation for the preterm infant. Research gaps remain in successfully implementing nutritional strategies to optimize fatty acid status in preterm infants.

> Hypoglycemia is a common condition in the newborn period. Several intrinsic and extrinsic factors play a role in the degree/duration of hypoglycemia. Multiple thresholds have been proposed as a potential point whereby hypoglycemia may have short and long-term adverse effects. Rather than a "numerical" threshold, treatment approaches should be individualized and tailored to the etiology, symptoms, and neonatal underlying conditions. Hyperglycemia in the newborn period is commonly seen in preterm infants and can exert gluco-toxic effects in organs at critical periods of development. Considering the peripheral insulin resistance (IR) of prematurity and contributing factors is key to achieving euglycemia.

> This article summarizes the available evidence reporting the relationship between perinatal dysglycemia and long-term neurodevelopment. We review the physiology of perinatal glucose metabolism and discuss the controversies surrounding definitions of perinatal dysglycemia. We briefly review the epidemiology of hypoglycemia and hyperglycemia in fetal, preterm, and term infants. We discuss potential pathophysiologic mechanisms contributing to dysglycemia and its effect on neurodevelopment. We highlight current strategies to prevent and treat dysglycemia in the context of neurodevelopmental outcomes. Finally, we discuss areas of future research and the potential role of continuous glucose monitoring.

1000 days from conception to a child's second birthday to optimize early development. Future research directed toward better biomarkers of malnutrition before acute clinical symptoms develop will help direct targeted efforts toward at-risk populations.

Mohan Pammi and Ravi M. Patel

Preterm infants are at higher risk of mortality and morbidity compared with those born at term. Nutrition-related morbidities include poor growth, immune deficiency, nutritional deficiencies, and adverse long-term neurodevelopment. In addition to macronutrients, many nutritional supplements have been used to enhance growth and development, and decrease infections. Nutrients can enhance preterm infants' immune status, optimize the microbiome, improve growth and development, and influence the risk of necrotizing enterocolitis, sepsis, and other outcomes.

Kathryn A. Hasenstab and Sudarshan R. Jadcherla

Infants in the neonatal intensive care unit (NICU) frequently have feeding difficulties with the root cause remaining elusive to identify. Evaluation of the provider/parent/infant feeding process may provide objective clues to sources of feeding difficulty. Specialized testing may be necessary to determine if the infant's swallowing skills are dysfunctional, immature, or maldeveloped, and to determine the risk of feeding failure or chronic tube feeding. Current evidence-based diagnostic and management approaches resulting in successful oral feeding in the NICU infant are discussed.

Muralidhar H. Premkumar

Due to recent advances, the mortality due to short bowel syndrome (SBS) has significantly decreased, but the morbidities are still high. Morbidities arising specifically due to dysmotility in SBS include feeding intolerance, prolonged dependence on parenteral nutrition, and associated complications such as intestinal failure associated liver disease, and bloodstream infections. The understanding of the pathogenesis of dysmotility in SBS has improved vastly. However, the tools to diagnose dysmotility in SBS in infants are restrictive, and the medical therapies to treat dysmotility are limited. Surgical techniques available for the treatment after failure of conservative management of dysmotility offer hope but carry their associated risks. The evidence to support either the medical therapies or the surgical techniques to treat dysmotility in SBS in children is scarce and weak. Development of newer therapies and efforts to build evidence to support currently available treatments in treating dysmotility in SBS is needed.

Jonathan Medernach and Jeremy P. Middleton

Feeding intolerance is ubiquitous in neonatal intensive care units with as many signs and symptoms as possible diagnoses. Optimizing nutrition is paramount in both preterm and term infants. Determining the cause of feeding intolerance and adjusting nutrition interventions is an important part of the daily care of newborns. This review discusses the role of malabsorption and food intolerance as possible causes of nutrition difficulties in the newborn.

Muralidhar H. Premkumar, Amuchou Soraisham, Nitasha Bagga, L. Adriana Massieu, and Akhil Maheshwarl

Short bowel syndrome (SBS) of infancy is a cause of prolonged morbidity with intolerance to enteral feeding, specialized nutritional needs, and partial/total dependence on parenteral nutrition. These infants can benefit from individualized nutritional strategies to support and enhance the process of intestinal adaptation. Early introduction of enteral feeds during the period of intestinal adaptation is crucial, even though the enteral feedings may need to be supplemented with an effective, safe, and nutritionally adequate parenteral nutritional regimen. Newer generation intravenous lipid emulsions can be effective in preventing and treating intestinal failure-associated liver disease. Prevention of infection(s), pharmaceutical interventions to enhance bowel motility and prevent/mitigate bacteria overgrowth, and specialized multidisciplinary care to minimize the injury to other organs such as the liver, kidneys, and the brain can assist in nutritional rehabilitation and lower the morbidity in SBS.

CLINICS IN PERINATOLOGY

SERIES OF RELATED INTEREST

Obstetrics and Gynecology Clinics of North America
https://www.obgyn.theclinics.com

THE CLINICS ARE AVAILABLE ONLINE!
Access your subscription at:
www.theclinics.com

PROGRAM OBJECTIVE

The goal of *Clinics in Perinatology* is to keep practicing perinatologists, neonatologists, obstetricians, practicing physicians and residents up to date with current clinical practice in perinatology by providing timely articles reviewing the state of the art in patient care.

TARGET AUDIENCE

Perinatologists, neonatologists, obstetricians, practicing physicians, residents and healthcare professionals who provide patient care utilizing findings from *Clinics in Perinatology*.

LEARNING OBJECTIVES

Upon completion of this activity, participants will be able to:

1. Recognize the identification of disorders that contribute to neonatal complications in the NICU setting using the appropriate assessment, screening, and diagnostic tools to assist in developing care management based on best practices and ethical considerations.
2. Discuss current controversies in perinatology and its impact on neonates, families, health care providers, and culture.
3. Review the efficacy, risks, and benefits of treatment and prevention strategies, including the use of assistive technology, surgical intervention, genomic testing, and pharmacotherapy.

ACCREDITATION

The Elsevier Office of Continuing Medical Education (EOCME) is accredited by the Accreditation Council for Continuing Medical Education (ACCME) to provide continuing medical education for physicians.

The EOCME designates this journal-based CME activity for a maximum of 16 *AMA PRA Category 1 Credit*(s)™. Physicians should claim only the credit commensurate with the extent of their participation in the activity.

All other health care professionals requesting continuing education credit for this enduring material will be issued a certificate of participation.

DISCLOSURE OF CONFLICTS OF INTEREST

The EOCME assesses conflict of interest with its instructors, faculty, planners, and other individuals who are in a position to control the content of CME activities. All relevant conflicts of interest that are identified are thoroughly vetted by EOCME for fair balance, scientific objectivity, and patient care recommendations. EOCME is committed to providing its learners with CME activities that promote improvements or quality in healthcare and not a specific proprietary business or a commercial interest.

The planning committee, staff, authors, and editors listed below have identified no financial relationships or relationships to products or devices they or their spouse/life partner have with commercial interest related to the content of this CME activity:

Belal Alshaikh, MD, MSc; Nitasha Bagga, MBBS, DNB; Cynthia L. Blanco, MD; Catherine O. Buck, MD; Susan Dai, MSc, RD; Keyur Donda, MD; Tanis R. Fenton, PhD, RD; Laura A. Gollins, MBA, RD, LD, CNSC; Amy B. Hair, MD; Kathryn A. Hasenstab, BS, BME; Sudarshan R. Jadcherla, MD, FRCPI, DCH, AGAF; Sangeeta Jain, MD; Sunil K. Jain, MD; Aamir Javaid, BS; Jennifer Kim, MD; Vikki Lalari, MSc, RD; Akhil Maheshwari, MD; Camilia R. Martin, MD, MS; L. Adriana Massieu, RD, LD, CNSC; Jonathan Medernach, DO; Stephanie Merlino Barr, MS, RDN; Jeremy P. Middleton, MD; Angela M. Montgomery, MD, MSEd; Mohan Pammi, MD, PhD, MRCPCH; Ravi M. Patel, MD; Megan E. Paulsen, MD; Patti H. Perks, MS, RDN, CNSC; Raghavendra B. Rao, MD; Kristin Santoro, MD; Amuchou Soraisham, MBBS, MD, DNB, DM, FRCPC; Jeyanthi Surendrakumar, BE; Sana Syed, MD, MSCR, MSDS; Doreen Thomas-Payne, MSN, BSN, RN, PMHNP-BC; Rachael Trotman, RD, CNSC; Jaclyn B. Wiggins, MD

The planning committee, staff, authors, and editors listed below have identified financial relationships or relationships to products or devices they or their spouse/life partner have with commercial interest related to the content of this CME activity:

Erynn M. Bergner, MD: Researcher: Prolacta Bioscience

Sharon Groh-Wargo, PhD, RDN: Consultant: Baxter

Muralidhar H. Premkumar, MBBS, DCH, DNB, MRCPCH, MS: Consultant: Fresenius Kabi USA

Jonathan R. Swanson, MD, MSc: Speaker: Prolacta Bioscience, Inc.

Sarah N. Taylor, MD: Researcher: Prolacta Bioscience

UNAPPROVED/OFF-LABEL USE DISCLOSURE

The EOCME requires CME faculty to disclose to the participants:

1. When products or procedures being discussed are off-label, unlabelled, experimental, and/or investigational (not US Food and Drug Administration [FDA] approved); and
2. Any limitations on the information presented, such as data that are preliminary or that represent ongoing research, interim analyses, and/or unsupported opinions. Faculty may discuss information about pharmaceutical agents that is outside of FDA-approved labelling. This information is intended solely for CME and is not intended to promote off-label use of these medications. If you have any questions, contact the medical affairs department of the manufacturer for the most recent prescribing information.

TO ENROLL

To enroll in the *Clinics in Perinatology* Continuing Medical Education program, call customer service at 1-800-654-2452 or sign up online at http://www.theclinics.com/home/cme. The CME program is available to subscribers for an additional annual fee of USD 265.00.

METHOD OF PARTICIPATION

In order to claim credit, participants must complete the following:

1. Complete enrolment as indicated above.
2. Read the activity.
3. Complete the CME Test and Evaluation. Participants must achieve a score of 70% on the test. All CME Tests and Evaluations must be completed online.

CME INQUIRIES/SPECIAL NEEDS

For all CME inquiries or special needs, please contact elsevierCME@elsevier.com.

Foreword

The Lifelong Imprint of Early Nutrition

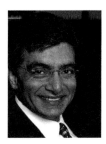

Lucky Jain, MD, MBA
Consulting Editor

A significant body of evidence indicates that the impact of maternal and fetal nutrition goes well beyond the neonatal period. Beginning with early gestation, the first 1000 days represent a time when nutritional factors can have a lasting impact for the rest of the life.[1] While the pathophysiologic effects of severe maternal undernutrition–induced intrauterine growth retardation are well described, severe gestational obesity and excessive nutrition have significant endocrine disruption effects, although the underlying mechanisms are not as well understood.[2] The Barker hypothesis provides a compelling mechanism for metabolic consequences of such perturbations and helps explain why too rapid nutritional recovery after birth can have detrimental consequences. Breast milk and breast-feeding provide a natural protective barrier to some of these consequences. In the end, it is a delicate balance between overnutrition and undernutrition. Supplementation of micronutrients has beneficial effects, but excessive use of these agents also can be detrimental.[3] Evidence points to an epigenetic role of vitamin C in neurodevelopment,[4] and role in cognitive development for folate and choline in addition to several other elements.[5] It is indeed a miracle that most babies do well despite these nutritional challenges and disruptions.

Recent years have also revealed the importance of the gut microbiome as a critical immune modulator in early life, and the impact breast-feeding has on it (**Fig. 1**).[1] As this figure shows, breast milk contains large amounts of bioactive molecules that improve immune defenses. Indeed, breast milk provides a unique pathway for immune modulation of the baby that goes well beyond passive transfer of immunoglobulins. These issues get complicated in the face of premature birth and neonatal complications associated with prolonged hospitalizations and nutritional challenges.

In this issue of the *Clinics in Perinatology*, Drs Swanson and Maheshwari have brought together an impressive lineup of authors and topics to address these critical

Clin Perinatol 49 (2022) xv–xvii
https://doi.org/10.1016/j.clp.2022.04.001
0095-5108/22/© 2022 Published by Elsevier Inc.

perinatology.theclinics.com

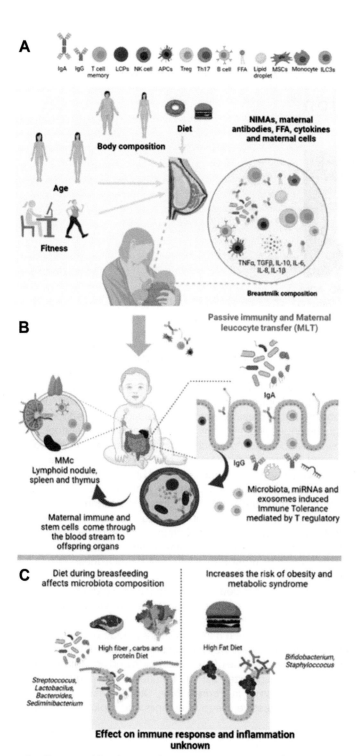

Fig. 1. Breast-feeding provides immunologic programming in the newborn. (*A*) Body weight, age, lifestyle, and diet quality influence breast milk composition, such as lipid

issues in maternal, fetal, and neonatal nutrition. As always, I am also thankful to the publishing staff at Elsevier, including Kerry Holland and Karen Justine Solomon, for their support in bringing this wonderful publication to you.

Lucky Jain, MD, MBA
Department of Pediatrics
Emory University School of Medicine
Children's Healthcare of Atlanta
Emory + Children's Pediatric Institute
2015 Uppergate Drive NE
Atlanta, GA 30322, USA

E-mail address:
ljain@emory.edu

REFERENCES

1. Camacho-Morales A, Caba M, Garcia-Juarez M, et al. Breastfeeding contributes to physiological immune programming in the newborn. Front Pediatr 2021;9:744104. https://doi.org/10.3389/fped2021.744104.
2. Barrea L, Vetrani C, Verde L, et al. Gestational obesity: an unconventional endocrine disruptor for the fetus. Biochem Pharmacol 2022;198:114974. https://doi.org/10.1016/j.bcp.2022.114974.
3. Ballestin SS, Gimenez Campos MI, Ballestin JB, et al. Is supplementation with micronutrients still necessary during pregnancy? A review. Nutrients 2021;13:3134. https://doi.org/10.3390/nu13093134.
4. Coker SJ, Smith-Diaz CC, Dyson RM, et al. The epigenetic role of vitamin C in neurodevelopment. Int J Mol Sci 2022;23:1208. https://doi.org/10.3390/ijms23031208.
5. Irvine N, England-Mason G, Field CJ, et al. Prenatal folate and choline levels and brain cognitive development in children: a critical narrative review. Nutrients 2022;14:364. https://doi.org/10.3390/nu14020364.

species, microbiota, cytokines, and accumulation of immune cell types. (*B*) Maternal antibodies, noninherited maternal antigens, and maternal leukocytes travel through the stomach and intestine of the offspring. Also, maternal immune and stem cells invade the newborn blood, leading to maternal microchimerism to generate immune tolerance. Finally, microbiota and exosomes provide immune tolerance by T-cell accumulation in gut of the offspring. (*C*) A high-fat, carbohydrates, and protein diet intake disrupts microbiota composition by promoting staphylococcus and Bifidobacterium accumulation, whereas high fiber, carbohydrates, and protein lead to lactobacillus microbiota. (*From* Camacho-Morales A, Caba M, Garcia-Juarez M, Caba-Flores MD, Viveros-Contreras R, Martinez-Valenzuela C. Breastfeeding Contributes to Physiological Immune Programming in the Newborn. Front Pediatr. 9:744104.)

Preface

Maternal, Fetal, and Neonatal Nutrition Has Lifelong Implications

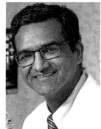
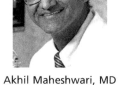

Akhil Maheshwari, MD   Jonathan R. Swanson, MD, MSc
Editors

Nutrition during the late perinatal and neonatal period is an important "environmental" modifier of long-term metabolic, growth, and developmental outcomes.[1-5] Preclinical and human clinical studies show that fetal undernutrition can occur due to maternal undernutrition, altered placental growth, or impaired uteroplacental vascular perfusion.[6,7] In animal models, maternal undernutrition can cause perinatal/neonatal metabolic derangements; cause anatomical/functional changes in the liver, pancreas, and the intestine; predispose to neurobehavioral changes, possible loss of cognitive potential; and even introduce risk factors for long-term outcomes, such as obesity, insulin resistance, and diabetes.[5,8,9] After birth, feeding has been known to influence the functional programming of the gastrointestinal tract, including metabolic, endocrine, and neurologic responses.[10-14] Nutrition can also alter the neonatal microbiome: it can change the timing and proportion in which the microbial flora gets established in the developing gut.[15,16] It can induce and maintain epigenetic changes, which can manifest with subtle interindividual variations in expression of isoforms of digestive enzymes and enterocyte receptors.[17-19] In at-risk premature infants, nutrition has a direct impact on developmental or nutritional anemia and influences the inflammatory milieu.[18,20-24] In some infants, conditions such as necrotizing enterocolitis may cause loss of intestine, both anatomically and functionally, and can set up the infant for further dysfunctional feed-forward loops.[25-27] In the medium/longer term, the loss of intestine can restrict later growth and metabolic health.[28,29] In short, there is good justification for continued investigation of the importance of nutrition during the late-fetal and early-neonatal periods for immediate, medium-, and long-term clinical outcomes.

In this issue, we have focused on the importance of maternal nutrition, metabolic/epigenetic impact of maternal milk lipids, systemic effects of milk-borne lipids and

https://doi.org/10.1016/j.clp.2022.03.001
0095-5108/22/© 2022 Published by Elsevier Inc.

glucose, and the impact of diet on the immune system. Some articles describe the potential benefits and systemic effects of milk fortification and nutritional supplements. An important section discusses the impact and therapeutic strategies to manage altered function/anatomy in infants with swallowing dysfunction, intestinal dysmotility, malabsorption, and short bowel syndrome. We have also evaluated the best methods for nutritional assessment. Finally, there are sections that inform about the impact of inadequate feeding, and the long-term impact of early nutritional management.

Irrespective of your role in the NICU, be it as a consultant or a bedside clinician, this issue of *Clinics in Perinatology* will be of interest. From full-term infants to micropremies, optimal nutrition plays a significant role in the health and well-being of all our little patients.

Akhil Maheshwari, MD
Global Newborn Society
6114 Lily Garden
Clarksville, MD 21029, USA

Jonathan R. Swanson, MD, MSc
University of Virginia Children's Hospital
Hospital Drive
Box 800386
Charlottesville, VA 22903, USA

E-mail addresses:
akhil@globalnewbornsociety.org (A. Maheshwari)
jrs3yc@virginia.edu (J.R. Swanson)

REFERENCES

1. Georgieff MK, Ramel SE, Cusick SE. Nutritional influences on brain development. Acta Paediatr 2018;107(8):1310–21.
2. Kuiper-Makris C, Selle J, Nusken E, et al. Perinatal nutritional and metabolic pathways: early origins of chronic lung diseases. Front Med (Lausanne) 2021;8:667315.
3. Filipouski GR, Silveira RC, Procianoy RS. Influence of perinatal nutrition and gestational age on neurodevelopment of very low-birth-weight preterm infants. Am J Perinatol 2013;30(8):673–80.
4. Fall CH. Fetal malnutrition and long-term outcomes. Nestle Nutr Inst Workshop Ser 2013;74:11–25.
5. Cortes-Albornoz MC, Garcia-Guaqueta DP, Velez-van-Meerbeke A, et al. Maternal nutrition and neurodevelopment: a scoping review. Nutrients 2021;13(10):1–18.
6. Mohan R, Baumann D, Alejandro EU. Fetal undernutrition, placental insufficiency, and pancreatic beta-cell development programming in utero. Am J Physiol Regul Integr Comp Physiol 2018;315(5):R867–78.
7. Reynolds LP, Caton JS, Redmer DA, et al. Evidence for altered placental blood flow and vascularity in compromised pregnancies. J Physiol 2006;572(Pt 1):51–8.
8. Belkacemi L, Nelson DM, Desai M, et al. Maternal undernutrition influences placental-fetal development. Biol Reprod 2010;83(3):325–31.
9. Fandino J, Toba L, Conzalez-Matias LC, et al. Perinatal undernutrition, metabolic hormones, and lung development. Nutrients 2019;11(12):1–18.

10. Lapillonne A, Griffin IJ. Feeding preterm infants today for later metabolic and cardiovascular outcomes. J Pediatr 2013;162(3 suppl):S7–16.
11. Agosti M, Tandoi F, Morlacchi L, et al. Nutritional and metabolic programming during the first thousand days of life. Pediatr Med Chir 2017;39(2):157.
12. Lucas A, Bloom SR, Green AA. Gastrointestinal peptides and the adaptation to extrauterine nutrition. Can J Physiol Pharmacol 1985;63(5):527–37.
13. Kitazawa T, Kaiya H. Regulation of gastrointestinal motility by motilin and ghrelin in vertebrates. Front Endocrinol (Lausanne) 2019;10:278.
14. Lebenthal A, Lebenthal E. The ontogeny of the small intestinal epithelium. JPEN J Parenter Enteral Nutr 1999;23(5 suppl):S3–6.
15. Ho TTB, Groer MW, Kane B, et al. Dichotomous development of the gut microbiome in preterm infants. Microbiome 2018;6(1):157.
16. Ma J, Li Z, Zhang W, et al. Comparison of gut microbiota in exclusively breast-fed and formula-fed babies: a study of 91 term infants. Sci Rep 2020;10(1):15792.
17. Mallisetty Y, Mukherjee N, Jiang Y, et al. Epigenome-wide association of infant feeding and changes in DNA methylation from birth to 10 years. Nutrients 2020;13(1):1–22.
18. Furness JB. Integrated neural and endocrine control of gastrointestinal function. Adv Exp Med Biol 2016;891:159–73.
19. Zhou X, Yang H, Yan Q, et al. Evidence for liver energy metabolism programming in offspring subjected to intrauterine undernutrition during midgestation. Nutr Metab (Lond) 2019;16:20.
20. Hellmuth C, Uhl O, Demmelmair H, et al. The impact of human breast milk components on the infant metabolism. PLoS One 2018;13(6):e0197713.
21. Jian C, Carpen N, Helve O, et al. Early-life gut microbiota and its connection to metabolic health in children: perspective on ecological drivers and need for quantitative approach. EBioMedicine 2021;69:103475.
22. Kiela PR, Ghishan FK. Physiology of intestinal absorption and secretion. Best Pract Res Clin Gastroenterol 2016;30(2):145–59.
23. Simeoni U, Yzydorczyk C, Siddeek B, et al. Epigenetics and neonatal nutrition. Early Hum Dev 2014;90(suppl 2):S23–4.
24. MohanKumar K, Namachivayam K, Song T, et al. A murine neonatal model of necrotizing enterocolitis caused by anemia and red blood cell transfusions. Nat Commun 2019;10(1):3494.
25. MohanKumar K, Namachivayam K, Cheng F, et al. Trinitrobenzene sulfonic acid-induced intestinal injury in neonatal mice activates transcriptional networks similar to those seen in human necrotizing enterocolitis. Pediatr Res 2017; 81(1–1):99–112.
26. Marquardt ML, Done SL, Sandrock M, et al. Copper deficiency presenting as metabolic bone disease in extremely low birth weight, short-gut infants. Pediatrics 2012;130(3):e695–8.
27. Maheshwari A, Patel RM, Christensen RD. Anemia, red blood cell transfusions, and necrotizing enterocolitis. Semin Pediatr Surg 2018;27(1):47–51.
28. Davis EC, Dinsmoor AM, Wang M, et al. Microbiome composition in pediatric populations from birth to adolescence: impact of diet and prebiotic and probiotic interventions. Dig Dis Sci 2020;65(3):706–22.
29. Ziegler MM. Short bowel syndrome in infancy: etiology and management. Clin Perinatol 1986;13(1):163–73.

Neonatal and Preterm Infant Growth Assessment

Tanis R. Fenton, PhD, RD[a,b,*], Susan Dai, MSc, RD[b,c], Vikki Lalari, MSc, RD[d],
Belal Alshaikh, MD, MSc[a,e]

KEYWORDS

- Preterm • Newborn • Infant • growth • Anthropometry • SGA • LGA • Nutrition
- z-scores • length • head circumference • weight

KEY POINTS

- Historically, the comparison of infant growth between sites has been difficult because consistent growth metrics have not been established for universal use.
- Infant growth assessments should include serial measurements for weight, head circumference, and length. These changes need to be evaluated with realistic goals that have been set with consideration of the infants' genetic potential, prenatal influences, nutritional history, and systemic illnesses.
- If an infant does not show weight gain or head or length growth parallel to established growth curves after the postnatal weight loss phase, first ensure that nutrition has been optimized, and evaluate for genetic and prenatal factors, social determinants, and biological disruptive factors, such as brain injury and other systemic illnesses.
- All anthropometric measures show normal biological variation, and therefore, an individual with size at an extreme (outside of the 3rd and 97th percentiles) and/or unusual growth rates for short periods of time could be normal for an individual.

Continued

[a] Community Health Sciences, O'Brien Institute of Public Health, Alberta Children's Hospital Research Institute, Cumming School of Medicine, University of Calgary, 3280 Hospital Drive NW, Calgary, Alberta T2N 4Z6, Canada; [b] Nutrition Services, Alberta Health Services, Calgary, Canada; [c] Alberta Children's Hospital Neonatal Follow-up Clinic, Alberta Health Services, 28 Oki Drive NW, Calgary, Alberta T3B 6A8, Canada; [d] Neonatal Intensive Care Unit, Neonatal Program, BC Women's Hospital and Health Centre, 4500 Oak Street, Vancouver, British Columbia V6H 3N, Canada; [e] Pediatrics, Cumming School of Medicine, University of Calgary, Room C211, Foothills Medical Centre, 1403 29th Street NW, Calgary, Alberta T2N 2T9, Canada
* Corresponding author. Community Health Sciences, O'Brien Institute of Public Health, Alberta Children's Hospital Research Institute, Cumming School of Medicine, University of Calgary, Nutrition Services, Alberta Health Services, 3280 Hospital Drive NW, Calgary, AB, T2N 4Z6, Canada.
E-mail address: tfenton@ucalgary.ca

Clin Perinatol 49 (2022) 295–311
https://doi.org/10.1016/j.clp.2022.02.001
perinatology.theclinics.com

Continued

- Many infants show brief periods of weight loss or slower weight gain during severe illness. If nutritional intake is appropriate per recommended intakes, then the infant should be assessed, as nutrition is appropriate and no changes would be needed in their care. Achievement of birth percentiles, or achievement of any other specific size, are not appropriate goals.
- Clinical and research needs to assess preterm infant growth differ. Growth assessments are used clinically to understand individuals' growth relative to their individual genetic potential and morbidity status. For research purposes, growth of groups needs to be quantified using meaningful metrics.

INTRODUCTION

Infants born at full term typically take about 3 to 4 months to double their weight. In contrast, preterm infants can double their birth weight in 8 weeks with growth rates per kilogram that are more than twice that of infants born at term gestation.[1,2] Neonatal researchers and practitioners now recognize that to achieve appropriate growth, preterm infants need to receive adequate nutrients intake throughout their neonatal intensive care unit (NICU) stay. Preterm infants commonly accumulate nutrient deficits during routine NICU care, which prevents them from achieving their growth potentials.[3,4] Growth assessment remains the most important key to assess nutrition adequacy of preterm infants.

Increasingly, there is evidence indicating a strong association between growth and neurodevelopmental outcomes of preterm infants.[5] Slower growth rates during the NICU stay and after hospital discharge have been associated with adverse outcomes.[5] Although growth at rates similar to intrauterine rates is necessary to achieve good neurodevelopmental outcomes in preterm infants, the attainment of superior growth cannot overcome adversities related to social determinants of health, maternal complications of pregnancy, and neonatal morbidities (**Table 1**). Preterm infants in NICUs face several challenges, such as neonatal stress, brain injury, necrotizing

Table 1 Contributors to altered infant growth	
Prenatal	Social determinants
	Maternal health (medical conditions, such as lupus, anemia, clotting problems, hypertension, diabetes, medications, smoking, alcohol, drugs)
	Infant genetic potential/inherited size
	Genetic disorders
	Multiple pregnancy
	TORCH infection (toxoplasmosis, rubella, cytomegalovirus, human immunodeficiency virus, syphilis)
	Maternal weight/weight gain
Neonatal/ postnatal	Social determinants of health
	Infant genetic potential/inherited size
	Morbidities: brain injury (which includes intraventricular hemorrhage and periventricular leukomalacia), patent ductus arteriosus, bronchopulmonary dysplasia, necrotizing enterocolitis, sepsis
	Neonatal stress
	Nutrition (inadequate nutrient intake, limited oral feeding ability)

enterocolitis, sepsis, and bronchopulmonary dysplasia (BPD). All these challenges can affect growth velocity. Therefore, it is critical to ensure that inadequate nutrition and suboptimal growth do not further contribute to the difficulties that preterm infants may face.

WHAT PRETERM INFANT GROWTH SHOULD WE AIM FOR?

Expert groups recommend that preterm infants should grow and accumulate nutrients similar to the best estimates of how the fetus grows and accretes nutrients.[6,7] Both the American Academy of Pediatrics (AAP) and the European Society for Pediatric Gastro-enterology, Hepatology, and Nutrition (ESPGHAN) also recommend that the nutrition goals for the preterm infant are to provide nutrients to achieve satisfactory neurodevelopment.[6,7]

For growth charts, the AAP endorses both intrauterine (those based on estimated fetal growth) and postnatal growth charts (those that show the actual growth of infants born prematurely). The Intergrowth 21st Project has developed a set of postnatal growth charts based on the patterns of how preterm infants with "an uncomplicated intrauterine life and low neonatal and infant morbidity" grew.[8] The project included growth data on only 28 infants born less than 34 weeks and 12 infants less than 33 weeks[9] Therefore, the AAP recommends that the Intergrowth Charts not be used for infants less than 36 weeks.[10] Preterm infant nutrition support and medical care have been changing over time, and so it is not clear which population in time and which medical and nutrition practices are the best ones to use as a goal to develop postnatal charts. Once adequate sample size postnatal growth charts are established, they will provide a useful adjunct for preterm infant growth monitoring so that health care providers can use both types of charts to compare each infant's growth patterns to both fetal and preterm infant references.

Low growth rates of preterm infants and small attained sizes after term age for weight, length, and head circumference have been repeatedly noted to be associated with adverse neurodevelopmental outcomes.[5] Experts do not recommend the achievement of any specific percentiles for weight, length, or head growth before or by 40 weeks, and they do not recommend return to birth weight percentile after the postnatal weight loss.[6,7] Preterm infants are not likely to gain lean mass more rapidly than fetal growth rates. Gaining weight to return to birth percentiles, which would require gaining at greater than estimated fetal rates, is often a gain of additional body fat only.

PRETERM INFANT GROWTH ASSESSMENT REQUIREMENTS

Adequate infant growth assessments require serial growth measurements, consideration of prebirth influences, respect of an infant's genetic potential, and consideration of influences of neonatal morbidities (see **Table 1**). For ideal growth monitoring, it is important to have realistic goals, try to understand the infant's genetic potential, evaluate nutritional needs, and ensure compliance with evidence-informed guidelines regarding daily nutrient intakes. Some infants may need additional investigations to understand causes of deviant growth patterns.

Health care providers need to focus on overall pattern of head and length growth and weight gain rather than striving to achieve a specific percentile by any specific age. There are normal biological variations in size for all anthropometric measures; therefore, an individual with size at an extreme could be normal for an individual.[35,38] Growth patterns for all anthropometric parameters (ie, weight, length, and head circumference) should be considered individually and in combination. Without serial measurements and an understanding of an infant's growth patterns and preterm infants' expected growth patterns, it is possible to make incorrect growth assessments. If an infant is assessed to be small or large but is already making appropriate catch-up or catch-down growth toward his or her genetic potential and nutrient intake meets the recommended intakes, then changes for his or her nutrition care might not be warranted. If an infants' growth pattern is as expected given the postnatal weight loss and their morbidities, and their nutrition is equal to recommended intakes, then the infant should be assessed as growing appropriately and no changes would be needed in their care. In contrast, if an infant is found to not be achieving recommended nutrition intakes, then regardless of their growth pattern, their nutritional care may need optimization. Some situations are challenging to assess individual infants' nutrition needs and intakes. Examples of challenges include estimating energy needs of infants with BPD and estimating human milk protein and energy content.

GROWTH ASSESSMENT IN LIGHT OF NEONATAL MORBIDITIES

Many neonatal morbidities have important influences on preterm infant growth. Franz and colleagues[11] found that growth to NICU discharge and development at 5 years of age were both associated with severe brain injury, duration of mechanical ventilation, retinopathy of prematurity, and the education of the mother. Of importance, rather than adjusting away the effects of these adversities the infants experienced, they reported the magnitude of different morbidities on neurodevelopmental outcomes to show their relative associations. They found that "the combined contribution of severe [brain injury] and of prolonged mechanical ventilation [on neurodevelopmental outcomes] was >9 times greater than the combined contribution of growth."[11] Others have also found brain injury to be among the most important predictors of adverse neurodevelopment.[12] Of note, Franz and colleagues[11] found head growth, both during NICU stay and after discharge, to be associated with neurodevelopment. Researchers in New Zealand found that early preterm infant protein intakes predicted head growth and neurodevelopmental outcomes.[13]

The actual causal pathway for poor neurodevelopment in units where good nutritional care is provided is likely primarily due to adverse events, including severe brain injury and prolonged mechanical ventilation, which cause both poor growth and poor development.[11,14-38] In units with good nutrition care, growth is more likely a marker for neonatal adversities than a simple reflection of poor nutrition.

PRETERM GROWTH PATTERNS: WHAT IS USUAL GROWTH AND INAPPROPRIATE GROWTH AND WHAT NEEDS TO BE DONE ABOUT IT?

To be able to assess preterm infant growth, it is important to have a good understanding of the usual patterns. Most, but not all, preterm infants lose weight in the first days of life due primarily to water loss as they transition from a water to an air environment (Fig. 1A–D). Many preterm infants do not grow in length or head circumference in the first week of life, so all 3 growth parameters often cross percentiles downwards on growth charts. If adequate nutrition is established, tolerated, and maintained, and when preterm infants avoid severe neonatal morbidities, they then tend to grow approximately parallel to growth chart curves, which shows growth tracking similar to estimates of fetal growth, as shown in growth charts, such as the Fenton preterm growth charts.[15] Prenatal factors, genetic potential, establishment of adequate nutrition, feeding tolerance, and neonatal morbidities will then play a role in the patterns of growth (see Table 1). The following examples of challenging preterm infant growth assessments may help understand the variables that need to be considered.

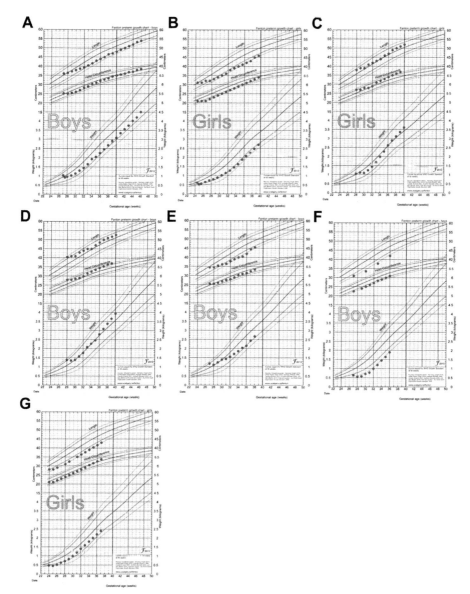

Fig. 1. Seven patterns of appropriate growth. (*A*) AGA baby with normal growth pattern. (*B*) AGA infant with "misnomer extrauterine growth restriction."[35]. (*C*) AGA infant with "upward crossing" due to genetic potential after in utero growth restriction. (*D*) LGA infant with good growth due to genetic potential. (*E*) LGA infant returning to normal growth, maternal diabetes. (*F*) SGA infant with growth parallel growth. (*G*) SGA infant regained birth weight percentile. (*Plotted using* Canadian Pediatric Endocrinology Group. Growth chart plotter for preterm infants 22 to 49 weeks based on Fenton 2013. https://cpeg-gcep.shinyapps.io/prem2013_DDE/ (last accessed Nov 10, 2021).)

ASSESSING SIZE AT BIRTH USING GROWTH CHARTS

There are 2 key purposes for which health care providers use growth charts for infants: (i) to assign size for gestational age as small (SGA), appropriate (AGA), or large (LGA), and (ii) to monitor growth. Perhaps the most immediate use for identifying infants by their SGA and LGA status is to identify infants at birth who need additional monitoring because SGA and LGA infants are at higher risk of hypoglycemia. Several tools are currently available to assess preterm infant's birth size and postnatal growth, such as Olson and Fenton growth charts. Olsen charts are made using American intrauterine size data up to 41 weeks' gestation,[16] whereas Fenton intrauterine size data are based on a 6-country meta-analysis of almost 4 million infants up to 42 weeks' gestation.[15] For assigning size for gestational age for term infants, the World Health Organization (WHO) growth standard[2] at birth could be used because infants born between 37 and 42 weeks were included in the WHO study.

THE VALUE OF ASSESSING Z-SCORES IN PRETERM INFANTS

How useful are the z scores to quantify preterm infant growth? What amount of z-score loss is too much? We do not really know. Z-score losses are variable in any cohort of preterm infants. At this point in time it is not clear how useful changes in z-scores are.

Z-scores define a person's anthropometric measurements (eg, weight, head circumference or length) compared with a growth chart in terms of the number of standard deviations below or above the growth chart median (50th percentile). Changes in z-scores provide information about whether the person's measurement is increasing, decreasing, or staying parallel. Z-scores are considered a good way to quantify a person's anthropometric measurements because they are meaningful for any size, whereas percentiles are not very meaningful at the extremes of size. Numerical values for percentiles at the extremes are small (for example, from −2 to −3 z-scores percentile equivalent values are 0.2 and 0.001, respectively), whereas z-scores remain the size of 1 standard deviation across the distributions.

Neonatal nutrition experts have recently recommended that preterm infant weight losses greater than 2 z-scores is an indicator of severe malnutrition.[17] They also suggest that preterm infant weight losses more more than 1.2 z-scores suggest moderate malnutrition, and losses greater than 0.8 z-scores suggest mild malnutrition. These cut points have not been validated, and there are 2 reasons these cut points need validation: they are arbitrary cut points, and even the healthiest well-nourished preterm infants sometimes lose up to 2 weight z-scores in their first weeks of life.[18]

Rochow and colleagues[18] found that the "healthiest" protocol-nourished less than 30-week gestation preterm infants weights decreased by an average of 0.8 z-scores by 3 weeks of age after their postnatal extracellular water weight loss. These healthy protocol-nourished infants had a considerable range and variability in their z-scores losses; some of these infants had a loss of 2 zscores, whereas others had a small gain in z-scores by 3 weeks of age. Although z-scores and changes in z-scores are useful to quantify infants' sizes, losses, and growth, any arbitrarily-defined growth metric will misclassify some individual infants. Determining an appropriate z-score weight loss guideline requires further validation work on z-score changes to determine whether there is a cutoff associated with adverse outcomes. Although changes in z-scores have the advantage that they adjust for sex and gestational age,[19] changes in z-score expectations may need to be different for SGA (**Fig. 1**F, G) infants and perhaps infants born to mothers who had diabetes (**Fig. 1**E). Because of the current lack of validation for using z-score changes as predictors of health and neurodevelopmental outcome, individuals should not be labeled to their parents as having poor growth owing to a large changes in z-scores.[20]

The figures in this article assume good measurement of length as well as head circumference and weight. Of these 3 parameters, length is the most poorly measured. To be able to adequately assess infant growth, their length needs to be measured periodically by 2 people using a length board and good technique.[6,21]

Appropriate Growth

AGA baby with normal growth pattern

Characterized by postnatal weight loss and slower head and length gain in early weeks, all 3 parameters often shift lower on growth chart curves **Fig. 1**A. Head circumference is first to show recovery toward the median, with final percentiles determined by genetic, nutritional, and medical variables. At week 35, this infant's weight gain velocity slowed to 9 g/kg/d (calculated using the average method)[22]; however, weight gain for the week before was 22 g/kg/d, and the overall pattern shows good growth in all 3 parameters at approximately the estimated intrauterine rate. Recommended weight gain velocity to 36 weeks based on fetal growth estimates is 15 to 20 g/kg/d.[22] The temporary slower rate of 9 g/kg/d is not a concern, because it was a short-term fluctuation and his growth remained appropriate. Weight and length recovery to genetically determined patterns usually occur after term age (40 weeks' postmenstrual age). This baby's birth percentiles were all approximately at the 60th percentile, which does not suggest any concerns. Head circumference has returned close to the 60th percentile at about 41 weeks, while weight is beginning to show some catch up at this age; the birth percentiles are not necessarily the goals because the baby's growth is no longer directly influenced by the uterine environment and so influences are different. This infant is growing appropriately.

AGA infant with "misnomer extrauterine growth restriction

This 24-week gestation baby had a typical growth pattern for a preterm infant, a growth pattern of no concerns **Fig. 1**B. Her weight might be categorized as growth failing because it is below the 10th percentile at 36 weeks; however, that age is too young to show much or any catch-up growth after the postnatal weight loss phase. Her growth is approximately good, parallel to growth chart curves after postnatal weight loss, which means she is meeting her growth goals. Her head and length growth suggest that she may be beginning catch-up growth. Being small (weight, length, head) after term (at 3 to 24 months corrected age) for preterm infants has been associated with poorer cognition.[1,5] Therefore, growth matters, but size at 36 weeks' postmenstrual age is not predictive of neurodevelopment.[1,5] This infant should be not be considered to be growth failing or growth restricted on the basis of weighing less than 10th percentile at 36 weeks[1] and should be nourished using preterm estimated nutrition recommendations.

Using a more comprehensive analysis regarding the diagnostic accuracy of the full range of percentile cut points at 36 weeks for cognitive outcomes, researchers found that across the full range of weight, length, and head circumference measures: no cut point was predictive of cognitive outcomes.[1] Infant growth is very important, as numerous studies have found that the AAP and ESPGHAN recommendation that preterm infants should grow at intrauterine rates is well supported by evidence.[5]

AGA infant with "up-ward crossing" due to genetic potential after in-utero growth restriction

This baby's birth percentiles were higher for length and head circumference than weight, which may suggest some in utero growth restriction **Fig. 1 C**. Her mother had preeclampsia. Both parents were taller than median heights. Health care providers and parents usually do not know an infant's genetic potential, although parental heights can assist making an estimate.[6] This baby shows high placement on the curves for all 3 parameters, with some early before-term catch-up in weight. She regained her weight and head percentiles before 40 weeks, likely because of the combination of being tall based on genetics and in utero growth restriction. SGA preterm infants are more likely to increase their weight percentile while in the NICU than AGA infants.[49] Babies in the AGA category can be growth restricted relative to their genetic potential.

Some neonatal researchers suggested that the expected goal of preterm infant growth is to have the infant return to their birth weight percentile before NICU discharge.[24] However, to regain birth weight percentile after the initial weight loss requires weight gain at rates that are faster than the fetus. Some preterm, particularly SGA, infants do more often than AGA infants regain their birth weight percentile as they catch-up to their lean mass growth potentials. Lean mass growth is influenced by genetics and requires less energy to grow than fat mass[25]; therefore, growth-restricted infants are able to gain weight faster on the same energy owing to their growing a higher proportion of lean mass.

Large-for-gestational-age infant with good growth due to genetic potential

This LGA 28-week preterm infant showed a growth pattern of a proportionate infant (**Fig 1** D). He followed the usual preterm infant pattern of losing some weight postnatally and having a lag in head and length growth, but all 3 of his anthropometric measures are in the upper percentiles. He has not returned to his birth size percentiles by 40 weeks. His growth does not suggest any concerns. Populations of infants of any gestational age are expected to have a wide distribution of percentiles for all anthropometric measures (weight, length, and head). Most of these infants are likely to measure between the 3rd and 97th percentiles. The probability of being smaller than the 3rd percentile or greater than the 97th percentile is small, occurring only among 6% of infants. After the postnatal weight loss that most infants achieve, they will place on the lower percentiles. Although having a birth weight greater than the 90th percentile has been associated with higher rates of hypoglycemia, some of those infants are genetically, not pathologically, greater than the 90th percentile at birth, and are not likely at higher risk of these adverse outcomes. However, some genetically small and large infants are likely to be misclassified by the small, large, and appropriate (SGA/LGA/AGA) categorization.

This infant should continue to be nourished based on evidence-informed nutrition recommendations. This child is not overweight despite weighing in the high percentiles, as his length and head are also in the high percentiles.

Even if this infant's length and head were not also in the high percentiles, it is good practice to continue to provide nutrition within recommended intakes because infants need nutrition support without too much concern about inducing overweight because at older ages preterm infants are at slightly lower risk of overweight.[26–28]

Large-for-gestational-age infant returning to normal growth, maternal diabetes

This LGA 27-week preterm infant had a higher percentile weight compared with his head and length at birth. His mother had poorly controlled diabetes during her pregnancy **Fig. 1**E. At 36 weeks, 9 weeks of age, his placement for weight, head, and length on growth chart curves was similar to a baby that did not have as high a birth weight percentile. His health care team thought that his weight had been elevated at birth because of his mother's diabetes. They were satisfied with his growth and thought he was adapting well. The infant was expected to gradually transition to his genetic potential for growth. This infant's birth weight was likely elevated by his mother's diabetes, and after birth, his weight gain curve was flatter than usual because of his genetic potential. His placement on the growth chart after 34 weeks was similar to the baby in **Fig. 1**A.

Fetal growth can be influenced by prenatal morbidities. Two well-known examples include gestational hypertension that can impede growth, and poorly controlled gestational diabetes that can lead to excess fetal weight gain. Once the infant is no longer in the in utero environment, these influences no longer influence infant growth.

Small-for-gestational-age infant with parallel growth
This SGA 27-week preterm infant had a growth pattern common among SGA infants **Fig. 1**F. His parents had short statures (mother: 150 cm, father: 163 cm), and their son will also likely have a short stature. His small size may be genetic and not pathologic or reflecting restricted growth.

Small infants who are constitutionally small and who have not had their growth restricted are likely to grow in a pattern similar to AGA infants, but they may be somewhat lower on growth chart curves. Although having a birth weight less than the 10th percentile has been associated with higher rates of hypoglycemia, necrotizing enterocolitis, and retinopathy, some of those infants are genetically, not pathologically, less than the 10th percentile at birth, and are not likely at higher risk of these adverse outcomes. This infant should continue to be nourished based on evidence-informed nutrition recommendations. Current nutrition recommendations are not different for SGA compared with AGA infants.

Small-for-gestational-age infant regained birthweight percentile
This SGA 27-week preterm infant regained her weight and head percentiles before term age **Fig. 1**G. Such recovery is seen more frequently in SGA infants than in AGA infants. This infant's regaining of her birth percentile likely reflects her genetic potential supported larger size that she likely would have achieved if her mother was healthy and nutrient delivery via the placenta had been appropriate. Among very preterm infants (<30 weeks) in the PreM Growth Study,[1] the rate of regaining birth percentiles by 36 weeks was greater among SGA infants, presumably because of these infants showing some catch-up growth toward their genetic potential. The rates of regaining birth percentiles by 36 weeks for weight were only 8% of AGA and LGA infants, but 14% among SGA infants.

Regaining head circumference birth percentiles is not a rare occurrence, presumably because of head sparing, that is due to the infant prioritizing head growth over weight gain as well as due in part to the deformational plagiocephaly that many early preterm infants experience, which can affect measurements.[29,30] By 36 weeks, 23% of AGA/LGA infants, but 31% of SGA infants of very preterm infants (<30 weeks) in the PreM Growth Study regained their birth head circumference percentiles. The cause of small birth weight for any given infant depends on their genetically determined size, maternal morbidities, the social determinants of health, and likely in many situations is a combination of all 3 of these factors.

Inappropriate Growth Patterns

Appropriate-for-gestational-age infant with poor growth
This AGA 28-week preterm infant showed a concerning growth pattern that did not keep up with the growth chart curves (**Fig. 2**A). After discharge at term age, his growth deviated further away from the normative data in the growth charts. Numerous prenatal and neonatal conditions contributed to slow his growth both in the hospital and after discharge (see **Table 1**). The health care team, including the dietitian and an

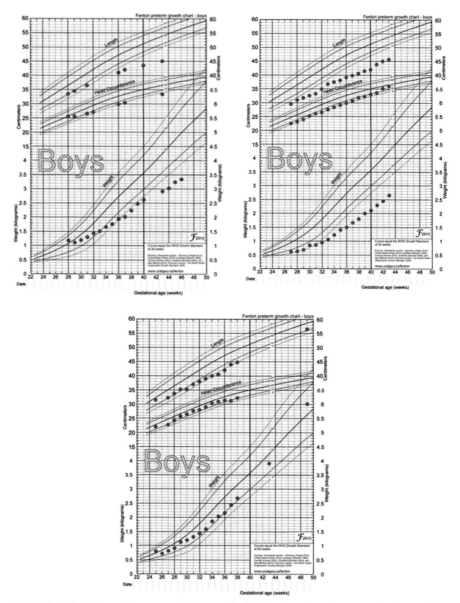

Fig. 2. Three patterns of inappropriate growth. (*A*) Appropriate-for-gestational-age infant with poor growth. (*B*) SGA infant who continues to grow poorly: needs investigation. (*C*) Excessive weight gain (*Plotted using* Canadian Pediatric Endocrinology Group. Growth chart plotter for preterm infants 22 to 49 weeks based on Fenton 2013. https://cpeg-gcep. shinyapps.io/prem2013_DDE/ (last accessed Nov 10, 2021).)

occupational therapist, needed to ensure that his nutrition was adequate, as suboptimum nutrition could further complicate his growth outcomes.

SGA infant who continues to grow poorly: needs investigation
This infant's prenatal history (maternal or fetal) did not provide any explanation for this infant's growth. His growth did not remain parallel to curves (**Fig. 2**B). He had some

feeding intolerance and needed time to adapt to enteral nutrition, but fortunately, he had no important morbidities. Although we need to accept, that even with good nutrition, some deviations from the growth curves can happen, this infant continued to deviate away from the growth chart curves for weight and length. This baby needed to be nourished based on evidence-informed nutrition recommendations (because we lack preterm evidence-informed guidance on how to adapt recommendations for situations of poor growth) with continued follow-up to ensure he is able to grow adequately after discharge and a workup to determine whether the infant has an undiagnosed morbidity.

Poor growth in SGA infants needs special attention, particularly in the absence of known causes of poor fetal growth (**Fig. 2**B). These infants may need further investigations to identify their cause for being SGA. Several rare genetic and endocrine disorders have been reported in preterm infants with severe growth restriction and slow growth velocity. These infants require careful examination of the growth patterns for weight, head, and length, nutrition care received, as well as consideration of additional factors that influence growth, including prenatal contributions (see **Table 1**). Each poorly growing infant (who does not show rates of fetal growth that fit the normative data) indicates the need for further investigation to determine whether poor growth is modifiable or explainable and to determine whether the infant requires more or different care. The goal of neonatal care is to support young infants to achieve the best they can be.

Excessive weight gain

These data are from an AGA 27-week preterm infant. His mother had poorly controlled diabetes during her pregnancy, and at birth he had a higher percentile weight compared (percentile: 67 z-score: 0.5) with his head (percentile: 29 z-score: −0.6) and length (percentile: 35 z-score: −0.4) **Fig. 2**C. At 36 weeks, the growth patterns seemed to be normalizing, and he was beginning to show good transition to oral feeding. At 2 months corrected age, the family informed their dietitian that they had been working very hard to feed him as much as they could manage to keep his weight gain high. She found that his weight was now at the 70th percentile (0.5 z-scores), and height at the 15th percentile (−1 z-scores) based on the growth chart.[15] The dietitian reassured the family that their son was doing well and advised that they focus instead on his feeding cues for hunger and satiety to avoid overfeeding. Inconsistent messaging about growth targets from health care providers and from within the caregiver's community can interfere with responsive feeding, overriding the infant's hunger and satiety, and contribute to overfeeding and excessive weight gain (**Fig. 2**C).

BODY MASS INDEX

Body mass index (BMI; defined as weight in kilograms divided by height in meters squared) has been suggested as a measure to identify appropriate preterm infant growth.[31] However, caution is needed when BMI is used since rising BMIs for preterm infants could easily be misinterpreted. Two groups of researchers have judged that a clinical application for the use of BMI among preterm infants has not been established.[32,33] Using BMI has the same limitations as weight assessments because it would not be clear whether increases are due to excess fat or improved lean mass gain; additionally, BMI measurements could increase in preterm infants because of typically slower length gain (see **Fig. 1**A) than weight gain. A further limitation of using BMIs for any population is that they do not assess body composition but rather simply express weight relative to height. Furthermore, any inaccuracies in length measurement, which are common for infants,[21] would be amplified. For populations other than preterm infants, higher and increasing BMIs are used as a crude screening tool to identify possible excess body weight. Usually, preterm infant weight catches up before length so their BMIs would be expected to increase. Rising preterm infant BMIs might be considered by some to indicate too rapid body mass gain when the actual reason for the higher values could be delayed length growth. Wells and colleagues[23] found that preterm infant discharge BMI z-scores were above the reference median because length z-scores were consistently lower than weight z-scores.

BODY COMPOSITION

Higher preterm infant body fat percent observed at term age has been a recent concern among neonatal health care providers; however, evidence suggests that it is temporaty and does not persist, so it is not a reason to restrict growth. A recent review summarized body composition data on preterm and term infants between 35 and 65 weeks postmenstrual age (PMA). At 40 weeks, preterm infants had a higher percentage body fat than term infants (16% vs 11%, respectively; $P<0.001$), but by 52 weeks PMA, percent fat mass was similar for preterm and term infants, averaging 24% to 25%.[34] It appears likely that all infants gain body fat over their first postnatal months,[35,36] and that this occurs at a younger postmenstrual age for preterm infants versus term infants, so it is only different in the short term.

Many are also concerned about lower lean mass for preterm infants at 40 weeks' PMA; however, body composition studies suggest that this is also a temporary phenomenon. The review by Hamatschek and colleagues[34] found that preterm infants compared with term newborn infants had significantly lower fat-free mass by 400 g on average at 40 weeks' PMA, but this difference decreased to less than 100 g when both groups were 60 weeks' PMA. It is worth realizing that preterm infants are not likely to gain lean mass beyond fetal growth rates. Therefore, for nonintrauterine growth-restricted infants to regain birth percentiles following their postnatal weight loss and to then continue to grow and reach body composition of a typical term infant would require gaining at greater than estimated fetal rates, which would likely require gaining additional body fat.

A recent study reinforces that NICU nutrition provision is important to achieve good outcomes. Researchers observed that higher energy and protein intakes in the first week of life and protein intakes throughout hospitalization were associated at discharge with higher fat-free mass z-scores but not higher percent body fat z scores. They also found that higher fat-free mass z-scores at discharge were associated with higher Bayley III scores.[37] This finding that preterm infant body fat percentage at discharge was not related to nutrition intakes reinforces that the frequently seen higher percent body fat at term age is likely a postnatal adaption.

NOURISHING INFANTS BASED ON GROWTH PATTERNS AND INFANT FEEDING CUES

Nutrition care support of preterm infants can be divided into 3 phases: parenteral, enteral, and oral feeding. Times of greatest risk of inadequate nutrition include getting established parenteral, enteral nutrition,[13] and oral feeding as well as the transitions between these phases. Optimizing nutrition during the transition periods is a key to prevent nutrition deficits.

Initially, preterm infants who are parenterally or enterally fed need to be nourished based on the best evidence-informed nutrition guidelines. None of the preterm nutrition guideline groups provide different guidance to nourish infants who are undersized or oversized.[6,7,38] Whether an infant's growth identifies a concern, nourishing these infants should undergo a transition from infants being provided evidence-informed recommended nutrient and energy amounts in the early weeks, to being supported to feed based on the infant's own cues of hunger and satiety. Many preterm infants will transition from prescribed volume enteral feedings to full oral feeding before discharge home. Some infants will require feeding strategies to support them to orally feed safely and adequately, and some may require some enteral tube feedings at discharge. Feeding protocols, which include infant-driven progression of oral feeding consider physiologic and neurologic maturity, infant skill, and development[39–41] and are associated with shorter time to transition to full oral feeding,[39,40] shorter length of stay,[40,42] and in one study, improved infant growth.[42]

Achievement of full oral feedings by 40 weeks PMA was associated with better neurodevelopmental outcomes at 18 to 26 months corrected age [12]. Inability to fully feed orally at 40 weeks' PMA may be a simple, clinically useful marker for risk of adverse neurodevelopmental outcomes.[12]

There is a paucity of studies or guiding algorithms to support families through the transition to on-demand feedings around discharge. Transition to cue-based feeding for timing and volumes requires caregivers who can sensitively respond to their infant to provide safe and pleasurable feeding that supports growth and provides a foundation for a positive feeding relationship. There are 2 reasons for allowing children to determine the amounts fed: (i) we never really know a childs individual genetic growth potential and (ii) we need to support them to trust and respond to their own appetite. Parents need support to trust their infant and to overcome the NICU emphasis on volumes consumed and short-term weight gains. The premise/goal of nourishing a child once the child is able should be based on infant cues of hunger and satiety and follow responsive feeding practices, which support the division of responsibility.[43] If a child is assessed as too small or too heavy or has growth that deviates from their usual pattern, the division of responsibility guidelines encourages caregivers to respect infant's hunger and satiety. There will be some exceptions for infants who may need supplemental tube feedings as well as those who have rare syndromes whereby hunger-satiety self-regulation is impaired.

RECOMMENDATIONS FOR PRETERM INFANT GROWTH MONITORING

The needs to assess preterm infant growth clinically differ from the needs to summarize growth for research. Clinically, growth assessments are used to understand individuals' growth relative to their individual genetic potential and morbidity status to be able to support the needs of each individual baby. Growth quantification for research purposes is used to quantify growth of groups using meaningful metrics. Historically, neonatology has lacked consistency in the use of growth metrics.[44,45]

CLINICAL GROWTH MONITORING

1. Aim to meet nutritional needs for all infants to support their growth.
2. Aim for growth approximately parallel to growth curves. Use the growth patterns of all 3 growth parameters (weight, length, and head circumference) plotted on growth charts to assess growth.[45] "Increasing weight out of proportion to length does not confer developmental benefits" or improve outcomes.[46,47]
3. Do not be concerned about preterm infant body fat proportion at 40 weeks, as it increases only temporarily as a postnatal event in preterm as well as term infants.[26,27,34]
4. Accept variability; remember biological variation: it is normal to see a range of sizes and growth rates. Do not aim to exceed any specific percentile or z-score because any infant's genetic potential is unknown and sizes within and, rarely, even outside of the 3rd to 97th percentiles are normal and expected in a population.
5. Do not aim for a return to the birth weight percentile after the extracellular fluid contraction weight loss.

6. Infants should not be considered growth restricted or failing just because their weight is less than 10th or 3rd percentile between 36 and 40 weeks' PMA.[1]
7. If nutrition is optimized and growth does not equal intrauterine rates, look for other potential causes (see **Table 1**).[14,20,38]
8. Do not label children to parents/caregivers as growth restricted, malnourished, stunted, wasted, underweight, overweight, or obese, as labels are not helpful for individuals.[20] It is better when talking with parents/caregivers to instead use less judgmental terms, when necessary, such as "weight is ahead of length" or "length is not as tall as expected."
9. When a child is able to self-feed, respect the child's appetite and satiety[43] and feeding abilities.

RESEARCH GROWTH MONITORING

The purpose of research growth monitoring is to summarize growth of groups of infants for research or audit purposes.

1. Report birth weight, length, and head circumference and z-scores for weight, length, and head circumference. Report the reference data set used to derive the z-scores.[45]
2. Growth velocity calculations (using grams per kilogram per day or changes in z-scores) to compare to intrauterine rates should begin at the nadir or day 7 (because the extracellular fluid contraction/postnatal weight loss phase is not growth, so it should be excluded). Growth velocity can be quantified using grams per kilogram per day up to 36 weeks (use the average or exponential method[22]); at ages older than 36 weeks, use grams per day[22]
3. For research summaries, z-score changes can be used at any age and for most time periods (after the postnatal weight loss phase), although short time periods are less likely to represent longer-term growth[48] (see **Fig. 1**A). For research, report z-score changes and/or growth velocity to 28 days and/or 36 weeks PMA or discharge, as relevant.[45]
4. Growth velocity from birth can also be useful to document in research, but when begun at birth, growth velocity should not be expected to equal intrauterine rates because of the postnatal weight loss phase.
5. Infants should not be considered growth restricted or failing just because their weight is less than 10th or 3rd percentile between 36 and 40 weeks PMA.[1]
6. Ideally, assess neurodevelopment at 2 years or older corrected age. Consider the numerous possible contributors to suboptimal development.[14,38]

Best Practices

- Without serial measurements and an understanding of preterm infants' expected growth patterns, it is possible to make incorrect growth assessments.

- If an infant is assessed to be small or large but is already making appropriate catch-up or catch-down growth toward his or her genetic potential, and nutrient intake meets the recommended intakes, then changes for his or her nutrition care might not be warranted.

- If an infants' growth pattern is as expected given their postnatal weight loss and morbidities, and their nutrition is equal to recommended intakes, then the infant should be assessed as growing appropriately and no changes would be needed in their care.

- If an infant's growth is slower than growth chart curves, further investigations are needed to explore for nutrition, morbidity, intrauterine or genetic reasons with the actions required depending on the cause.

DISCLOSURE

The authors declare no commercial or financial conflicts of interest and received no funding for this work.

REFERENCES

1. Fenton TR, Nasser R, Creighton D, et al. Weight, length, and head circumference at 36 weeks are not predictive of later cognitive impairment in very preterm infants. J Perinatol 2020;41(3):606–14.
2. World Health Organization. Growth standards. 2021. Available at: https://www. who.int/tools/child-growth-standards. Accessed May 16, 2021.
3. Fenton TR, McMillan DD, Sauve RS. Nutrition and growth analysis of very low birth weight infants. Pediatrics 1990;86(3):378–83.
4. Embleton NE, Pang N, Cooke RJ. Postnatal malnutrition and growth retardation: an inevitable consequence of current recommendations in preterm infants? Pediatrics 2001;107(2):270–3.
5. Fenton TR, Cormack B, Goldberg D, et al. Extrauterine growth restriction" and "postnatal growth failure" are misnomers for preterm infants. J Perinatol 2020; 40(5):704–14.
6. American Academy Pediatrics Committee on Nutrition. Nutritional needs of preterm infants. In: Kleinman RE, Greer FR, editors. Pediatric nutrition handbook. 8th edition. Itasca Il; 2020.
7. Agostoni C, Buonocore G, Carnielli VP, et al. Enteral nutrient supply for preterm infants: commentary from the European Society of Paediatric Gastroenterology, Hepatology and Nutrition Committee on Nutrition. J Pediatr Gastroenterol Nutr 2010;50(1):85–91.
8. Villar J, Giuliani F, Barros F, et al. Monitoring the postnatal growth of preterm infants: a paradigm change. Basel(Switserland): Pediatrics 2018;141(2): e20172467.
9. Villar J, Giuliani F, Bhutta ZA, et al. Postnatal growth standards for preterm infants: the preterm postnatal follow-up study of the INTERGROWTH-21(st) project. Lancet Glob Heal 2015;3(11):e681–91.
10. American Academy Pediatrics Committee on Nutrition. Assessment of Nutritional status. In: Kleinman RE, Greer FRE, editors. Pediatric Nutrition Handbook. 8th edition. Itasca Il; 2020.
11. Franz AR, Pohlandt F, Bode H, et al. Intrauterine, early neonatal, and postdischarge growth and neurodevelopmental outcome at 5.4 years in extremely preterm infants after intensive neonatal nutritional support. Pediatrics 2009;123(1): e101–9.
12. Lainwala S, Kosyakova N, Power K, et al. Delayed achievement of oral feedings is associated with adverse neurodevelopmental outcomes at 18 to 26 months follow-up in preterm infants. Am J Perinatol 2020;37(5).
13. Cormack BE, Jiang Y, Harding JE, et al. Relationships between neonatal nutrition and growth to 36 weeks' corrected age in ELBW babies–secondary cohort analysis from the provide trial. Nutrients 2020;12(3):760.
14. Fenton TR, Goldberg D, Alshaikh B, et al. A holistic approach to infant growth assessment considers clinical, social and genetic factors rather than an assessment of weight at a set timepoint. J Perinatol 2021;41(3):650–1.
15. Fenton TR, Kim JH. A systematic review and meta-analysis to revise the Fenton growth chart for preterm infants. BMC Pediatr 2013;13(1):59.

16. Olsen IE, Groveman SA, Lawson ML, et al. New intrauterine growth curves based on United States data. Pediatrics 2010;125(2):e214–24.
17. Goldberg DL, Becker PJ, Brigham K, et al. Identifying malnutrition in preterm and neonatal populations: recommended indicators. J Acad Nutr Diet 2018;118(9): 1571–82.
18. Rochow N, Raja P, Liu K, et al. Physiological adjustment to postnatal growth trajectories in healthy preterm infants. Pediatr Res 2016;79(6):870–9.
19. Fabrizio V, Shabanova V, Taylor SN. Factors in early feeding practices that may influence growth and the challenges that arise in growth outcomes research. Nutrients 2020;12(7):1939.
20. Fenton CJ, Elmrayed S, Fenton TR. Growth standards. In: Koletzko B, Bhutta ZA, Dhansay MA, et al, editors. Pediatric nutrition in practice, 124, 3rd ed. 2021.
21. Foote JM, Brady LH, Burke AL, et al. Development of an evidence-based clinical practice guideline on linear growth measurement of children. J Pediatr Nurs 2011;26(4):312–24.
22. Fenton TR, Griffin IJ, Hoyos A, et al. Accuracy of preterm infant weight gain velocity calculations vary depending on method used and infant age at time of measurement. Pediatr Res 2019;85(5):650–4.
23. Wells N, Stokes TA, Ottolini K, et al. Anthropometric trends from 1997 to 2012 in infants born at $\not\geq$28 weeks' gestation or less. J Perinatol 2017;37(5):521–6.
24. Ehrenkranz RA, Dusick AM, Vohr BR, et al. Growth in the neonatal intensive care unit influences neurodevelopmental and growth outcomes of extremely low birth weight infants. Pediatrics 2006;117(4):1253–61.
25. National Academies Press. Dietary reference intakes for energy, carbohydrate, fiber, fat, fatty acids, cholesterol, protein, and amino acids 2005.
26. Giannì ML, Roggero P, Piemontese P, et al. Boys who are born preterm show a relative lack of fat-free mass at 5 years of age compared to their peers. Acta Paediatr 2015;104(3):e119–23.
27. Forsum E, Flinke E, Olhager E. Premature birth was not associated with increased body fatness in four-year-old boys and girls. Acta Paediatr 2020;109(2). https://doi.org/10.1111/APA.14990.
28. Hack M, Schluchter M, Andreias L, et al. Change in prevalence of chronic conditions between childhood and adolescence among extremely low-birth-weight children. JAMA 2011;306(4):394–401.
29. Nuysink J, Eijsermans MJC, van Haastert IC, et al. Clinical course of asymmetric motor performance and deformational plagiocephaly in very preterm infants. J Pediatr 2013;163(3):658–65.
30. Ifflaender S, Rüdiger M, Konstantelos D, et al. Prevalence of head deformities in preterm infants at term equivalent age. Early Hum Dev 2013;89(12):1041–7.
31. Olsen IE, Lawson ML, Ferguson AN, et al. BMI curves for preterm infants. Pediatrics 2015;135(3):e572–81.
32. Lorch SA. The clinical and policy implications of new measures of premature infant growth. Pediatrics 2015;135(3):e703–4.
33. Kiger JR, Taylor SN, Wagner CL, et al. Preterm infant body composition cannot be accurately determined by weight and length. J Neonatal Perinatal Med 2016;9(3): 285–90.
34. Hamatschek C, Yousuf EI, Möllers LS, et al. Fat and fat-free mass of preterm and term infants from birth to six months: a review of current evidence. Nutrients 2020; 12(2):288.
35. Griffin IJ, Cooke RJ. Development of whole body adiposity in preterm infants. Early Hum Dev 2012;88(Suppl 1):S19–24.

36. Fields DA, Gilchrist JM, Catalano PM, et al. Longitudinal body composition data in exclusively breast-fed infants: a multicenter study. Obesity 2011;19(9): 1887–91.

37. Ramel SE, Haapala J, Super J, et al. Nutrition, illness and body composition in very low birth weight preterm infants: implications for nutritional management and neurocognitive outcomes. Nutrients 2020;12(1):145.

38. Fenton TR, Elmrayed S, Alshaikh B. Nutrition, growth and long-term outcomes. In: Koletzko B, Cheah F, Domellöf M, et al, editors. Nutr Care Preterm Infants, Scientific Basis Pract Guidel122. World Rev Nutr Diet; 2021. p. 12–31. Available at. https://www.karger.com/Article/Abstract/514745.

39. McCain GC, Gartside PS, Greenberg JM, et al. A feeding protocol for healthy preterm infants that shortens time to oral feeding. J Pediatr 2001;139(3):374–9.

40. Wellington A, Perlman JM. Infant-driven feeding in premature infants: a quality improvement project. Arch Dis Child - Fetal Neonatal Ed 2015;100(6):F495–500.

41. Dalgleish SR, Kostecky LL, Blachly N. Eating in "SINC": safe individualized nipple-feeding competence, a quality improvement project to explore infant-driven oral feeding for very premature infants requiring noninvasive respiratory support. Neonatal Netw 2016;35(4):217–27.

42. Celen R, Arslan FT, Soylu H. Effect of SINC feeding protocol on weight gain, transition to oral feeding, and the length of hospitalization in preterm infants: a randomized controlled trial. JPEN J Parenter Enteral Nutr 2021;45(3).

43. Satter E. The ellyn satter. 2019. Available at: https://www.ellynsatterinstitute.org. Accessed May 31, 2021.

44. Fenton TR, Chan HT, Madhu A, et al. Preterm infant growth velocity calculations: a systematic review. Pediatrics 2017;139(3):e20162045.

45. Cormack BE, Embleton ND, van Goudoever JB, et al. Comparing apples with apples: it is time for standardized reporting of neonatal nutrition and growth studies. Pediatr Res 2016;79(6):810–20.

46. Belfort MB, Gillman MW, Buka SL, et al. Preterm infant linear growth and adiposity gain: trade-offs for later weight status and intelligence quotient. J Pediatr 2013; 163(6):1564–9, e2.

47. Belfort MB, Rifas-Shiman SL, Sullivan T, et al. Infant growth before and after term: effects on neurodevelopment in preterm infants. Pediatrics 2011;128(4): e899–906.

48. Fenton TR, Senterre T, Griffin IJ. Time interval for preterm infant weight gain velocity calculation precision. Arch Dis Child - Fetal Neonatal Ed 2019;104(2): F218–9.

49. Molony CL, Growth trajectory of preterm small-for-gestational-age neonates, J Matern Fetal Neonatal Med, 2021, PMID: 34503371, https://doi.org/10.1080/14767058.2021.1974835, In preparation.

Maternal Nutrition and Fetal/Infant Development

Sangeeta Jain, MD[a], Akhil Maheshwari, MD[b,*], Sunil K. Jain, MD[c]

KEYWORDS

- Pregnancy • Fetal outcome • Fetal programming • Obesity • Perinatal outcomes
- Gestational weight gain • Reproductive-age women • Euglycemia

KEY POINTS

- Maternal nutrition.
- Fetal programming.
- Reproductive age women.
- Pregnancy and obesity.

Nutrition in pregnant women has long been known to be an important determinant of fetal/maternal outcomes. With increasing information on fetal programming, there is renewed interest in evaluating the effects of the quality/availability of nutrition on short- and long-term fetal growth and development. The impact of recent obesity epidemic has had a profound effect both on women's health and the overall field of medicine. There is a need for a better understanding of the medical, financial, and social costs, and possible remedies of malnutrition during pregnancy.

In general, the typical American diet shows opportunities for improvement. The intake of fruits, vegetables, whole grains, and fiber may be below recommended levels, but the relative proportion of sodium, fats, and carbohydrates is high.[1] The consumption of high fructose corn syrup increased greater than 1000% between 1970 and 1990.[2] During the 20th century, inadequate gestational weight gain (GWG) contributed to suboptimal perinatal outcomes. These problems may have now reversed; 56% of reproductive-age women are overweight and 35% are obese.[3] Excessive GWG contributes to suboptimal health outcomes during and after pregnancy, and possibly to the long-term risk of metabolic and cardiovascular diseases.[4] The concepts of the fetal origin of adult diseases also emphasizes that maternal

[a] Division of Maternal-Fetal Medicine, University of Texas Medical Branch, 301 University Boulevard, Galveston, TX 77555, USA; [b] Global Newborn Society, Clarksville, MD 21029, USA; [c] Division of Neonatology, University of Texas Medical Branch, 301 University Boulevard, Galveston, TX 77555, USA
* Corresponding author.
E-mail address: akhil@globalnewbornsociety.org

Clin Perinatol 49 (2022) 313–330
https://doi.org/10.1016/j.clp.2022.02.005
0095-5108/22/© 2022 Elsevier Inc. All rights reserved.
perinatology.theclinics.com

nutrition and metabolic status during pregnancy may affect neonatal outcomes.[5] There is a need for intervention; 27% of pregnant women reported that they received no guidance about weight gain during pregnancy.[6] Clearly, there is a need to strengthen these efforts. Clinicians taking care of reproductive-age women need to educate themselves as well as their patients about the importance of nutritional health before, during, and after pregnancy.

MATERNAL NUTRITION AT THE TIME OF CONCEPTION

Maternal nutritional and metabolic status at the time of conception may be more important for fetal development than nutrition during pregnancy. Organogenesis occurs early in the first trimester before many women are aware of the pregnancy. In planned pregnancy, preconceptional optimization of nutritional and metabolic status is very important. Women with pregestational diabetes mellitus (GDM) should strive to achieve euglycemia before conception, as higher levels of hemoglobin A1C (a marker for hyperglycemia) is associated with progressively higher rates of miscarriages and congenital deformities. Intake of 4 mg of folic acid in women on antiepileptic medications or prior history of a child with neural tube defects (NTDs), can reduce the incidence of NTDs in the current fetus. Women who are underweight at the beginning of pregnancy are seen to be at increased risk for preterm delivery and small for gestational age (SGA) infants, when compared with those who have a normal BMI.

FETAL NUTRITION *IN UTERO*
Role of the Placenta

The nutrient supply to the fetus is dependent on placental transport (**Fig. 1**). The human placenta grows rapidly until 32 weeks gestational age, but the capacity for nutritional transport capacity continues to grow during later gestation. Uterine and umbilical blood flow continues to increase in the third trimester, indicating that the growth and maturation of the placenta are geared toward nutrient requirements for the growing fetus.[7] The placenta lies between the maternal and fetal vascular beds, whereby it mediates nutrient and waste exchange. Nutrient transportation across the placenta to the umbilical circulation depends on the permeability of the placenta, the maternal to fetal concentration gradient, and uterine, placental, and umbilical

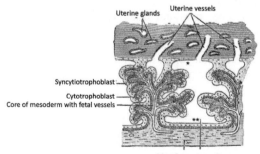

Fig. 1. Sectional diagram of the first-trimester human placenta. A basal plate intervillous space lining is covered with chorionic ectodermal tissue in the form of syncytiotrophoblast continuous with that of the chorionic villous tree. The chorionic plate lining is identified (**). It lies on the opposite side of the intervillous space from the basal plate lining (*).as depicted. Modified from Ockleford CD. The allo-epi-endothelial lining of the intervillous space. Placenta. 2010 Dec;31(12):1035 to 42.

blood flow. The large surface area of the placental transport interface allows for efficient diffusion of the nutrients and waste across the placenta.[8]

The maternal blood is separated from the fetal capillary endothelium only by an epithelial monolayer.[9] Hydrophilic molecules do not readily cross-plasma membranes because of their poor lipid solubility, and transporter protein–mediated mechanisms are generally necessary for transporting these molecules. Transport can also occur passively across concentration gradients, or actively as in the case of calcium and amino acids.[10] Nutritional status before and during pregnancy affects placental formation and function and altered placental development can influence the offspring after birth.[11]

Fetal Nutrient Requirements

Fetal nutrient requirements are determined by the rate of growth, the composition of new tissues, and the metabolic rate. The process of growth is complex because of the ongoing turnover and remodeling of tissues in addition to net accretion. The human fetus grows at an average of 1.5% per day from mid-gestation to term. The caloric accretion rates are considerably high, reaching up to 40 kcal/kg/d.

Carbohydrate
Placental glucose transport occurs by facilitated diffusion. Net placenta to fetus glucose transport depends on both maternal glucose concentration and the transplacental glucose concentration gradient up to a maximum rate of uptake.[12] In fetal lambs, the glucose uptake rate under normal conditions is about 4 mg/kg/min, which is similar to the use rate of glucose by preterm and term human infants as measured by isotope dilution techniques.[13] The fetal glucose pool has both exogenous (from maternal circulation) and endogenous (from fetal glycogen breakdown) sources. Glucose is an important but not the sole metabolic fuel for the fetus. The human fetus depends on glucose for oxidative metabolism due to the large brain to body weight ratio (3–4 times compared with other species) and a significant amount of glucose is consumed by the brain.[14]

Protein and amino acids
Fetal plasma contains higher amino acid concentrations than maternal plasma; the transplacental transfer of maternal amino acids to the fetus involves active transport mechanisms besides those driven by concentration gradients. High fetal urea production rate suggests a role for amino acids as metabolic fuel. In undernourished/fasting mothers, the fetus diverts amino acids from protein synthesis to synthesize glucose as a metabolic fuel. Amino acids such as alanine, glycine, lysine, and tyrosine are also directly oxidized. Amino acids thus may be important in supplying energy both for basal metabolism and as alternate fuels during energy deficiency.[15]

Fat
Placental permeability regulates fetal lipid uptake. Fat is transported to the fetus from the placenta via fatty acid carrier-mediated diffusion, by synthesis de novo and by the hydrolysis of triglycerides, lipoproteins, and phospholipids. Fats are unlikely to contribute to fetal energy balance as plasma and tissue concentrations of carnitine are relatively low. Immediately after birth, milk feeding and associated fat intake/metabolism results in decreased respiratory quotients.

Essential fatty acids
Omega-6 and ω-3 fatty acids, the essential fatty acids, are needed for fetal development.[16] Studies show that populations with a high intake of seafood containing long-

chain ω-3 fatty acids during pregnancy may have longer durations of gestation with better fetal growth.[17] ω-3 fatty acids play an important role in neurodevelopment and inflammatory pathways, thus impacting childhood neurologic outcomes and inflammation-mediated conditions such as preterm birth (PTB), allergy, asthma, and eczema.

Iron

Nutritional iron deficiency is highest in reproductive age group women, especially during pregnancy. Increased iron requirement of the developing fetus and an increase in red cell mass in the mother may cause the mother with low iron stores to develop iron deficiency anemia. The World Health Organization (WHO) reports 56% and 18% of pregnant women in developing and developed countries, respectively, are anemic.[18] Iron deficiency is associated with impaired fetal growth, prematurity, and maternal and infant mortality. There is a need for monitoring and if needed, supplementation.[19]

Folate

Folate, a methyl-group donor, is a key nutrient during pregnancy. It is essential for nucleic acid synthesis, erythropoiesis, and fetal and placental growth. The effects of folate consumption during pregnancy have been extensively investigated. A recent study of SGA (<10th percentile birthweight) and large for gestational age (LGA; >10th percentile birthweight) infants showed lower expression of genes associated with folate transport and related proteins than in controls.[20] Gene ontology analysis showed its associations with biological adhesion, biological regulation, cell proliferation, development, metabolism, and signaling, in which regulators of decidua formation were observed.[21] In human placental cells, folate supplementation increased the cellular proliferation.[22] Folate is also needed for decidual angiogenesis.[23,24] There seems to be an association between maternal folate sufficiency, placental development, and fetal growth.

Maternal folic acid deficiency can cause NTDs in the fetus and other congenital anomalies. The US Centers for Disease Control and Prevention recommends 0.4 mg/d of folic acid from diet or supplements for all women capable of becoming pregnant to reduce the risk for NTDs. In 1998, the United States started mandatory folic acid fortification of cereal and grain products which significantly improved the folate status of US childbearing age women and reduced the incidence of NTDs by 25%. Women with a previous pregnancy affected by an NTD should take higher amounts of daily folic acid (4 mg/d) starting 4 weeks before planning pregnancy and throughout the first trimester.[25] Folate levels are lower in obese women and they are also at increased risk for NTDs. The relationship between obesity and NTDs is not clear; it may be related to a higher hemoglobin A1C rather than folate deficiency specifically.[26]

Iodine

Iodine is an essential component of the thyroid hormone which is required during fetal development for appropriate neuronal migration and myelination.[27] During pregnancy, the daily recommended requirement of iodine increases to 220 mg/d. Severe maternal iodine deficiency is associated with fetal and neonatal hypothyroidism along with impaired cognitive development in the infant.[28]

CONTRIBUTION OF MATERNAL DIETARY FACTORS IN FETAL OUTCOMES
Diets Inadequate in Key Nutrients

There is a considerable change in the nutritional needs of women during pregnancy (**Table 1**). According to a population-based National Health and Nutrition Examination

Table 1
Dietary Reference Intakes: Recommended Daily Intakes for Individuals

Vitamin/Mineral	Age (yr)	Nonpregnant	Pregnant	Upper Intake Levels
Vitamin A (μg)	<18	700	750–1200	2800
	19–30	700	770–1300	3000
	31–50	700	770–1300	3000
Vitamin C (mg)	<18	65	80	1800
	19–30	75	85	2000
	31–50	75	85	2000
Vitamin D (μg)	<18	15	15	100
	19–30	15	15	100
	31–50	15	15	100
Vitamin E (mg)	<18	15	15	800
	19–30	15	15	1000
	31–50	15	15	1000
Vitamin K (μg)	<18	75	75	ND
	19–30	90	90	ND
	31–50	90	90	ND
Thiamin (mg)	<18	1.1	1.4	ND
	19–30	1.1	1.4	ND
	31–50	1.1	1.4	ND
Riboflavin (mg)	<18	1.1	1.4	ND
	19–30	1.1	1.4	ND
	31–50	1.1	1.4	ND
Niacin (mg)	<18	14	18	30
	19–30	14	18	35
	31–50	14	18	35
Vitamin B 6 (mg)	<18	1.2	1.9	80
	19–30	1.3	1.9	100
	31–50	1.3	1.9	100
Folate (μg)	<18	400	600	800
	19–30	400	600	1000
	31–50	400	600	1000
Vitamin B 12 (μg)	<18	2.4	2.6	ND
	19–30	2.4	2.6	ND
	31–50	2.4	2.6	ND
Pantothenic acid (mg)	<18	5	6	ND
	19–30	5	6	ND
	31–50	5	6	ND
Biotin (μg)	<18	25	30	ND
	19–30	30	30	ND
	31–50	30	30	ND
Choline (mg)	<18	400	450	3000
	19–30	425	450	3500
	31–50	425	450	3500
Calcium (mg)	<18	1300	1300	3000
	19–30	1000	1000	2500
	31–50	1000	1000	2500

(continued on next page)

Vitamin/Mineral	Age (yr)	Nonpregnant	Pregnant	Upper Intake Levels
Chromium (μg)	<18	24	29	ND
	19–30	25	30	ND
	31–50	25	30	ND
Copper (μg)	<18	890	1000	8000
	19–30	900	1000	10,000
	31–50	900	1000	10,000
Fluoride (mg)	<18	3	3	10
	19–30	3	3	10
	31–50	3	3	10
Iodine (μg)	<18	150	220	900
	19–30	150	220	1100
	31–50	150	220	1100
Iron (mg)	<18	15	27	45
	19–30	18	27	45
	31–50	18	27	45
Magnesium (mg)	<18	360	400	350
	19–30	310	350	350
	31–50	320	360	350
Phosphorus (mg)	<18	1250	1250	4000
	19–30	700	700	4000
	31–50	700	700	4000
Selenium (μg)	<18	55	60	400
	19–30	55	60	400
	31–50	55	60	400
Zinc (mg)	<18	9	12	34
	19–30	8	11	40
	31–50	8	11	40

Table 1
(continued)

DRIs are included for calcium, phosphorus, magnesium, vitamin D, and fluoride (1997); for thiamin, riboflavin, niacin, vitamins B 6 and B 12, folate, pantothenic acid, biotin, and choline (1998); for vitamins C and E, selenium, and the carotenoids (2000); for vitamins A and K, arsenic, boron, chromium, copper, iodine, iron, manganese, molybdenum, nickel, silicon, vanadium, and zinc (2001); and for calcium and vitamin D (2011).
Abbreviation: ND, non-determined
Data from http://www.iom.edu/Activities/Nutrition/SummaryDRIs/DRI-Tables.aspx.

Survey (2007–2008), 2.1% of the US population consider themselves vegetarian.[29] The primary concern about vegetarian diets is vitamin B12 deficiency, as animal food is the main source of vitamin B12. Pregnant women who consume eggs and/ or dairy products may have adequate B12 intake. Those who completely exclude all animal products (vegans) generally require a B12 supplement or B12-fortified vegetarian foods for adequate intake. The vegan diet may also be too high in fibers and low in fat that the caloric intake may be insufficient for pregnancy. Intakes of calcium, vitamin D, riboflavin, and iron may also need evaluation. In 2009 the American Dietetic Association stated that "appropriately planned vegetarian diets, including total vegetarian or vegan diets, are healthful, nutritionally adequate, and may provide health benefits in the prevention and treatment of certain diseases." The American Dietetic

Association added that with appropriate planning, vegetarian diets are safe for all life stages, including pregnancy. A 2015 systematic review and meta-analysis of 13 observational studies reported no convincing evidence that vegetarian diets were associated with major birth defects, preeclampsia, length of gestation, or infant birth weight. However, these women need careful assessment and counseling.

Seafood Consumption: Mercury

Studies conducted in the Faroe Islands and in New Zealand showed worse performance on neurobehavioral tests among children exposed to higher levels of mercury-contaminated fish.[30] In 2004, a US health advisory recommended that pregnant women limit fish consumption to avoid exposure to methyl mercury, heavy metal and industrial pollutant that accumulates in some seafood. Mercury is neurotoxic, and the developing fetus is especially vulnerable. Subsequent to the fish advisories, fish consumption in the United States dropped among women of reproductive age.[31] In 2017, the Environmental Protection Agency (EPA) revised recommendations to balance the health benefits with the concern for methyl mercury. They categorized more than 60 fish into 3 categories—Best choices, Good choices, and Choices to avoid. The advisory recommended pregnant women eat 8 to 12 oz of fish from Best choices category weekly and no more than 6 oz from the Good choices category.

Impact of Inborn Errors of Metabolism on Pregnancy

Inborn errors of metabolisms (IEMs) were once considered incompatible with a successful pregnancy. However, increasing reports now suggest that some IEMs might not completely exclude the possibility of a successful pregnancy.[32] IEMs are rare with a collective prevalence of greater than 1:800.[33] Early diagnosis has improved by universal newborn screening programs. However, the biological stresses of pregnancy, delivery, and the postpartum period produce significant challenges. Protein requirements increase in early pregnancy and increase throughout gestation.[34] Maternal gluconeogenesis depends on lipolysis and 50% of maternal glucose is used by the growing fetus. Estrogen-induced reduction in hepatic lipoprotein lipase activity increases maternal cholesterol and triglyceride levels, which release free fatty acids for fetal growth.[35] Prolonged and significant muscular contractions during labor increase energy requirements, and these limitations might be accentuated by the altered cellular metabolism. After childbirth, the mother remains in a catabolic state and is at risk of metabolic decompensation because of the diversion of energy and amino acid pools to milk production. The outcomes are better if the IEM is exactly known which might improve the feasibility of preventive and pre-emptive management.[32] In this review, we will discuss some common IEMs and their effect on the maternal-fetal dyad.

Urea cycle disorders in pregnancy

Pregnancy increases metabolic demands, and requirements for protein, amino acids, and energy. Urea cycle defects increase the risk of decompensation as these increased demands may be difficult to meet and the excessive catabolism may overwhelm the needs of ureagenesis and ammonia consumption. Chances of decompensation are highest when the diagnosis is unrecognized and/or treatment is delayed or not given. In 1990, a case series reported postpartum coma and death of a female carrier with a previously undiagnosed urea cycle disorder.[36] The tolerance to protein may be higher in the third trimester because of increasing fetal utilization of protein, but the risk of metabolic decompensation remains high in mothers with inadequate nutritional intake and/or catabolic stressors.[37] The risk of decompensation continues after childbirth as additional catabolic stressors may arise following cesarean section, birth trauma, or postoperative wound infections. Even blood transfusions may add to the protein load. Breastfeeding is possible so long as caloric intake is adequate.

The outcomes are better if the specific urea cycle disorder is known before pregnancy. Multidisciplinary planning includes clinical observation, monitoring of ammonia levels, and avoidance of prolonged fasting; and careful use of protein-free nutrition orally or parenterally. In neonates, most decompensations tend to occur during the first few weeks after birth as the catabolic drive increases from postnatal days 3 to 11 and can cause metabolic instability.

Phenylketonuria

Phenylketonuria (PKU) occurs due to absent or dysfunctional phenylalanine hydroxylase enzyme with decreased conversion of phenylalanine to tyrosine. Untreated, PKU can cause developmental delay, mood disorders, and behavioral disturbances. Excess phenylalanine is toxic to the developing brain and competes with tryptophan in crossing the blood–brain barrier. The deficiency of tyrosine along with excessive phenylalanine alters the balance of neurotransmitters in the brain leading to deficiencies of dopamine, noradrenaline, and serotonin. Hyperphenylalaninemia also increases oxidative stress, impairs cholesterol synthesis, and activates osteoclasts.

The clinical outcome in PKU was revolutionized by Horst Bickel's therapeutic diet, natural protein restriction and supplementation with micronutrient fortified phenylalanine-free amino acid-based supplements to meet nutritional requirements. Close blood-spot monitoring of phenylalanine levels maintained throughout the development, has enabled the attainment of near-potential developmental indices in the fetus. Unfortunately, many women of childbearing age are lost to follow-up, often in adolescence. This is concerning as high blood phenylalanine levels can be teratogenic. Infections, antenatal steroids, and unsuitable diets can worsen phenylalanine control. Breastfeeding is not contraindicated in women with PKU.[38]

Homocystinuria

Genetic causes of hyperhomocysteinemia include the deficiency of cystathionine beta-synthase enzyme deficiency (classical homocystinuria), and cobalamin C disease which results in combined methylmalonic acidemia and homocystinuria due to deficient adenosyl-cobalamin. These conditions may differ in clinical features and severity but all are associated with elevated homocysteine levels and an increased risk of thrombosis. Management includes the replacement of cofactors such as B6 for classical homocystinuria, folate for MTHFR deficiency, B12 for cobalamin C disease, and betaine to enhance remethylation to methionine. Protein restriction with the provision of methionine-free amino acid supplementation may help. The management of these conditions resembles that of thrombophilic conditions, with anticoagulation throughout pregnancy and the puerperium. As protein requirements increase during pregnancy, protein restrictions need adjustment to meet nutritional requirements.[39]

Mitochondrial energy metabolism

In mitochondrial disorders, energy supply may be further compromised during pregnancy by altered ketogenesis, fatty acid oxidation, and respiratory chain function. In fetal long-chain hydroxy acyl CoA dehydrogenase deficiency (LCHAD), incomplete beta-oxidation can generate peroxide radicals that enter the maternal circulation and impair hepatic mitochondrial function and cause acute fatty liver of pregnancy.[40] Placental mitochondrial dysfunction may also be seen in many pathologic conditions such as preeclampsia or HELLP syndrome.[41]

During pregnancy, undiagnosed IEMs should be considered in women with unexplained, prolonged hyperemesis gravidarum, liver failure, or neuropsychiatric disturbances. Even though uncommon, milder versions of many IEMs have been linked to preeclampsia, HELLP syndrome, gestational diabetes, neuropsychiatric conditions, and intra-uterine growth restriction (IUGR).

WEIGHT GAIN DURING PREGNANCY

In 2009, the Institute of Medicine (IOM) issued revised guidelines for weight gain during pregnancy and recommended 28 to 40, 25 to 35, 15 to 25 and 11 to 20 lbs weight gain during whole pregnancy in underweight (BMI <18.5), normal weight (18.5–24.9), overweight (25–29.9) and obese (≥30) women, respectively.[4] The Agency on Healthcare Research and Quality showed that GWG above recommendations is associated with an increased incidence of cesarean delivery, maternal postpartum weight retention, preeclampsia, and LGA fetus.[42]

Low GWG is also linked to low birth weight and SGA infants. There is a growing consensus that both inadequate and excessive GWG contribute to childhood obesity, cardiovascular and metabolic disorders.[43]

The IOM recommends that it is important for clinicians to (a) assess prepregnancy BMI and to recommend the appropriate target GWG, (b) normalize maternal weight before conception, (c) assist individualized dietary and physical activity patterns for optimal GWG, and (d) help women return to their prepregnancy BMI after pregnancy. It is important to recognize that measuring and discussing weight gain alone is not sufficient. Individualized care, particularly for obese women, is required. A multidisciplinary team approach including a dietitian and physical activity trainer should be part of the strategy to prevent excessive GWG. There is evidence that women, including obese women, who exercise or are more physically active during pregnancy gain less weight.[44]

Maternal Obesity

In the United States, the average BMI is increasing in all age categories. Women are entering pregnancy with higher body weights. In a recent study, 39.7% of reproductive-age women were noted to be obese and 55.8% were overweight. The mean maternal weight of women at their first prenatal visit increased by 20% during the period from 1980 to 1999. The percentage of women weighing greater than 200 lbs at the first visit increased from 7.3% to 24%, and those who weighed greater than 300 lbs increased from 2% to 11%[3]

Women who were obese before pregnancy are at higher risk of spontaneous abortions and intrauterine fetal deaths. These fetuses may also have congenital anomalies such as NTDs, cardiac, and gastrointestinal anomalies.[45] Obese women are also more likely to have cesarean sections, perioperative thromboembolic disease, and other complications including an increase in morbidity and mortality.[46]

Diabetes During Pregnancy

Worldwide, one in seven pregnancies is complicated by diabetes and is associated with fetal overgrowth (**Fig. 2**). These women may have had diabetes before the onset of pregnancy or it may develop during mid- or late-gestation. Prevalence of gestational diabetes is higher in Hispanic, African American, and Native Americans pregnant women.[47] In normal pregnancies, fetal and maternal glycemic fluctuations are limited hence fetal insulin levels also don't change significantly. However, sustained hyperglycemia in a diabetic mother results in persistently increased fetal insulin secretion and

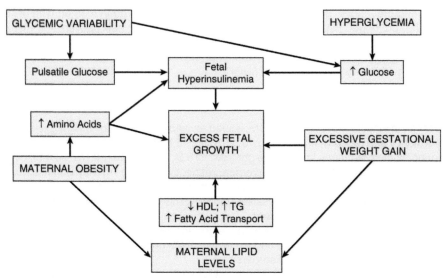

Fig. 2. Contribution of maternal factors to fetal overgrowth in type 1 diabetes in pregnancy and possible mechanisms of action. Additional cross-talk between pathways may occur through as-yet-unidentified mechanisms. *HDL*, High-density lipoprotein; *TG*, triglyceride.

beta-cell hyperplasia which predisposes to neonatal macrosomia because of accelerated fetal growth and fat deposition.[48] Once there is fetal hyperinsulinemia, high glucose transfer from the mother persists which is why early optimization of maternal glycemic control is important to prevent LGA infants in gestational diabetes.[49]

Preconceptional obesity and GDM are associated with the largest fetal weight and abdominal circumference at 20 weeks gestation. In this subset of pregnant women, early diagnosis (16–18 weeks gestation) of gestational diabetes could normalize fetal growth more effectively.[50] About 85% of GDM can be controlled solely with nutrition and physical activity [48] while the remaining 15% require pharmacologic treatment.[51]

The highest risk for neonatal large-for-gestation status and a higher percentage of body fat is with diabetes appearing later in life.[52] Maternal obesity may also possibly augment childhood obesity, asthma, and metabolic syndrome.[53] However, some women with diabetic vasculopathy may have chronic hypertension, and their infants may be under-weight and at risk of preterm delivery and IUGR[43,54,55]

Fetal Growth Restriction

Fetal growth restriction (FGR) is defined as a fetus with an estimated fetal weight or abdominal circumference less than the 10th percentile for gestational age. It can occur from a multitude of maternal, fetal, placental, and uterine factors (**Fig. 3**). It is a risk factor for perinatal morbidity and mortality proportionate to the growth restriction. It is not clear if generalized caloric intake reduction or specific substrate limitation (like protein or key minerals), or both are important for FGR. There is little gluconeogenesis in a normally developing fetus, and hence fetal glucose uptake is critical for growth. In growth-restricted fetuses, the maternal–fetal glucose concentration difference is increased as a function of the severity of the growth restriction, which facilitates glucose transfer across the small placenta.[56] In some cases, FGR may be associated with low zinc content in peripheral blood leukocytes as maternal serum zinc concentrations less

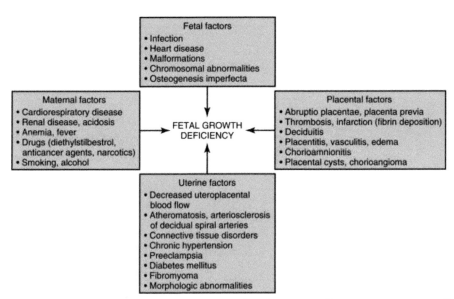

Fig. 3. Causes of fetal growth restriction. (*Modified from* Fanaroff AA, Lissauer T, Fanaroff JM. Physical Growth: Physical Examination of the Newborn Infant and the Physical Environment. In: Fanaroff AA, Fanaroff JM, editors. Klaus and Fanaroff's Care of the High-Risk Neonate. United States: Elsevier; 2019. p. 58 to 79.e2.)

than 60 μg/dL in the third trimester are associated with a 5-fold increase in low birth weight.[57] Similarly, an association between low serum folate levels and FGR has been reported.[58]

The growth-restricted fetus is at risk of asphyxia, meconium aspiration, hypoglycemia and other metabolic abnormalities, and polycythemia during the neonatal period. After correction for gestational age, it has been shown that the premature infant with FGR is at increased risk of mortality, necrotizing enterocolitis, and need for respiratory support at 28 days of age.[59] FGR has long term effects as almost 50% of infants with FGR have learning deficits at ages 9 to 11 years. Blair and Stanley[60] reported a strong association between FGR and spastic cerebral palsy in infants born after 33 weeks gestation. This association was highest in FGR infants who were short, thin, with a small head circumference.

There is a known epidemiologic association between FGR and disorders of adulthood (**Fig. 4**). Barker's Hypothesis suggested that adults with a history of FGR had a higher frequency of chronic hypertension, ischemic heart disease, type 2 diabetes, and obstructive lung disease.[61] A recent echocardiographic study of 5-year-old children born with FGR showed altered myocardial function with higher heart rates and blood pressures, lower stroke volumes, and a higher frequency of globular cardiac ventricles.[62] There was also a higher risk of various metabolic disorders.[63]

The epidemiologic data in the Dutch famine study,[64] the Hertfordshire Cohort Study, and the Helsinki Birth Cohort Study also showed that infants born during unfavorable nutritional deprivation periods frequently developed metabolic disorders.[65] During the Dutch famine, epidemiologic studies showed low placental size.[66] Infants who were in mid-to-late gestation during the famine had lower birth weights than those who were in early gestation during the famine or conceived after the famine ended. These data

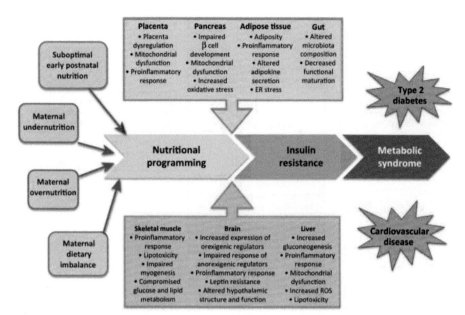

Fig. 4. Causes and consequences of insulin resistance in nutritional programming. Different types of maternal nutrition cause systemic insulin resistance in the offspring through several molecular mechanisms in different organs and tissues. Consequently, systemic insulin resistance triggers the offspring to have metabolic syndrome (MetS) or metabolic diseases such as type 2 diabetes (T2D) and cardiovascular disease. ER, endoplasmic reticulum; ROS, reactive oxygen species. (*Modified from* Duque-Guimarães DE, Ozanne SE. Nutritional programming of insulin resistance: causes and consequences. Trends Endocrinol Metab. 2013 Oct;24(10):525 to 35.)

suggested that there may be critical epochs when the maternal nutritional status was more likely to affect fetal health. Consistently, animal studies have also shown that altered maternal diet and weight gain during pregnancy can trigger placental inflammation and oxidative stress, and alter nutrient transport across the placenta.[67] In humans, nutritional factors during the process of placental formation can affect the offspring even several decades after birth.

Maternal Nutritional Status During Later Pregnancy

Unbalanced maternal diets
Nutrition during pregnancy can alter the metabolic balance in the fetus. Late gestation maternal diets with excessive protein and low carbohydrate content may not alter the placental weight, but these may increase the risk of future hypertension in the children born to these mothers. These children may continue to have high cortisol levels into adulthood.[68] Similar results have been seen in pregnant pigs, whereby excessive protein intake compared with carbohydrates altered the expression of glucocorticoid-related genes and carbohydrate metabolism in the liver, and the hormonal balance through the placenta.[69] On the other extreme, inadequate protein intake during pregnancy may also affect the metabolic/autonomic profiles in the offspring and needs further study.

Fasting during pregnancy
Ramadan fasting is frequently observed in Islamic communities. Although pregnant and lactating women are not required to do Ramadan fasting per religion, many still choose to fast. Ramadan fasting during pregnancy did not show significant effects on the biophysical profile, amniotic fluid index, reactivity of the nonstress test, Doppler indices of the umbilical and middle cerebral arteries, or fetal growth.[70] Azizi and colleagues[71] did not find a significant effect of Ramadan fasting on intelligence quotient scores in 4 to 13 years old children.

Pregnancy in adolescent mothers
Adolescence (age <20 years) is a distinct and unique physical and developmental stage in a woman's life. Adolescent pregnancy has distinct risks and hence understanding of this risk is important for better outcomes for the mother and the infant. Worldwide, 10% of infants are born to adolescent mothers but they are responsible for 23% of maternal morbidity and mortality.[72] Adolescents have a significantly lower attendance of prenatal classes and first-trimester antenatal visits due to perceived lack of importance of the prenatal visit, to hide pregnancy, judgmental attitudes from health care providers, financial barriers and many other reasons. Adolescents who are pregnant have higher rates of smoking and substance abuse.[73] Anemia (hemoglobin < 10.5 g/dL) is commonly seen in pregnant adolescents (prevalence of 50% to 66%) usually attributed to inadequate nutrition.[74] Soares and colleagues showed significantly lower body iron stores and ferritin in pregnant adolescents than in pregnant adults.[75] Care for the pregnant adolescent should, therefore, incorporate nutritional care to both optimize weight gain and manage potential nutritional deficiencies.[76]

The depression rate in this age group varies from 16% to 44%, almost twice as high as in adult pregnant women and nonpregnant adolescents. There is also an increased association with adverse maternal, neonatal outcome, and postpartum depression.[77] Adolescent pregnancies have a higher risk of PTB (<37 weeks), early PTB, (<32 weeks), and extremely early PTB (<28 weeks), as well as low birth weight (<2500 g) and very low birth weight (<1500 g) infants,[78] IUGR (<3rd centile for gestational age), stillbirths, and neonatal-intensive-care-unit admissions and neonatal deaths.[79] Teen pregnancies are also associated with an increase in congenital anomalies of the face (cleft lip, cleft palate), digits (polydactyly, syndactyly), central nervous system (anencephaly, spina bifida, hydrocephaly, microcephaly), and the gastrointestinal system (gastroschisis, omphalocele).[80] Antenatal ultrasound is recommended at 18 to 20 weeks gestation to rule out congenital anomalies. Another assessment at 32 to 34 weeks is recommended to evaluate for IUGR.

Adolescent mothers are at increased risk for recurrence of pregnancy at short interval, with 25% becoming pregnant again within 2 years of delivery. Intra-uterine contraceptive devices,intramuscular formulation of medroxyprogesterone acetate and the etonorgestrel implant are better at preventing pregnancy than oral contraception, contraceptive patch, or barrier methods.[81] Postpartum care programs should be available to support adolescent parents and their children, to improve the mothers' knowledge of parenting, to increase breastfeeding rates, to screen for and manage postpartum depression, to increase birth intervals, and to decrease repeat pregnancy rates.

Future Studies

There is a need for continued studies in human cohorts and animal models to evaluate nutritional interventions for fetal growth and development in undernourished as well as overweight/obese mothers. It seems that many nutrients can possibly alter vasoregulation in the utero-placental circulation. Amino acids may affect not only protein synthesis and tissue growth but also serve as major donors of methyl groups to affect DNA and histone modifications. Understanding the functional role(s) of specific amino acids and micronutrients as metabolic regulators during gestation will be highly desirable. Finally, multidisciplinary efforts are required to develop effective solutions for prevention, timely diagnosis, and treatment of gestational diabetes and fetal/neonatal macrosomia, and IUGR.

Best Practices

- Maternal nutrition needs close study to determine the optimum daily intake of carbohydrates, proteins, lipids, trace elements, and vitamins.
- Fetal nutrition and growth need close monitoring throughout the pregnancy.
- Maternal age, nutritional status, and conditions such as obesity and diabetes can have long-term implications on fetal outcomes. There is also a need for vigilance for the intake of toxins such as mercury.

CLINICS CARE POINTS

- Nutrition in pregnant women may be an important determinant of fetal/maternal outcomes. Maternal obesity, diabetes, and many genetic disorders can affect fetal growth and development.
- The nutrient supply to the fetus is dependent on placental transport; the capacity for nutritional transport capacity continues to grow throughout gestation.
- Fetal nutrient requirements are determined by the rate of growth, the composition of new tissues, and the metabolic rate.
- There is a need for continued study of the transplacental transport of various nutrients, including carbohydrates, proteins, lipids, iron, folate, iodine, and various vitamins.
- The impact of various toxins such as mercury needs study.

DISCLOSURE

The authors have nothing to disclose.

REFERENCES

1. Guenther PM, Dodd KW, Reedy J, et al. Most Americans eat much less than recommended amounts of fruits and vegetables. J Am Diet Assoc 2006;106(9): 1371–9.
2. Nielsen SJ, Popkin BM. Changes in beverage intake between 1977 and 2001. Am J Prev Med 2004;27(3):205–10.
3. Flegal KM, Carroll MD, Kit BK, et al. Prevalence of obesity and trends in the distribution of body mass index among US adults, 1999-2010. JAMA 2012;307(5): 491–7.
4. Rasmussen KM, Yaktine AL, editors. Weight gain during pregnancy: reexamining the guidelines. National Institutes of Health; 2009. The National Academies Collection: Reports funded by.
5. Catalano PM. Obesity, insulin resistance, and pregnancy outcome. Reproduction 2010;140(3):365–71.

6. Cogswell ME, Scanlon KS, Fein SB, et al. Medically advised, mother's personal target, and actual weight gain during pregnancy. Obstet Gynecol 1999;94(4): 616–22.

7. Battaglia FC, Hay WW Jr. Energy and substrate requirements for fetal and placental growth and metabolism. In: Beard RW, Nathanielsz PW, editors. Fetal physiology and medicine. Marcel Dekker; 1984. p. 601–28.

8. Dilworth MR, Sibley CP. Review: transport across the placenta of mice and women. *Placenta*. 2013;34(Suppl):S34–9.

9. Simmons DG, Natale DN, Bogay V, et al. Early patterning of the chorion leads to the trilaminar trophoblast cell structure in the placental labyrinth. Development 2008;135(12):2083–91.

10. Dilworth MR, Kusinski LC, Cowley E, et al. Placental-specific Igf2 knockout mice exhibit hypocalcemia and adaptive changes in placental calcium transport. Proc Natl Acad Sci U S A 2010;107(8):3894–9.

11. Tarrade A, Panchenko P, Junien C, et al. Placental contribution to nutritional pro-gramming of health and diseases: epigenetics and sexual dimorphism. J Exp Biol 2015;218(Pt 1):50–8.

12. Widdas WF. Inability of diffusion to account for placental glucose transfer in the sheep and consideration of the kinetics of a possible carrier transfer. J Physiol 1952;118(1):23–39.

13. W.W. H. Glucose metabolism in the fetal-placental unit. In: R.M. C, editor. Princi-ples of perinatal-neonatal metabolism. Springer; 1991.

14. Cross KW. Review lecture. La chaleur animale and the infant brain. J Physiol 1979;294:1–21.

15. Gresham EL, James EJ, Raye JR, et al. Production and excretion of urea by the fetal lamb. Pediatrics 1972;50(3):372–9.

16. Hornstra G. Essential fatty acids in mothers and their neonates. Am J Clin Nutr 2000;71(5 Suppl):1262S–9S.

17. van Eijsden M, Hornstra G, van der Wal MF, et al. Maternal n-3, n-6, and trans fatty acid profile early in pregnancy and term birth weight: a prospective cohort study. Am J Clin Nutr 2008;87(4):887–95.

18. Allen LH. Anemia and iron deficiency: effects on pregnancy outcome. Am J Clin Nutr 2000;71(5 Suppl):1280S–4S.

19. Scholl TO. Iron status during pregnancy: setting the stage for mother and infant. Am J Clin Nutr 2005;81(5):1218S–22S.

20. Caviedes I, Iniguez G, Hidalgo P, et al. Relationship between folate transporters expression in human placentas at term and birth weights. *Placenta*. 2016; 38:24–8.

21. Geng Y, Gao R, Chen X, et al. Folate deficiency impairs decidualization and alters methylation patterns of the genome in mice. Mol Hum Reprod 2015;21(11): 844–56.

22. Ahmed T, Fellus I, Gaudet J, et al. Effect of folic acid on human trophoblast health and function in vitro. *Placenta*. 2016;37:7–15.

23. Li Y, Gao R, Liu X, et al. Folate deficiency could restrain decidual angiogenesis in pregnant mice. Nutrients 2015;7(8):6425–45.

24. Ge J, Wang J, Zhang F, et al. Correlation between MTHFR gene methylation and pre-eclampsia, and its clinical significance. Genet Mol Res 2015;14(3):8021–8.

25. Mosley BS, Cleves MA, Siega-Riz AM, et al. Neural tube defects and maternal folate intake among pregnancies conceived after folic acid fortification in the United States. Am J Epidemiol 2009;169(1):9–17.

26. Ray JG, Wyatt PR, Vermeulen MJ, et al. Greater maternal weight and the ongoing risk of neural tube defects after folic acid flour fortification. Obstet Gynecol 2005; 105(2):261–5.

27. Vanderpas J. Nutritional epidemiology and thyroid hormone metabolism. Annu Rev Nutr 2006;26:293–322.

28. Zimmermann MB. The effects of iodine deficiency in pregnancy and infancy. Paediatr Perinat Epidemiol 2012;26(Suppl 1):108–17.

29. Farmer B, Larson BT, Fulgoni VL 3rd, et al. A vegetarian dietary pattern as a nutrient-dense approach to weight management: an analysis of the national health and nutrition examination survey 1999-2004. J Am Diet Assoc 2011; 111(6):819–27.

30. Grandjean P, White RF, Weihe P, et al. Neurotoxic risk caused by stable and variable exposure to methylmercury from seafood. Ambul Pediatr 2003;3(1):18–23.

31. Oken E, Kleinman KP, Berland WE, et al. Decline in fish consumption among pregnant women after a national mercury advisory. Obstet Gynecol 2003; 102(2):346–51.

32. Langendonk JG, Roos JC, Angus L, et al. A series of pregnancies in women with inherited metabolic disease. J Inherit Metab Dis 2012;35(3):419–24.

33. Mak CM, Lee HC, Chan AY, et al. Inborn errors of metabolism and expanded newborn screening: review and update. Crit Rev Clin Lab Sci 2013;50(6):142–62.

34. Elango R, Ball RO. Protein and amino acid requirements during pregnancy. Adv Nutr 2016;7(4):839S–44S.

35. Cetin I, Alvino G, Cardellicchio M. Long chain fatty acids and dietary fats in fetal nutrition. J Physiol 2009;587(Pt 14):3441–51.

36. Arn PH, Hauser ER, Thomas GH, et al. Hyperammonemia in women with a mutation at the ornithine carbamoyltransferase locus. a cause of postpartum coma. N Engl J Med 1990;322(23):1652–5.

37. Lipskind S, Loanzon S, Simi E, et al. Hyperammonemic coma in an ornithine transcarbamylase mutation carrier following antepartum corticosteroids. J Perinatol 2011;31(10):682–4.

38. van Spronsen FJ, van Wegberg AM, Ahring K, et al. Key European guidelines for the diagnosis and management of patients with phenylketonuria. Lancet Diabetes Endocrinol 2017;5(9):743–56.

39. Morris AA, Kozich V, Santra S, et al. Guidelines for the diagnosis and management of cystathionine beta-synthase deficiency. J Inherit Metab Dis 2017;40(1): 49–74.

40. Natarajan SK, Ibdah JA. Role of 3-hydroxy fatty acid-induced hepatic lipotoxicity in acute fatty liver of pregnancy. Int J Mol Sci 2018;19(1). https://doi.org/10.3390/ijms19010322.

41. Illsinger S, Janzen N, Sander S, et al. Preeclampsia and HELLP syndrome: impaired mitochondrial function in umbilical endothelial cells. Reprod Sci 2010; 17(3):219–26.

42. Viswanathan M, Siega-Riz AM, Moos MK, et al. Outcomes of maternal weight gain. Evid Rep Technol Assess (Full Rep) 2008;168:1–223.

43. Poston L, Harthoorn LF, Van Der Beek EM. Contributors to the IEW. Obesity in pregnancy: implications for the mother and lifelong health of the child. a consensus statement. Pediatr Res 2011;69(2):175–80.

44. Olson G, Blackwell SC. Optimization of gestational weight gain in the obese gravida: a review. Obstet Gynecol Clin North Am 2011;38(2):397–407, xii.

45. Salihu HM, Dunlop AL, Hedayatzadeh M, et al. Extreme obesity and risk of stillbirth among black and white gravidas. Obstet Gynecol 2007;110(3):552–7.

46. Bujold E, Hammoud A, Schild C, et al. The role of maternal body mass index in outcomes of vaginal births after cesarean. Am J Obstet Gynecol 2005;193(4): 1517–21.

47. Chiefari E, Arcidiacono B, Foti D, et al. Gestational diabetes mellitus: an updated overview. J Endocrinol Invest 2017;40(9):899–909.

48. Beardsall K, Ogilvy-Stuart AL, et al. Developmental physiology of carbohydrate metabolism and the pancreas. In: Kovacs CS, Deal CL, editors. Maternal-fetal and neonatal endocrinology. Academic Press; 2020. p. 587–97.

49. Li M, Hinkle SN, Grantz KL, et al. Glycaemic status during pregnancy and longitudinal measures of fetal growth in a multi-racial US population: a prospective cohort study. Lancet Diabetes Endocrinol 2020;8(4):292–300.

50. Chiefari E, Quaresima P, Visconti F, et al. Gestational diabetes and fetal overgrowth: time to rethink screening guidelines. Lancet Diabetes Endocrinol 2020; 8(7):561–2.

51. American Diabetes A. 14. management of diabetes in pregnancy: standards of medical care in diabetes-2021. Diabetes Care 2021;44(Suppl 1):S200–10.

52. Sewell MF, Huston-Presley L, Super DM, et al. Increased neonatal fat mass, not lean body mass, is associated with maternal obesity. Am J Obstet Gynecol 2006;195(4):1100–3.

53. Tam WH, Ma RC, Yang X, et al. Glucose intolerance and cardiometabolic risk in adolescents exposed to maternal gestational diabetes: a 15-year follow-up study. Diabetes Care 2010;33(6):1382–4.

54. Stothard KJ, Tennant PW, Bell R, et al. Maternal overweight and obesity and the risk of congenital anomalies: a systematic review and meta-analysis. JAMA 2009; 301(6):636–50.

55. Abenhaim HA, Kinch RA, Morin L, et al. Effect of prepregnancy body mass index categories on obstetrical and neonatal outcomes. Arch Gynecol Obstet 2007; 275(1):39–43.

56. Marconi AM, Paolini C, Buscaglia M, et al. The impact of gestational age and fetal growth on the maternal-fetal glucose concentration difference. Obstet Gynecol 1996;87(6):937–42.

57. Neggers YH, Cutter GR, Alvarez JO, et al. The relationship between maternal serum zinc levels during pregnancy and birthweight. Early Hum Dev 1991; 25(2):75–85.

58. Goldenberg RL, Tamura T, Cliver SP, et al. Serum folate and fetal growth retardation: a matter of compliance? Obstet Gynecol 1992;79(5):719–22.

59. Garite TJ, Clark R, Thorp JA. Intrauterine growth restriction increases morbidity and mortality among premature neonates. Am J Obstet Gynecol 2004;191(2): 481–7.

60. Blair E, Stanley F. Intrauterine growth and spastic cerebral palsy. I. Association with birth weight for gestational age. Am J Obstet Gynecol 1990;162(1):229–37.

61. Barker DJ. The fetal and infant origins of adult disease. Br Med J 1990;301(6761): 1111.

62. Crispi F, Bijnens B, Figueras F, et al. Fetal growth restriction results in remodeled and less efficient hearts in children. Circulation 2010;121(22):2427–36.

63. Barker DJ, Osmond C. Infant mortality, childhood nutrition, and ischaemic heart disease in England and Wales. Lancet 1986;1(8489):1077–81.

64. Painter RC, de Rooij SR, Bossuyt PM, et al. Early onset of coronary artery disease after prenatal exposure to the Dutch famine. Am J Clin Nutr 2006;84(2):322–7 ; quiz 466-7.

65. Syddall HE, Sayer AA, Simmonds SJ, et al. Birth weight, infant weight gain, and cause-specific mortality: the Hertfordshire Cohort Study. Am J Epidemiol 2005; 161(11):1074–80.
66. Roseboom TJ, Painter RC, de Rooij SR, et al. Effects of famine on placental size and efficiency. Placenta. 2011;32(5):395–9.
67. Thornburg KL, O'Tierney PF, Louey S. Review: the placenta is a programming agent for cardiovascular disease. Placenta. 2010;31(Suppl):S54–9.
68. Kanitz E, Otten W, Tuchscherer M, et al. High and low proteinratio carbohydrate dietary ratios during gestation alter maternal-fetal cortisol regulation in pigs. PLoS One 2012;7(12):e52748.
69. Metges CC, Gors S, Lang IS, et al. Low and high dietary protein:carbohydrate ratios during pregnancy affect materno-fetal glucose metabolism in pigs. J Nutr 2014;144(2):155–63.
70. Abd-Allah Rezk M, Sayyed T, Abo-Elnasr M, et al. Impact of maternal fasting on fetal well-being parameters and fetal-neonatal outcome: a case-control study. J Matern Fetal Neonatal Med 2016;29(17):2834–8.
71. Azizi F, Sadeghipour H, Siahkolah B, et al. Intellectual development of children born of mothers who fasted in Ramadan during pregnancy. Int J Vitam Nutr Res 2004;74(5):374–80.
72. UNFPA annual report: Available at: https://www.unfpa.org/publications/unfpa-annual-report-2007. Accessed April 14, 2022.
73. Organization DoCaAHaDotWH. Child and adolescent health and development. 2007. Available at: https://apps.who.int)iris)9789241595384_eng. Accessed April 14, 2022.
74. Chang SC, O'Brien KO, Nathanson MS, et al. Hemoglobin concentrations influence birth outcomes in pregnant African-American adolescents. J Nutr 2003; 133(7):2348–55.
75. Soares NN, Mattar R, Camano L, et al. Iron deficiency anemia and iron stores in adult and adolescent women in pregnancy. Acta Obstet Gynecol Scand 2010; 89(3):343–9.
76. Briggs MM, Hopman WM, Jamieson MA. Comparing pregnancy in adolescents and adults: obstetric outcomes and prevalence of anemia. J Obstet Gynaecol Can 2007;29(7):546–55.
77. McClanahan KK. Depression in pregnant adolescents: considerations for treatment. J Pediatr Adolesc Gynecol 2009;22(1):59–64.
78. Malabarey OT, Balayla J, Klam SL, et al. Pregnancies in young adolescent mothers: a population-based study on 37 million births. J Pediatr Adolesc Gynecol 2012;25(2):98–102.
79. de Vienne CM, Creveuil C, Dreyfus M. Does young maternal age increase the risk of adverse obstetric, fetal and neonatal outcomes: a cohort study. Eur J Obstet Gynecol Reprod Biol 2009;147(2):151–6.
80. Chen XK, Wen SW, Fleming N, et al. Teenage pregnancy and adverse birth outcomes: a large population based retrospective cohort study. Int J Epidemiol 2007;36(2):368–73.
81. Tocce K, Sheeder J, Python J, et al. Long acting reversible contraception in postpartum adolescents: early initiation of etonogestrel implant is superior to IUDs in the outpatient setting. J Pediatr Adolesc Gynecol 2012;25(1):59–63.

Human Milk Lipids Induce Important Metabolic and Epigenetic Changes in Neonates

Keyur Donda, MD[a], Akhil Maheshwari, MD[b],*

KEYWORDS

- Fatty acids • DNA methylation • Infant nutrition • Breast milk • Lipid receptors
- Intrauterine growth restriction • Extrauterine growth restriction
- Polyunsaturated fatty acids

KEY POINTS

- Lipids are a major source of energy in neonates. However, in addition to the known nutritional roles, lipids are now also known to activate a range of metabolic pathways and regulate gene expression.
- The perinatal period may be particularly important for long-term metabolic, cardiovascular, and cognitive health because the initial nutritional exposures may set up patterns of nutrient utilization.
- The composition of lipids ingested/administered in young infants can influence the expression of regulatory genes that determine long-term health and disease.
- Early recognition of nutritional programming can help in the identification of potential therapeutic targets and timely intervention to prevent adult-onset chronic diseases.

INTRODUCTION

Recent years have shown major advances in the care of premature and critically ill neonates with decreased morbidity and mortality. However, growth failure remains a frequent problem in these patients, and there is a clear need to evaluate nutritional practices. Growth failure in neonates and young infants is usually categorized based on intrauterine and extrauterine onset. Infants with anthropometric measurements less than the 10th percentile at birth are recognized to have had intrauterine growth restriction (IUGR) and are known to be at increased risk of adverse clinical outcomes.[1] However, increasing information now shows that many neonatal intensive care unit

Funding: NIH awards HL133022 and HL124078 (to A.M.).
a Department of Pediatrics, University of South Florida Health Morsani College of Medicine, Tampa, FL, USA; b Global Newborn Society, Clarksville, MD, USA
* Corresponding author.
E-mail address: akhil@globalnewbornsociety.org

Abbreviations	
IUGR	intrauterine growth restriction
MFG	milk-fat globules
CLD	cytoplasmic lipid droplet
MLG	membrane encapsulated milk lipid globules
MCFA	medium-chain fatty acids
SV	sectory vesicles
ARA	Arachidonic acid
DHA	Docosahexaenoic acid
PUFA	polyunsaturated fatty acid
LA	linoleic acid
EPA	eicosapentaenoic acid
LCPUFA	long-chain polyunsaturated fatty acids
MUFA	monounsaturated FA
SFA	saturated FA
SNP	single nucleotide polymorphisms
FADS	fatty desaturase cluster
LDL	low-density lipoprotein

patients and graduates also have extrauterine growth restriction; some studies show prevalence rates as high as 90%.[2,3] After premature birth, the continuous supply of nutrients from placenta ceases, and even best efforts to maintain nutrition at high levels do not always succeed in achieving postnatal growth rates similar to those in utero. To correct IUGR and/or suboptimal postnatal growth owing to feeding intolerance or high metabolic rates related to illness, caloric supplementation in enteral feedings or with parenteral nutrition is frequently used. Lipids are an essential source of calories in both strategies and need evaluation for both the optimization of doses and the identification of any adverse effects. The importance of dietary lipids has also been emphasized in 2 other articles, one by Santoro and Martin, and another by Groh-Wargo and Barr, within this issue of the Clinics in Perinatology.

In this article, the authors reviewed lipids as a main building block and explored the major molecular pathways. They have also attempted to evaluate the lipid-related epigenetic changes and the clinical implications as a result. This article combines peer-reviewed evidence from the authors' own studies with an extensive literature search in the databases PubMed, EMBASE, and Scopus.

HUMAN MILK LIPIDS

Fats constitute about 2.5% to 5% of human milk and contribute to more than 50% of the infant's daily energy requirement (**Table 1**). A major fraction is contained in the phospholipid membrane-bound spherical droplets, the milk-fat globules (MFGs), that range between 0.1 and 15 μm in diameter.[4] The MFG membrane contains high concentrations of physiologically important lipids that might be important for preventing infections, promoting colonization with friendlier commensal microflora, neurologic and cognitive development, and maturation of the immune system.[5] The MFG membrane prevents the MFGs from aggregating and keeps these dispersed in the aqueous fraction of milk; there are large amounts of phosphatidylcholine, phosphatidylethanolamine, and sphingomyelin, but relatively less phosphatidylserine and phosphatidylinositol.[6] Ultrastructural and biochemical studies show a triglyceride core enclosed in a protein-rich electron-dense material, likely comprising the peripheral proteins and cytoplasmic domains of the integral membrane proteins, just below the outer

Table 1
Lipid class composition of human milk during lactation

Lipid Class	Percentage of Total Lipids at Lactation Day					
	3	7	21	42	84	Immediate Extraction
Total lipid, % in milk[a]	2.04 ± 1.32	2.89 ± 0.31	3.45 ± 0.37	3.19 ± 0.43	4.87 ± 0.62	
Phospholipid	1.1	0.8	0.8	0.6	0.6	0.81
Monoacylglycerol	—	—	—	—	—	ND
Free fatty acids	—	—	—	—	—	0.08
Cholesterol (mg/dL)[b]	1.3 (34.5)	0.7 (20.2)	0.5 (17.3)	0.5 (17.3)	0.4 (19.5)	0.34
1,2-Diacylglycerol	—	—	—	—	—	0.01
1,3-Diacylglycerol	—	—	—	—	—	ND
Triacylglycerol	97.6	98.5	98.7	98.9	99.0	98.76
Cholesterol esters (mg)[c]						
Number of women	39	41	25	18	8	6

Abbreviation: ND, not done.
[a] Mean ± SEM.
[b] Total cholesterol content ranges from 10 to 20 mg/dL after 21 d in most milks.
[c] Not reported, but in Bitman et al (Bitman J, Wood DL, Mehta NR, et al. Comparison of the cholesteryl ester composition of human milk from preterm and term mothers. J Pediatr Gastroenterol Nutr 1986;5:780), it was 5 mg/dL at 3 d and 1 mg/dL at 21 d and thereafter.
From Jensen RG, Bitman J, Carlson SE. Milk lipids. In: Jensen RG, ed. *Handbook of Milk Composition*. San Diego: Academic Press; 1995.

phospholipid layers.[7] The adipophilin protein is an important regulator of milk lipid production and is present in high concentrations in the membranes of milk-secreting cells.[8,9]

The formation of MFGs begins in the cytoplasm with the packaging of triacylglycerols into microlipid droplets that bud from the endoplasmic reticulum of mammary gland alveolar epithelial cells[6,9] (**Fig. 1**). These cytoplasmic lipid droplets are surrounded by a lipid monolayer and migrate to the apical pole of the epithelial cell to fuse with the plasma membrane, where an outer phospholipid bilayer containing many bioactive proteins is added (**Fig. 2**). The fully fledged MFG is then secreted outside the cell to become part of the milk.[10,11]

The aqueous fraction of milk contains some phospholipids and also vitamin A esters, vitamin D, vitamin K, alkyl glyceryl ethers, and glyceryl ether diesters. More than 400 fatty acids are carried within milk fat. There are about 50 biologically active proteins and polypeptides.[10]

There is considerable interindividual and intraindividual variability in the lipid content, both in the MFGs and in the aqueous fraction, in human milk. The interindividual factors include duration of gestation (milk from mothers who deliver prematurely contains more polyunsaturated fatty acids [PUFAs]), parity (high parity is associated with less lipids), maternal diet (low-fat diets increase medium-chain fatty acids [MCFAs]), and maternal nutritional status (higher weight gain during pregnancy is associated with more milk-fat content).[12]

Considering the interindividual variability, there has been interest in comparison of studies done across geographic areas. The milk-fat content has been noted to vary with geographic location in various parts of the world. Milk fat is known to change with diet and maternal adipose stores. Yuhas and colleagues[13] studied milk samples

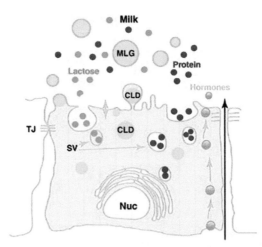

Fig. 1. Lipid secretion in milk. The lipids are packaged in cytoplasmic lipid droplets (CLD; highlighted in yellow) in milk-secreting cells, which are then secreted into milk as membrane encapsulated milk lipid globules (MLG). Milk also contains several other important components, including proteins such as casein, oligosaccharides, and nutrients such as lactose and citrate, which are packaged in secretory vesicles (SV) and transported into milk by exocytosis. In some species, serum and interstitial substances can be transferred into milk before tight junctions (TJs) are formed. (*Modified from* Chong BM, Reigan P, Mayle-Combs KD, Orlicky DJ, McManaman JL. Determinants of adipophilin function in milk lipid formation and secretion. Trends Endocrinol Metab. 2011 Jun;22(6):211-7.)

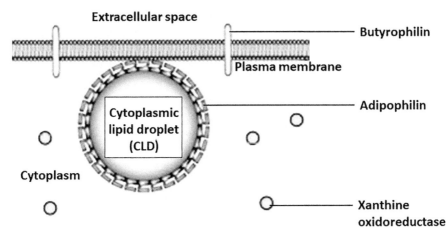

Fig. 2. Putative mechanism of exocytosis of CLDs that contain lipids. Specialized proteins, such as adipophilin, function as adaptors to couple CLDs to the apical plasma membrane. Factors, such as butyrophilin and xanthine oxidoreductase, which are presumably essential for development and secretion of droplets, are recruited to the site. (*From* Chong BM, Reigan P, Mayle-Combs KD, Orlicky DJ, McManaman JL. Determinants of adipophilin function in milk lipid formation and secretion. Trends Endocrinol Metab. 2011 Jun;22(6):211-7.).

from 9 countries (Australia, Canada, Chile, China, Japan, Mexico, Philippines, the United Kingdom, and the United States). The study was fairly well standardized; the timing of collections was comparable in all countries. All samples were collected by electric pump, except in Japan where they were hand expressed. They noted that saturated fatty acids were constant across countries, and monounsaturated fatty acids varied minimally. Arachidonic acid (ARA; C20: 4 $n-6$) was also similar. Docosahexaenoic acid (DHA; 22: 6 $n-3$), however, was variable everywhere, but was dramatically different with milk from Japan, having the highest values, and the United States and Canada, having the lowest values.

Many intraindividual variables have been identified in the lipid content/composition in human milk. Milk lipids show diurnal variations (higher fat content during the day than in the night), and also change with the stage of lactation (higher lipid content in the colostrum), duration of feeding (hind milk has 3 times more lipid content that foremilk), and the type of feeding (on-demand feeding leads to short interfeeding interval and is associated with higher lipid content than "by clock" feeding).

Glycerolipids

Human milk contains a diverse group of lipids, including glycerolipids, phospholipids, free fatty acids, sterols, fat-soluble vitamins, and human MFGs.[14,15] Glycerolipids (monoacylglycerols, diacylglycerols, triacylglycerols) comprise a large proportion, up to 99%, of all human milk lipids. The glycerol backbones are linked to a variable number of fatty acids and are described as short- ($\leq$5 carbon), medium- (6–12 carbons), long- (13–21 carbons), and very-long chain ($\geq$22 carbons) glycerolipids. The fatty acids are further identified as saturated and unsaturated based on the lack or presence, respectively, of carbon-carbon double bonds. Unsaturated fatty acids have one (mono-) or more (PUFAs) of these carbon-carbon double bonds. Finally, depending on the distance of the carbon double bonds from the methyl end of the chain, PUFAs can be classified as omega (ω)-3, ω-6, or ω-9. This nomenclature

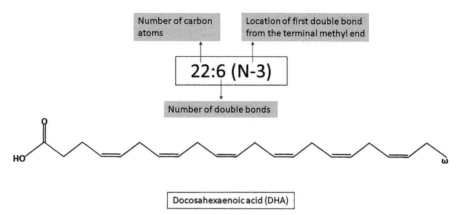

Fig. 3. Nomenclature of fatty acids.

system built on number of carbon atoms, number of double bonds, and the location of the first double bond, is depicted in **Fig. 3**.

Fatty acids

The human body can synthesize most fatty acids except 2 essential fatty acids (EFAs) and derivatives that have to be acquired from the external environment.The EFAs contain double bonds at ω-3 (α-linolenic acid [ALA]) and ω-6 (linoleic acid [LA]) positions. When metabolized, LA is broken down to ARA and ALA to eicosapentaenoic acid (EPA) and DHA. At least 167 fatty acids have been identified in human milk; possibly others are present in trace amounts (**Fig. 4**). Milk from vegetarians (lacto-ovo) contained a lower proportion of fatty acids derived from animal fat and a higher proportion of PUFAs derived from dietary vegetable fat. Women who consumed 35 g or more of animal fat per day had higher C10:0, C12:0, and C18:3 (ALA) but lower levels of unsaturated fats C16:0 and C18:0. Many characteristics of milk-borne lipids and long-chain PUFAs have been described in detail in an article by Santoro and Martin within this issue of the *Clinics in Perinatology*.

Fatty acid composition varies depending on the geographic location, maternal diet during pregnancy and lactation, gestational age, and circadian rhythm (**Fig. 5**). Milk from American and European mothers typically contain 35% to 40% saturated fatty acids as compared with 55% to 60% in Filipino mothers. The dramatic variation is seen in DHA content, with milk from Japanese and Filipino mothers having the highest level and American and Canadian mothers having the lowest level.[13] Maternal diet is another important factor that has extensive impact on the fat component alteration in breast milk, but not on the total fat amount. In the United States, dietary changes with increased consumption of vegetable oils have led to a steady increase of LA content in breast milk, from 6% to 16%, whereas ALA content has remained unchanged.[16] Provision of LA or LA-rich fat to lactating mothers increased LA content of breast milk.[17,18]

The ω-3 fatty acids are important components of milk. DHA (22 carbons, ω-3) is detectable in infantile nerve and brain tissue, retina, and testes.[19] Human milk contains DHA in large amounts. EPA (20 carbons; ω-3) is part of another group of ω-3 fatty acids, the eicosanoids. These comprise 2 families, the prostanoids (prostaglandins, prostacyclins, and thromboxanes) and the leukotrienes. Both are known primarily as inflammatory mediators, but in many situations, the eicosanoids provide cytoprotection and vasoactivity.

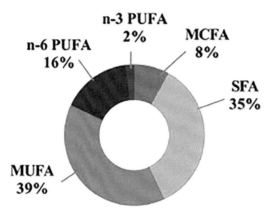

Fig. 4. Diversity of fatty acid (FA) categories and individual FA in term mature human milk after pooled data analysis of worldwide milk samples. The figure highlights the distribution per FA category and particular FAs predominantly contributing to the total HMFA fraction. The overall contribution of LCPUFAs is relatively low compared with the other FA categories and mainly comes from linoleic acid (C18:2 *n* −6). MCFA, (saturated) medium-chain FA (C6–C12); MUFA, monounsaturated FA (1 double-bond); SFA, saturated FA (FA without double-bond). (*From* Floris LM, Stahl B, Abrahamse-Berkeveld M, Teller IC. Human milk fatty acid profile across lactational stages after term and preterm delivery: A pooled data analysis. Prostaglandins Leukot Essent Fatty Acids. 2020 May;156:102023.)

Coastal populations with high fish consumption show higher DHA content in breast milk. The impact of a fish-rich diet has been confirmed in a randomized controlled trial (RCT).[20] On the other hand, a vegan and vegetarian diet is rich in ω-6, LA, and ω-6 PUFAs but is deficient in ω-3 fatty acids and monounsaturated fatty acids. Milk from vegan and vegetarian mothers contains 4 times higher ω-6, LA content than cow's milk.[21–23] Maternal fat intake, regardless of source (animal vs. plant based), also determines the fatty acid composition of human breast milk. Lactating mothers with low-fat intake have breast milk with higher MCFAs and ARA content.[24] The milk composition differs between mothers of premature full-term neonates, with higher levels of MCFAs and DHA in premature milk. Moreover, ARA and DHA seemed to decrease, and short- and MCFAs increased over time[25–27] (**Fig. 6**).

Polyunsaturated Fatty Acids

PUFAss include C18:2 and C18:3, or linoleic and linolenic acid. The ratio of polyunsaturated to saturated fats (P/S ratio) in bovine milk is 4, but the ratios in human milk are approximately 1.2 to 1.3. The essentiality of PUFAs in brain and retinal development has received prime attention of researchers for years, and therefore, has been studied extensively. The nervous system is the one of the largest lipid-containing tissues after the adipose tissue. The human brain grows exponentially between the third trimester and 18 months of life. At full growth, the average brain contains approximately 50% to 60% of its dry weight as lipids.[19] PUFAs are also determinants of proper myelination, an essential process for optimal brain function.[28] Furthermore, PUFAs are essential drivers of immunologic development, adipocyte differentiation, and other biological processes, including organogenesis and angiogenesis. DHA and ARA are the principal long-chain polyunsaturated fatty acids (≥C18 and more than one double-bond) (LCPUFAs) supplied by breast milk. Human breast milk worldwide contains 0.32% + 0.22% weight/weight (wt/wt) and 0.47% + 0.13% wt/wt DHA and ARA,

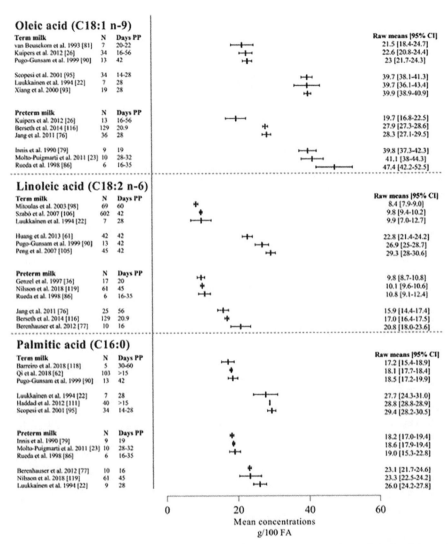

Fig. 5. Human milk contains variable amounts of key fatty acids, such as oleic, linoleic, and palmitic acid. The data show results from 3 studies reporting the highest and lowest mean levels in both term and preterm mature milk (16 to ≤60 days postpartum) for each. The interstudy variation was higher for oleic and linoleic at 7.9% to 30.6% and 18.4% to 52.5% of total fatty acids, than for palmitic acid that ranged between 15.4% and 31% of the total fatty acid content. (*Modified from* Floris LM, Stahl B, Abrahamse-Berkeveld M, Teller IC. Human milk fatty acid profile across lactational stages after term and preterm delivery: A pooled data analysis. Prostaglandins Leukot Essent Fatty Acids. 2020 May;156:102,023.)

respectively, with geographic variation.[29] The LCPUFAs in breast milk are derived from 2 sources, maternal diet and maternal hepatic and adipose tissue stores. Most ARA in breast milk comes from body stores, and hence, the level in breast milk remains constant regardless of maternal diet. In contrast, milk DHA content has a linear relationship with dietary DHA. The amount of LCPUFA supplementation and the need for such a supplementation in any infant to achieve neurodevelopmental benefits are a

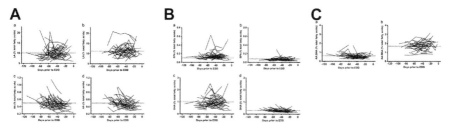

Fig. 6. (*A*) Longitudinal variability in ω-6 PUFA concentrations in human milk from mothers of preterm neonates. Temporal changes in the concentration of LA (*top panel*) and AA (*lower panel*) in human milk (% total fatty acids) from mothers of preterm infants in the high-DHA group (*left column*) or control (*right column*). (*B*) Longitudinal variability in ω-3 PUFA concentrations in human milk from the same mothers. Graph shows temporal changes in the concentration (% total fatty acids) of EPA (*top panel*) and DHA (*lower panel*) in human milk from mothers of preterm infants in the high-DHA group (*left column*) or control (*right column*). (*C*) Longitudinal variation in the ratio AA/DHA present in human milk samples from mothers of preterm neonates. The temporal changes in the ratio AA/DHA in human milk from mothers of preterm infants in the high-DHA group (*left column*) or control (*right column*). Each solid black line represents human milk samples collected from individual women at approximately 2-week intervals from enrollment until the infant's expected term delivery date. Dashed gray lines show the mean for the group. Multiple samples were collected for many women with n = 42, 34, 22, 17, and 6 mothers from the high-DHA group providing 2 to 6 samples, respectively, during the intervention period, whereas n = 44, 27, 19, 9 and 5 mothers in the control group provided 2 to 6 samples during the intervention period. AA-DHA, arachidonic acid-docohexaenoic acid ; EDD, expected delivery date. (*From* Smithers LG, Markrides M, Gibson RA. Human milk fatty acids from lactating mothers of preterm infants: a study revealing wide intra- and inter-individual variation. Prostaglandins Leukot Essent Fatty Acids. 2010 Jul;83(1):9 to 13.)

matter of intense discussion, particularly when the most recent Cochrane review analyzed 11 RCTs exploring the neurodevelopmental outcomes after LCPUFA supplementation.[30] The results are inconclusive, showing no benefits or harms of LCPUFA supplementation in formula-fed full-term infants. There are at least 4 determinants for LCPUFA availability at site of action in infants: (a) maternal dietary preferences; (b) genetic and environmental factors determining maternal body stores; (c) infant's diet (mother's milk vs formula); and (d) genetic and environmental factors determining infant's endogenous production. The rate-limiting step in LCPUFA biosynthetic pathway is fatty desaturase cluster (*FADS*) on chromosome 11q12.2, which includes 3 genes: *FADS1, FADS2,* and *FADS3*[31] (**Fig. 7**). There are racial differences in allelic frequencies in the FADS genotype; the African American population shows higher production of ARA.[31,32] Similarly, breast-milk LCPUFA content is influenced by maternal genotype. For example, single nucleotide polymorphisms (SNPs) have been described determining LCPUFA in breast milk.[33,34] Interestingly, in a population-based study, breast feeding benefited infants carrying rs174575 SNP in *FADS2* gene with 6.8 higher intelligent quotient points.[35] Together, these findings provide insight of a complex interaction between environment and genotype determining long-term outcomes of a newborn.

The importance of PUFAs is now being recognized increasingly because of the role of these nutrients in brain growth. During the first year of life, the human brain more than doubles in size, and the cortical total phospholipid fatty acid composition in both term and preterm infants is greatly influenced by dietary fat intake. Phospholipids make up about 25% of the solid matter. Brain growth is associated with incorporation

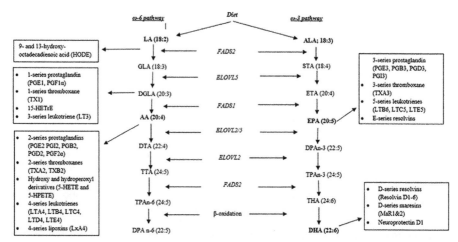

Fig. 7. Metabolically important derivatives of ω-6 and ω-3 PUFAs. AA, arachidonic acid; DGLA, Dihomo gamma linoleic acid; DPA, docosapentaenoic acid; DTA, docosatetraenoic acid; ELVOL, elongase; ETA, eicosatetraenoic acid; GLA, gamma-linoleic acid; STA, steardonic acid; THA, tetrahexaenoic acid; TPA, tetracosapentaenoic acid; TTA, tetracosatetraaenoic acid. (*Modified from* Panda C, Varadharaj S, Voruganti VS. PUFA, genotypes and risk for cardiovascular disease. Prostaglandins Leukot Essent Fatty Acids. 2022 Jan;176:102377.)

of long-chain PUFAs, ARA, and DHA into the phospholipid in the cerebral cortex. The transition from colostrum to mature milk leads to an increase in sphingomyelin and a decrease in phosphatidylcholine in the milk of mothers who deliver prematurely, along with a decrease in phospholipid content. Phospholipids are essential to brain growth, especially in a premature infant. Sphingomyelin and phosphatidylcholine are sources of choline, a major constituent of membranes in the brain and nervous tissue. Extreme dietary alterations in animal experiments have demonstrated an altered PUFA composition of the developing brain. The fatty acids characteristic of gray matter (C20:4 and C22:6) accumulate before the appearance of fatty acids characteristic of myelin (C20:1, paullinic acid; and C24:1, nervonic acid) in the developing brain. ARA (C20:4) and DHA (C22:6) are synthesized from linoleic and linolenic acids, respectively, but the latter two must be obtained in the diet.

Cholesterol

Cholesterol is an essential, consistent component of breast milk that is not affected by maternal dietary changes. It is a key building block for cell membranes, and therefore, important for cell maintenance. In addition to substrate for bile acids, lipoproteins, and vitamin D, cholesterol also derives oxysterols, which serve as ligands for cholesterol, lipid, and glucose homeostasis pathways.[36] The breast milk contains substantial amounts of cholesterol as compared with formula (90–150 mg/L vs 0 to 4 mg/L in formula).[7] Neonatal plasma cholesterol levels are low (50–100 mg/dL) at birth but increase rapidly in breastfed infants over the first few days after birth. These elevated cholesterol levels suppress endogenous cholesterol synthesis.[37,38] In a systematic review including 17 studies, cholesterol was found to be lower in adolescents and adults who received exclusive breast milk during infancy.[39,40] Exclusively breastfed infants seem to be protected against metabolic syndromes in adult life, including dyslipidemia, although the mechanisms are yet to be identified. Early exposure to high cholesterol levels in breast milk could possibly program the cholesterol production and metabolism mechanisms to efficiently regulate cholesterol later in life, and therefore, may provide protection. Animal investigations indicated that high dietary cholesterol early in life was better able to cope with cholesterol in later life and maintained a lower cholesterol level.[41,42] In a study of 6 breastfed and 12 formula-fed infants, ages 4 to 5 months, Wong and colleagues[38] measured the fractional synthesis rate. The breastfed infants had higher cholesterol intakes (18.4 ± 4.0 mg/kg per day) than formula-fed infants (only 3.4 ± 1.8 mg/kg per day). Plasma cholesterol levels were 183 ± 47 versus 112 ± 22 mg/dL; low-density lipoprotein (LDL)-cholesterol levels were 83 ± 26 versus 48 ± 16 mg/dL. An inverse relationship existed between the fractional synthesis rate of cholesterol and dietary intake of cholesterol. The investigators concluded that the greater cholesterol intake of breastfed infants is associated with elevated plasma LDL-cholesterol concentrations. In addition, cholesterol synthesis in human infants may be efficiently regulated by coenzyme A reductase when challenged with dietary cholesterol. A carefully designed, well-controlled longitudinal study is needed exploring how fetal and neonatal programming from early exposure to cholesterol determines the long-term cardiovascular diseases risk in adult life.

SIGNALING PATHWAYS AND RELATED MECHANISMS

Naturally, breast milk is the first source of nutrition for an infant after birth. Even for a premature infant, the goal is to introduce human milk as early as possible after the commencement of the extrauterine life. The aggressive promotion of exclusive breast feeding in any infant stems from many well-documented benefits. It reduces the risk of gastrointestinal as well as respiratory tract infections, sudden infant death syndrome, allergies, necrotizing enterocolitis in premature infants, and overall mortality.[43,44] In addition, breast milk determines long-term health "programming" that protect against many disorders of adulthood, such as obesity, type 2 diabetes, hypertension, hyperlipidemia, cancers, and neurocognitive impairment.[39,45–49] Therefore, breast milk may not only be a source of nutrition but also an evolutionary way of communication between the mother's and the infant's bodies that shapes with both short- and long-term health of the offspring. In this section, the authors review how interplay between various signaling pathways, in utero environment, infant's genotype, and various ligands in breast milk affects fetal and neonatal programming.

LIPIDS AND EPIGENETIC CHANGES

Nutritional development of a neonate is a complex and critical journey that begins in utero and continues in the "outer world" after birth, with contributions from various factors broadly divided into maternal, fetal, and placental categories. Interactions between clinical, molecular, and/or cellular events during this critical perinatal period of nutritional development may determine the lifelong health of the premature neonate. A "two-hit model" with environmental factors in the presence of genetic predisposition may explain individual variability of early nutritional status and disease state later in life, particularly chronic conditions, such as cardiovascular diseases, type 2 diabetes, insulin resistance, and obesity.

Lipid promotion of genomic variation in fetal and neonatal growth/development regulation may involve 2 basic mechanisms: (a) inherited genetic variations encoded in DNA that controls the metabolism of lipids; and (b) epigenetic changes that may explain the effect of lipids on gene expression.[50] The phenomenon of fetal and infant origins of adult disease was first elucidated by the "Barker hypothesis."[51] The hypothesis states that the events in early life "program" the fetus to better prepare for similar situations in later life. The programming can be subtle with normal phenotypic appearance at birth but different metabolic traits that may become apparent after exposure to additional stressors later in life. Such events may have started even in early life of the mother herself. As evidenced by many studies, maternal malnutrition, both underweight and overweight, directly impacts offspring during fetal life, childhood, as well as later life.[52–55] There is a possibility that maternal malnutrition may induce inheritable genetic changes affecting the lifetime health of a child as well as the subsequent generations and provides a basis for "epigenetics." More importantly, these epigenetic changes are modifiable, and therefore, there is an urgent need for in-depth understanding of fatty acid–induced epigenetic changes in neonates that will empower the neonatologist with greater responsibility to make a lifetime difference not only in any human being but also in the upcoming generations.

Epigenetic programming may play a crucial role in gene regulation by chromatin remodeling without changing the underlying DNA sequence. Chromatin consists of double-stranded DNA, histone, and nonhistone proteins. Core histone proteins, H2A, H2B, H3, and H4, form an organizational unit of chromatin, the nucleosome. Epigenetic changes involve core histone modifications by various processes, such as methylation, acetylation, phosphorylation, ADP-ribosylation, monoubiquitylation, and SUMOylation (the acronym SUMO stands for small ubiquitin-like modifier). DNA cytosine methylation (C_pG) and histone posttranslational modifications are the most studied epigenetic mechanisms.

LIPID RECEPTORS AND LIGANDS

The benefits of human milk in neonatal growth and development are undisputable. Fat is an essential macronutrient of human milk. Apart from calorie-dense energy and carbon sources, lipids are crucial gene regulators and impact growth, neural and retinal development as well as immune modulation.[19,56,57] Ongoing research has identified the gene regulatory ability of lipids through various nuclear receptors on top of its nutritional and structural properties.[58] The major lipid-regulated nuclear receptors are peroxisome proliferator activated receptors (PPARs), the liver X receptor (LXR), hepatocyte nuclear factor 4 alpha (HNF4α), and retinoid X receptor (RXR) among which epigenetic modifications of PPARs have been studied. In this section, the authors review the current knowledge of various lipid receptors and ligands, inducible epigenetic changes of the receptors, and the effect on gene regulation and phenotype.

Peroxisome Proliferator Activated Receptors

PPARs are an important superfamily of nuclear receptors that regulate adipogenesis and lipogenesis by modulating cellular development, differentiation, metabolism, and immune response. These contain DNA-binding domains that are agonist-dependent or -independent. Once activated by binding specific ligands, the PPARs undergo conformational changes that permit dissociation of corepressors and binding with coactivators.[59] PPARs heterodimerize with RXRs and bind the PPAR response elements in promoters of the target genes. PPARs are thought to regulate gene expression through either "transactivation" or "transrepression." Transactivation is characterized by ligand-activated PPARs directly acting as transcription factors and regulating gene expression. Transrepression is characterized by ligand-activated PPARs modulating gene regulation indirectly by binding and releasing other transcription regulators that suppress the target genes.[60,61]

There are 3 different subtypes of PPARs with unique tissue expression patterns: PPARα, PPARβ/δ, and PPARγ. **Table 2** describes these PPARs and their activating ligands. PPARα is mainly found in oxidative tissues, such as liver, heart, kidney,

Table 2
Types of peroxisome proliferator activated receptors and activating ligands

Receptor	Endogenous Activating Ligands	Synthetic Activating Ligands
PPARα	Saturated fatty acids, unsaturated fatty acids, leukotriene B4, 8-hydroxyeicosatetraenoic acid (HETE)	Fibrates (clofibrate, fenofibrate, gemfibrozil, Wy-14643)
PPARγ	Polyunsaturated fatty acids (PUFA), 15-HETE, 15-deoxy-Δ12,14-prostaglandinJ2 (15d-PGJ2), 9- and 13-hydroxyoctadecadienoic acid (HODE), components of oxidized low-density lipoprotein (oxLDL)	Thiazolidinediones (rosiglitazone, pioglitazone, troglitazone, ciglitazone)
PPARβ/δ	Saturated fatty acids, PUFA, 15-HETE, prostacyclin	GW-501516

muscle, and brown adipose tissue. It maintains energy homeostasis during fasting and regulates hepatic lipid catabolism by modulating fatty acid oxidation and ketogenesis.[60,61] In addition, it promotes thermogenesis and insulin sensitization and also regulates inflammation.[62–64] PPARγ has 3 subtypes: PPARγ1 is ubiquitously expressed, whereas PPARγ2 and PPARγ3 are expressed mainly in macrophages and white adipose tissue.[65,66] PPARγ is a crucial regulator of adipose tissue development and maintenance, lipogenesis, and insulin sensitization. PPARγ is also vital for establishing the uteroplacental villous circulation and maintaining uterine vascular function (vasoprotective properties), improves endothelium-dependent vasorelaxation by suppressing ET-1 synthesis and prepro-ET-1 expression in vascular endothelial cells.[67–71] PPARβ/δ is the least studied subtype. It is universally expressed but is most abundant in adipose tissue, liver, muscle, and heart. Similar to PPARα, it regulates genes controlling lipid metabolism, glucose homeostasis, thermogenesis, and inflammation. However, different from PPARα and PPARγ, the anti-inflammatory action of PPARβ/δ is mediated by ligand-independent transpression.[72]

The role of PPARs in maternal malnutrition- and placental insufficiency-related IUGR has received attention. PPARγ is highly expressed in human placental tissues, such as the labyrinth zone, trophoblasts, and the vascular smooth muscles,[67,73–75] and helps establish the structure for uteroplacental villous circulation. It also regulates blood flow by modulating vasoreactivity of uterine artery and placental circulation.[68,69,76,77] Fetal programming during the period of malnutrition and placental insufficiency involves PPARγ as evidenced by sex- and tissue-specific deranged expression of PPARγ as well as its corepressors, such as sirtuin 1, and the small ubiquitous nuclear corepressor (Cor-nuclear receptor corepressor), silencing mediator for retinoid and thyroid hormone receptor and coactivators steroid receptor coactivator 1 and the transcriptional intermediary factor 1.[78–81] Early changes in PPARγ signaling mechanisms persist even during childhood and may be responsible for metabolic syndrome later in life.[82] These changes in PPAR expression are thought to be due to epigenetic modifications. Lillycrop and colleagues[83,84] first described epigenetic modification of PPARα in IUGR rat pups induced by maternal protein restriction; the protein-restricted diets led to PPARα gene hypomethylation. The expression of DNA methyltransferase 1 decreased with higher PPARα levels. Like PPARα, epigenetic changes in PPARγ-dependent transcription in adipogenesis have been described. PPARγ regulates the genes encoding SET-domain histone lysine methyltransferase Setd8, which methylates histone H3 and H4. Methylated H3 and H4 are characteristic epigenetic changes implicated in gene silencing.[85] PPARγ gene modifications may also affect lung alveolarization.[86–88] Because PPARγ can be activated by natural ligands, such as the LCPUFAs, as well as synthetic ligands, such as thiazolidinediones, fatty acid supplementation and medications are attractive interventions to reverse these epigenetic changes and clinical consequences.[88–90]

Hepatocyte Nuclear Factor 4α

The HNF4α is a highly conserved nuclear receptor expressed in liver, intestines, pancreas, and kidney. It is a key regulator of hepatocyte function, including lipid homeostasis, and has been linked with several metabolic changes seen in obesity, diabetes, atherosclerosis, and cancer.[91,92] Hertz and colleagues[93] showed that dietary fatty acids can modulate HNFα receptor function. Yuan and colleagues[94] demonstrated that HNF4α binds LA (C18:2ω6), although the functional implications were unclear. In later studies, McCurdy and colleagues[95] showed that it may reprogram fetal hepatic gluconeogenesis, which persisted in postnatal life.[96,97] Prematurity may also epigenetically influence HNF4α expression.[98] There may be decreased methylation of HNF4α at 4 CpG sites in the P1 promoters that correlated with higher triglyceride levels.[99] The hypomethylation of HNF4A-CpG4 in P1 and hypermethylation of HNF4α-CpG3 in P2 may be associated with higher total cholesterol levels.[100] Together, these findings are important, as they highlight in utero epigenetic programming that persists through childhood as well as through adult life and correlates with metabolic phenotypes. However, the mechanisms need further elucidation.

Liver X Receptor

LXRs are nuclear receptors that mediate the effects of fatty acids on gene transcription. There are 2 subtypes of LXRs: LXRα and LXRβ. LXRα is mainly expressed in liver, adipose tissue, and macrophages, whereas LXRβ is more ubiquitous. The best-known endogenous LXR ligands are oxysterols, such as 22-hydroxy-cholesterol, 24(S)-hydroxycholesterol and 24(S), and 25-epoxycholesterol.[101] Although not confirmed, LXRs seem to promote cholesterol homeostasis by promoting its elimination when the tissue concentrations are high.[102–105] These findings differ from those in adults. Fetal and early postnatal programming of LXRs upon exposure to maternal protein-restricted diets may alter histone H3 (K9, 14) methylation and suppress LXRα expression into adulthood.[106] These findings bring up exciting possibilities for research into fetal onset of metabolic diseases of adulthood, with the possibility of modification via diet or methylation inhibitors.

Sterol Regulatory Element Binding Protein-1

Sterol regulatory element binding proteins (SREBPs) are a membrane-bound basic-helix-loop-helix leucine zipper class of transcription factors that are involved in biosynthesis and uptake of cholesterol and fatty acids.[64] There are 2 SREBP genes, SREBP1 and SREBP2, which differ in tissue-specific expression and target gene. SREBP1 has 2 isoforms, SREBP-1a and SREBP-1c, and are responsible for de novo lipogenesis regulation, whereas SREBP-2 regulates cholesterol synthesis. SREBPs bind SREBP cleavage-activating protein (SCAP) and insulin-induced proteins. Depending on the sterol levels, SCAP determines whether to retrain or release SREBPs from the endoplasmic reticulum.[107] Once in the nucleus, SREBP regulates fatty acids and cholesterol synthesis. PUFAs are natural ligands and selectively suppress SREBP1 through proteolytic processing.[108] DHA regulates SREBP1 degradation by proteosome-dependent pathway. There is need for further study to understand the impact of maternal diet and of PUFAs in breast milk on the epigenetic regulation of SREBPs.

Toll-like Receptor-4

Toll-like receptors (TLRs) are important pattern recognition receptors that identify the invading pathogens to activate immune inflammatory responses. TLR4 binds lipopolysaccharide (LPS) from gram-negative bacteria, particularly the fatty acyl chains in the lipid A moiety. Removal of fatty acyl chains from lipid A renders LPS nontoxic.[109,110] Saturated fatty acids may activate, whereas PUFAs can inhibit the TLR4 complex to alter the inflammatory responses.[111,112] Recent studies suggest that TLRs contribute to insulin resistance and the development of metabolic syndrome.[113,114] However, the effects of intrauterine and extrauterine nutrition, particularly the exposure to fatty acids exposure on epigenetic modifications of the TLR4 complex and metabolic syndrome later in life, still need to be studied.

G Protein-Coupled Receptors

G protein-coupled receptors (GPRs) are the largest superfamily of transmembrane receptors with extracellular and intracellular components modulating myriads of physiologic processes, including cell differentiation and growth, inflammation, microbiome, secretion of insulin, and various gastrointestinal hormones.[115–118] There are more than 800 types of GPRs, and only around 200 have been characterized. Here, the authors review only relevant GPRs related to lipids. GPR41 and GPR43 are well expressed in enteroendocrine L cells, white adipocytes, and pancreatic β cells.

Once activated by short-chain fatty acids (SCFAs), such as butyrate, propionate, acetate, valerate, GPP41 and GPR43 are involved in the regulation of glucagon-like peptide (GLP)-1 secretion, leptin production, and insulin secretion.[119] In addition, they also seem to modulate SCFA-induced microbiota-led inflammatory response.[64,120] SCFAs are produced by gut microbiota and play a major role in inflammation regulation via GPRs modulation, particularly, GPR41, GPR43, and GPR109A.[121,122] GPR109A is expressed in colonic epithelial cells, where they suppress inflammation and carcinogenesis by regulating T cells.[119] In contrast, GPR40 and GPR120 are activated by medium- and long-chain, saturated and unsaturated FAs. GPR40 is expressed in pancreatic β-cells and enteroendocrine cells, where it potentiates glucose-stimulated insulin secretion and gastric inhibitor polypeptide and GLP-1, respectively. GPR120 is expressed in hypothalamus and adipose tissues, where it modulates inflammation and adipocyte differentiation, respectively. Because breast milk is the prime source of FAs, its role in GPR-mediated intestinal inflammation modulation needs to be studied.

CLINICAL IMPLICATIONS

Breast milk is the obvious choice for nutrition after birth. However, many situations, including insufficient milk production, medical contraindications for breast feeding, and extreme prematurity, demand alternatives for lipid provision to newborns. Such alternatives include pasteurized donor breast milk (PBM), formula, and intravenous lipid emulsions. There exist major qualitative and quantitative differences in lipid composition as well as long-term outcomes between mother's own milk (MOM) and alternative lipid sources. PBM-fed infants are more likely to encounter growth failure and worse neurodevelopment as compared with MOM.[123–126] The worse outcomes in PBM-fed infants can be explained by significantly less fat content,[126,127] pasteurization-induced inactivation of bile salt-stimulated lipase,[128] and antioxidants such as glutathione,[129] inadequate LC-PUFA, particularly DHA and ARA.[130–132] Similarly, infant formulas and traditional intravenous lipid emulsions contain none or negligible DHA and ARA as compared with MOM. Omegaven is a fish oil–derived lipid preparation that contains DHA and ARA; however, the Food and Drug Administration has approved it only for infants with intestinal failure-associated liver disease.[133] DHA and ARA are important fatty acids for fetal development, particularly for brain growth. Because of biomagnification, there is an exponential increase in LCPUFA transfer to the fetus during the third trimester, and after birth, the newborn continues to receive those LCPUFAs via MOM.[134] However, many infants may have to rely on PBM, formula, and/or intravenous lipid emulsions for lipids, which are deficient in LCPUFAs. Such situations have birthed research studies exploring LCPUFA supplementation in the neurodevelopment of infants. In a Cochrane review including 15 RCTs (n = 1889) evaluating LCPUFA supplementation in term infants, Jasani and colleagues[30] found no favorable effect on growth, visual acuity, and neurodevelopment. Because prematurity cuts the third trimester short, it would be logical to supplement the preterm infants with LCPUFA with expectations of better outcomes. However, the Cochrane review, including 17 RCTs (n = 2260), showed no long-term benefits of LCPUFA supplementations in preterm infants.[135] These systematic reviews are limited by marked heterogeneity owing to variations in dosing and duration of supplementation as well as differences in outcome measures (different endpoints, different evaluation methods). It warrants large, multicenter RCTs teasing out the dose of LCPUFA supplementation, duration, DHA-to-ARA ratio, in conjugation with genetic factors (epigenetic changes in receptors induced by in utero environment, FADS genotype determining availability of LCPUFAs at end organ). In addition, LCPUFAs are one of the many key lipid components of breast milk. We really need to dissect breast milk and roles of the different ingredients in determining the lifetime health. In the future, with more clinical data at our disposal, we may be able to match the infant formula and/or intravenous lipid emulsion composition to MOM.

SUMMARY

The authors have reviewed current literature on lipids and their mechanistic pathways that may broaden the vision of looking at lipids as biologically active signaling molecules. There are important gaps in clinical data and in the understanding of the impact of various components of breast milk. There is a need for large multicenter studies to explore the effects of maternal and neonatal dietary modifications, including breast milk/formula/intravenous lipids with custom-tailored lipid components, on the infant's neurodevelopment and long-term outcomes of metabolic health.

BEST PRACTICES

- Lipids are an essential source of calories for premature infants receiving enteral/parenteral nutrition.
- Careful optimization of lipid doses can promote growth and development, but these dietary modifications need careful monitoring for adverse effects.
- Fats constitute about 2.5-5% of human milk and contribute to more than 50% of the infant's daily energy requirement. Continued examination of these lipid constituents can help develop useful treatment strategies for premature and critically-ill infants.
- The inter-individual and longitudinal variability in the amount/types of lipids in mother's milk needs to be noted.
- The cellular signaling pathways activated by lipids need to be studied for clinical implications.

AUTHOR CONTRIBUTION

K. Donda wrote the article. A. Maheshwari reviewed and made important revisions.

CONFLICTS OF INTEREST

The authors disclose no conflicts.

ACKNOWLEDGMENTS

The authors appreciate all the encouragement given by Dr Benjamin Torres.

REFERENCES

1. Fanaroff, A.A. and R.J. Martin, Fanaroff and Martins Neonatal-Perinatal Medicine.
2. Miller M, et al. Transitioning preterm infants from parenteral nutrition: a comparison of 2 protocols. J Parenter Enteral Nutr 2017;41(8):1371–9.
3. Dusick AM, et al. Growth failure in the preterm infant: can we catch up? Semin Perinatol 2003;27(4):302–10.
4. Lopez C, Menard O. Human milk fat globules: polar lipid composition and in situ structural investigations revealing the heterogeneous distribution of proteins and the lateral segregation of sphingomyelin in the biological membrane. Colloids Surf B Biointerfaces 2011;83(1):29–41.
5. Brink LR, Lönnerdal B. Milk fat globule membrane: the role of its various components in infant health and development. J Nutr Biochem 2020;85:108465.
6. Silva RCD, Colleran HL, Ibrahim SA. Milk fat globule membrane in infant nutrition: a dairy industry perspective. J Dairy Res 2021;88(1):105–16.
7. Koletzko B. Human milk lipids. Ann Nutr Metab 2016;69(Suppl 2):28–40.
8. Lee H, et al. Compositional dynamics of the milk fat globule and its role in infant development. Front Pediatr 2018;6:313.
9. Chong BM, et al. Determinants of adipophilin function in milk lipid formation and secretion. Trends Endocrinol Metab 2011;22(6):211–7.
10. Majid, S., Bioactive components in milk and dairy products. 2009.
11. Smoczyński M. Role of phospholipid flux during milk secretion in the mammary gland. J Mammary Gland Biol Neoplasia 2017;22(2):117–29.
12. Picciano MF. Nutrient composition of human milk. Pediatr Clin North America 2001;48(1):53–67.
13. Yuhas R, Pramuk K, Lien EL. Human milk fatty acid composition from nine countries varies most in DHA. Lipids 2006;41(9):851 8.
14. Wei W, Jin Q, Wang X. Human milk fat substitutes: past achievements and current trends. Prog Lipid Res 2019;74:69–86.
15. Demmelmair H, Koletzko B. Lipids in human milk. Best Pract Res Clin Endocrinol Metab 2018;32(1):57–68.
16. Ailhaud G, et al. Temporal changes in dietary fats: role of n-6 polyunsaturated fatty acids in excessive adipose tissue development and relationship to obesity. Prog Lipid Res 2006;45(3):203–36.
17. Demmelmair H, et al. Metabolism of U13C-labeled linoleic acid in lactating women. J Lipid Res 1998;39(7):1389–96.
18. Harzer G, Dieterich I, Huag M. Effects of the diet on the composition of human milk. Ann Nutr Metab 1984;28.
19. Lauritzen L. The essentiality of long chain n-3 fatty acids in relation to development and function of the brain and retina. Prog Lipid Res 2001;40(1–2):1–94.

20. Dunstan JA, et al. The effects of fish oil supplementation in pregnancy on breast milk fatty acid composition over the course of lactation: a randomized controlled trial. Pediatr Res 2007;62(6):689–94.

21. Sanders TAB, Reddy S. The influence of a vegetarian diet on the fatty acid composition of human milk and the essential fatty acid status of the infant. J Pediatr 1992;120(4):S71–7.

22. Finley DA, et al. Breast milk composition: fat content and fatty composition in vegetarians and non-vegetarians. J Clin Nutr 1985;41(4):787–800.

23. Karcz K, Krolak-Olejnik B. Vegan or vegetarian diet and breast milk composition - a systematic review. Crit Rev Food Sci Nutr 2021;61(7):1081–98.

24. Nasser R, et al. The effect of a controlled manipulation of maternal dietary fat intake on medium and long chain fatty acids in human breast milk in Saskatoon, Canada. Int Breastfeed J 2010;5(1):3.

25. Floris LM, et al. Human milk fatty acid profile across lactational stages after term and preterm delivery: a pooled data analysis. Prostaglandins Leukot Essent Fatty Acids 2020;156:102023.

26. Thakkar SK, et al. Temporal progression of fatty acids in preterm and term human milk of mothers from Switzerland. Nutrients 2019;11(1):112.

27. Iranpour R, et al. Comparison of long chain polyunsaturated fatty acid content in human milk in preterm and term deliveries and its correlation with mothers' diet. J Res Med Sci 2013;18(1):1–5.

28. Chiurazzi M, et al. Human milk and brain development in infants. Reprod Med 2021;2(2):107–17.

29. Brenna JT, et al. Docosahexaenoic and arachidonic acid concentrations in human breast milk worldwide. Am J Clin Nutr 2007;85(6):1457–64.

30. Jasani B, et al. Long chain polyunsaturated fatty acid supplementation in infants born at term. Cochrane Database Syst Rev 2017;3:CD000376.

31. Mathias RA, Pani V, Chilton FH. Genetic variants in the FADS gene: implications for dietary recommendations for fatty acid intake. Curr Nutr Rep 2014;3(2):139–48.

32. Sergeant S, et al. Differences in arachidonic acid levels and fatty acid desaturase (FADS) gene variants in African Americans and European Americans with diabetes or the metabolic syndrome. Br J Nutr 2012;107(4):547–55.

33. Xie L, Innis SM. Genetic variants of the FADS1 FADS2 gene cluster are associated with altered (n-6) and (n-3) essential fatty acids in plasma and erythrocyte phospholipids in women during pregnancy and in breast milk during lactation. J Nutr 2008;138(11):2222–8.

34. Lattka E, et al. Genetic variants in the FADS gene cluster are associated with arachidonic acid concentrations of human breast milk at 1.5 and 6 mo post-partum and influence the course of milk dodecanoic, tetracosenoic, and trans-9-octadecenoic acid concentrations over the. The Am J Clin Nutr 2011;93(2):382–91.

35. Caspi A, et al. Moderation of breastfeeding effects on the IQ by genetic variation in fatty acid metabolism. Proc Natl Acad Sci 2007;104(47):18860–5.

36. Björkhem I. Do oxysterols control cholesterol homeostasis? J Clin Invest 2002;110(6):725–30.

37. Cruz MLA, et al. Effects of infant nutrition on cholesterol synthesis rates. Pediatr Res 1994;35(2):135–40.

38. Wong WW, et al. Effect of dietary cholesterol on cholesterol synthesis in breast-fed and formula-fed infants. J Lipid Res 1993;34(8):1403–11.

39. Owen CG, et al. Infant feeding and blood cholesterol: a study in adolescents and a systematic review. Pediatrics 2002;110(3):597–608.
40. Owen CG, et al. Does initial breastfeeding lead to lower blood cholesterol in adult life? A quantitative review of the evidence. The Am J Clin Nutr 2008; 88(2):305–14.
41. Li JR, Bale LK, Kottke BA. Effect of neonatal modulation of cholesterol homeostasis on subsequent response to cholesterol challenge in adult Guinea pig. J Clin Invest 1980;65(5):1060–8.
42. Mott GF, et al. Cholesterol metabolism in juvenile baboons. Influence of infant and juvenile diets. Arteriosclerosis 1985;5(4):347–54.
43. Agostoni C, et al. Breast-feeding: a commentary by the ESPGHAN committee on nutrition. J Pediatr Gastroenterol Nutr 2009;49(1):112–25.
44. Molbak K, et al. Prolonged breast feeding, diarrhoeal disease, and survival of children in Guinea-Bissau. BMJ 1994;308(6941):1403–6.
45. Owen CG, et al. Effect of infant feeding on the risk of obesity across the life course: a quantitative review of published evidence. Pediatrics 2005;115(5): 1367–77.
46. Owen CG, et al. The effect of breastfeeding on mean body mass index throughout life: a quantitative review of published and unpublished observational evidence. The Am J Clin Nutr 2005;82(6):1298–307.
47. Martin RM. Breastfeeding in infancy and blood pressure in later life: systematic review and meta-analysis. Am J Epidemiol 2005;161(1):15–26.
48. Owen CG, et al. Does breastfeeding influence risk of type 2 diabetes in later life? A quantitative analysis of published evidence. The Am J Clin Nutr 2006; 84(5):1043–54.
49. Anderson JW, Johnstone BM, Remley DT. Breast-feeding and cognitive development: a meta-analysis. Am J Clin Nutr 1999;70(4):525–35.
50. Finch, C.E., The biology of human longevity inflammation, nutrition, and aging in the evolution of lifespans.
51. Barker DJP. Fetal and infant origins of adult disease. Monatsschrift Kinderheilkunde 2001;149(0):S2–6.
52. Castillo H, Santos IS, Matijasevich A. Relationship between maternal pre-pregnancy body mass index, gestational weight gain and childhood fatness at 6–7 years by air displacement plethysmography. Matern Child Nutr 2015;11(4): 606–17.
53. Fall CHD. Fetal malnutrition and long-term outcomes. Basel, Switzerland: S. Karger AG; 2013. p. 11–25.
54. Mangel L, et al. The effect of maternal habitus on macronutrient content of human milk colostrum. J Perinatology 2017;37(7):818–21.
55. Williams CB, Mackenzie KC, Gahagan S. The effect of maternal obesity on the offspring. Clin Obstet Gynecol 2014;57(3):508–15.
56. Serhan CN, Chiang N. Endogenous pro-resolving and anti-inflammatory lipid mediators: a new pharmacologic genus. Br J Pharmacol 2008;153(S1): S200–15.
57. Patole, S., Nutrition for the preterm neonate A clinical perspective.
58. Bravo-Ruiz I, Medina MA, Martinez-Poveda B. From food to genes: transcriptional regulation of metabolism by lipids and carbohydrates. Nutrients 2021;13(5).
59. Aranda, A. and A. Pascual, Aranda 2001_Nuclear hormone receptors and gene expression. 2001.

60. SzéLes L, et al. Research resource: transcriptome profiling of genes regulated by RXR and its permissive and nonpermissive partners in differentiating monocyte-derived dendritic cells. Mol Endocrinol 2010;24(11):2218–31.

61. Varga T, Czimmerer Z, Nagy L. PPARs are a unique set of fatty acid regulated transcription factors controlling both lipid metabolism and inflammation. Biochim Biophys Acta 2011;1812(8):1007–22.

62. Goto T. A review of the studies on food-derived factors which regulate energy metabolism via the modulation of lipid-sensing nuclear receptors. Biosci Biotechnol Biochem 2019;83(4):579–88.

63. Rachid TL, et al. Fenofibrate (PPARalpha agonist) induces beige cell formation in subcutaneous white adipose tissue from diet-induced male obese mice. Mol Cell Endocrinol 2015;402:86–94.

64. Georgiadi A, Kersten S. Mechanisms of gene regulation by fatty acids. Adv Nutr 2012;3(2):127–34.

65. Escher P, et al. Rat PPARs: quantitative analysis in adult rat tissues and regulation in fasting and refeeding. Endocrinology 2001;142(10):4195–202.

66. Bookout AL, et al. Anatomical profiling of nuclear receptor expression reveals a hierarchical transcriptional network. Cell 2006;126(4):789–99.

67. Parast MM, et al. PPARγ regulates trophoblast proliferation and promotes labyrinthine trilineage differentiation. PLoS ONE 2009;4(11):e8055.

68. McCarthy FP, et al. PPAR-γ - a possible drug target for complicated pregnancies. Br J Pharmacol 2013;168(5):1074–85.

69. Gokina NI, et al. Inhibition of PPARgamma during rat pregnancy causes intrauterine growth restriction and attenuation of uterine vasodilation. Front Physiol 2013;4:184.

70. Delerive P, et al. Peroxisome proliferator-activated receptor activators inhibit thrombin-induced endothelin-1 production in human vascular endothelial cells by inhibiting the activator protein-1 signaling pathway. Circ Res 1999;85(5):394–402.

71. Ketsawatsomkron P, et al. Does peroxisome proliferator-activated receptor-γ (PPARγ) protect from hypertension directly through effects in the vasculature? J Biol Chem 2010;285(13):9311–6.

72. Vázquez-Carrera M. Unraveling the effects of PPARβ/δ on insulin resistance and cardiovascular disease. Trends Endocrinol Metab 2016;27(5):319–34.

73. Meher A, Sundrani D, Joshi S. Maternal nutrition influences angiogenesis in the placenta through peroxisome proliferator activated receptors: a novel hypothesis. Mol Reprod Dev 2015;82(10):726–34.

74. Barak Y, Sadovsky Y, Shalom-Barak T. PPAR signaling in placental development and function. PPAR Res 2008;1–11.

75. Fournier T, et al. PPARs and the placenta. Placenta 2007;28(2–3):65–76.

76. Waite LL, Louie RE, Taylor RN. Circulating activators of peroxisome proliferator-activated receptors are reduced in preeclamptic pregnancy. J Clin Endocrinol Metab 2005;90(2):620–6.

77. Díaz M, et al. Placental expression of peroxisome proliferator-activated receptor γ (PPARγ): relation to placental and fetal growth. The J Clin Endocrinol Metab 2012;97(8):E1468–72.

78. Sreekantha S, et al. Maternal food restriction-induced intrauterine growth restriction in a rat model leads to sex-specific adipogenic programming. FASEB J 2020;34(12):16073–85.

79. Lane SL, et al. Pharmacological activation of peroxisome proliferator-activated receptor γ (PPAR-γ) protects against hypoxia-associated fetal growth restriction. FASEB J 2019;33(8):8999–9007.
80. Lane SL, et al. Peroxisome proliferator-activated receptor gamma blunts endothelin-1-mediated contraction of the uterine artery in a murine model of high-altitude pregnancy. FASEB J 2020;34(3):4283–92.
81. Desai M, et al. Programmed regulation of rat offspring adipogenic transcription factor (PPARγ) by maternal nutrition. J Developmental Origins Health Dis 2015; 6(6):530–8.
82. Desai M, et al. Programmed upregulation of adipogenic transcription factors in intrauterine growth-restricted offspring. Reprod Sci 2008;15(8):785–96.
83. Lillycrop KA, et al. Dietary protein restriction of pregnant rats induces and folic acid supplementation prevents epigenetic modification of hepatic gene expression in the offspring. J Nutr 2005;135(6):1382–6.
84. Lillycrop KA, et al. Feeding pregnant rats a protein-restricted diet persistently alters the methylation of specific cytosines in the hepatic PPAR alpha promoter of the offspring. Br J Nutr 2008;100(2):278–82.
85. Wakabayashi K, et al. The peroxisome proliferator-activated receptor gamma/retinoid X receptor alpha heterodimer targets the histone modification enzyme PR-Set7/Setd8 gene and regulates adipogenesis through a positive feedback loop. Mol Cell Biol 2009;29(13):3544–55.
86. Joss-Moore LA, et al. IUGR decreases PPARγ and SETD8 expression in neonatal rat lung and these effects are ameliorated by maternal DHA supplementation. Early Hum Dev 2010;86(12):785–91.
87. Joss-Moore LA, et al. IUGR differentially alters MeCP2 expression and H3K9Me3 of the PPARγ gene in male and female rat lungs during alveolarization. Birth Defects Res A Clin Mol Teratol 2011;91(8):672–81.
88. Zana-Taieb E, et al. Impaired alveolarization and intra-uterine growth restriction in rats: a postnatal genome-wide analysis. J Pathol 2015;235(3):420–30.
89. Morales E, et al. Nebulized PPARγ agonists: a novel approach to augment neonatal lung maturation and injury repair in rats. Pediatr Res 2014;75(5): 631–40.
90. Takeda K, et al. Peroxisome proliferator-activated receptor-g agonist treatment increases septation and angiogenesis and decreases airway hyperresponsiveness in a model of experimental neonatal chronic lung disease. Anat Rec (Hoboken) 2009;292(7):1045–61.
91. Walesky C, Apte U. Role of hepatocyte nuclear factor 4α (HNF4α) in cell proliferation and cancer. Gene Expr 2015;16(3):101–8.
92. Hayhurst GP, et al. Hepatocyte nuclear factor 4alpha (nuclear receptor 2A1) is essential for maintenance of hepatic gene expression and lipid homeostasis. Mol Cell Biol 2001;21(4):1393–403.
93. Hertz R, et al. Fatty acyl-CoA thioesters are ligands of hepatic nuclear factor-4α. Nature 1998;392(6675):512–6.
94. Yuan X, et al. Identification of an endogenous ligand bound to a native orphan nuclear receptor. PLoS One 2009;4(5):e5609.
95. McCurdy CE, et al. Maternal high-fat diet triggers lipotoxicity in the fetal livers of nonhuman primates. J Clin Invest 2009;119(2):323–35.
96. Sandovici I, et al. Maternal diet and aging alter the epigenetic control of a promoter-enhancer interaction at the Hnf4a gene in rat pancreatic islets. Proc Natl Acad Sci 2011;108(13):5449–54.

97. Einstein F, et al. Cytosine methylation dysregulation in neonates following intra-uterine growth restriction. PLoS ONE 2010;5(1):e8887.

98. Kwon EJ, et al. DNA methylations of MC4R and HNF4alpha are associated with increased triglyceride levels in cord blood of preterm infants. Medicine (Baltimore) 2016;95(35):e4590.

99. Kwon EJ, et al. Association between the DNA methylations of POMC, MC4R, and HNF4A and metabolic profiles in the blood of children aged 7–9 years. BMC Pediatr 2018;18(1):121.

100. Ribel-Madsen R, et al. Genome-wide analysis of DNA methylation differences in muscle and fat from monozygotic twins discordant for type 2 diabetes. PLoS ONE 2012;7(12):e51302.

101. Lehmann JM, et al. Activation of the nuclear receptor LXR by oxysterols defines a new hormone response pathway. J Biol Chem 1997;272(6):3137–40.

102. Gabbi C, Warner M, Gustafsson J-AK. Minireview: liver X receptor β: emerging roles in physiology and diseases. Mol Endocrinol 2009;23(2):129–36.

103. Pawar A, et al. The role of liver X receptor-α in the fatty acid regulation of hepatic gene expression. J Biol Chem 2003;278(42):40736–43.

104. Ou J, et al. Unsaturated fatty acids inhibit transcription of the sterol regulatory element-binding protein-1c (SREBP-1c) gene by antagonizing ligand-dependent activation of the LXR. Proc Natl Acad Sci 2001;98(11):6027–32.

105. van Straten EM, et al. The liver X-receptor gene promoter is hypermethylated in a mouse model of prenatal protein restriction. Am J Physiol Regul Integr Comp Physiol 2010;298(2):R275–82.

106. Vo TX, et al. Maternal protein restriction leads to enhanced hepatic gluconeogenic gene expression in adult male rat offspring due to impaired expression of the liver X receptor. J Endocrinol 2013;218(1):85–97.

107. Yang T, et al. Crucial step in cholesterol homeostasis. Cell 2002;110(4):489–500.

108. Takeuchi Y, et al. Polyunsaturated fatty acids selectively suppress sterol regulatory element-binding protein-1 through proteolytic processing and autoloop regulatory circuit. J Biol Chem 2010;285(15):11681–91.

109. Munford RS, Hall CL. Detoxification of bacterial lipopolysaccharides (endotoxins) by a human neutrophil enzyme. Science 1986;234(4773):203–5.

110. Kitchens RL, Ulevitch RJ, Munford RS. Lipopolysaccharide (LPS) partial structures inhibit responses to LPS in a human macrophage cell line without inhibiting LPS uptake by a CD14-mediated pathway. J Exp Med 1992;176(2):485–94.

111. Lee JY, et al. Differential modulation of Toll-like receptors by fatty acids: preferential inhibition by n-3 polyunsaturated fatty acids. J Lipid Res 2003;44(3):479–86.

112. Lee JY, et al. Saturated fatty acid activates but polyunsaturated fatty acid inhibits Toll-like receptor 2 dimerized with Toll-like receptor 6 or 1. J Biol Chem 2004;279(17):16971–9.

113. Tilich M, Arora R. Modulation of toll-like receptors by insulin. Am J Ther 2011;18(5):e130–7.

114. Zhu Y-J, et al. Toll-like receptor-2 and -4 are associated with hyperlipidemia. Mol Med Rep 2015;12(6):8241–6.

115. Vieira WA, Sadie-Van Gijsen H, Ferris WF. Free fatty acid G-protein coupled receptor signaling in M1 skewed white adipose tissue macrophages. Cell Mol Life Sci 2016;73(19):3665–76.

116. Moran BM, Flatt PR, McKillop AM. G protein-coupled receptors: signalling and regulation by lipid agonists for improved glucose homoeostasis. Acta Diabetol 2016;53(2):177–88.

117. Ge Y-J, et al. Anti-inflammatory signaling through G protein-coupled receptors. Acta Pharmacol Sin 2020;41(12):1531–8.
118. Sun M, et al. Microbiota metabolite short chain fatty acids, GPCR, and inflammatory bowel diseases. J Gastroenterol 2017;52(1):1–8.
119. Kimura I, et al. Free fatty acid receptors in health and disease. Physiol Rev 2020; 100(1):171–210.
120. Zhou W, et al. Implication of gut microbiota in cardiovascular diseases. Oxidative Med Cell Longevity 2020;2020:1–14.
121. Tan J, et al. The role of short-chain fatty acids in health and disease. Adv Immunol 2014;121:91–119.
122. Zheng N, et al. Short chain fatty acids produced by colonizing intestinal commensal bacterial interaction with expressed breast milk are anti-inflammatory in human immature enterocytes. PLoS One 2020;15(2):e0229283.
123. Montjaux-Régis N, et al. Improved growth of preterm infants receiving mother's own raw milk compared with pasteurized donor milk. Acta Paediatr 2011; 100(12):1548–54.
124. Madore LS, et al. Effects of donor breastmilk feeding on growth and early neurodevelopmental outcomes in preterm infants: an observational study. Clin Ther 2017;39(6):1210–20.
125. Brownell EA, et al. Dose-response relationship between donor human milk, mother's own milk, preterm formula, and neonatal growth outcomes. J Pediatr Gastroenterol Nutr 2018;67(1):90–6.
126. Hård AL, et al. Review shows that donor milk does not promote the growth and development of preterm infants as well as maternal milk. Acta Paediatr 2019; 108(6):998–1007.
127. Underwood MA. Human milk for the premature infant. Pediatr Clin North Am 2013;60(1):189–207.
128. Baro C, et al. Effect of two pasteurization methods on the protein content of human milk. Front Biosci (Elite Ed) 2011;3:818–29.
129. Silvestre D, et al. Antioxidant capacity of human milk: effect of thermal conditions for the pasteurization. Acta Pdiatrica 2008;97(8):1070–4.
130. Valentine CJ, et al. Docosahexaenoic acid and amino acid contents in pasteurized donor milk are low for preterm infants. J Pediatr 2010;157(6):906–10.
131. Baack ML, et al. Long-chain polyunsaturated fatty acid levels in US donor human milk: meeting the needs of premature infants? J Perinatology 2012;32(8): 598–603.
132. Henderson TR, Fay TN, Hamosh M. Effect of pasteurization on long chain polyunsaturated fatty acid levels and enzyme activities of human milk. J Pediatr 1998;132(5):876–8.
133. Calkins KL, Robinson DT. Intravenous lipid emulsions in the NICU. NeoReviews 2020;21(2):e109–19.
134. Haggarty P. Fatty acid supply to the human fetus. Annu Rev Nutr 2010;30(1): 237–55.
135. Moon K, Rao SC, Schulzke SM, et al. Longchain polyunsaturated fatty acid supplementation in preterm infants. Cochrane Database Syst Rev 2016;12(12): Cd000375.

Parenteral Nutrition

Sharon Groh-Wargo, PhD, RDN[a], Stephanie Merlino Barr, MS, RDN[b],*

KEYWORDS

- Neonatal • Parenteral nutrition • Energy • Protein • Fat • Micronutrients • Calcium
- Phosphorus

KEY POINTS

- Parenteral nutrition is a necessary therapy for high-risk newborns.
- Balanced neonatal parenteral nutrition regimens require daily provision of adequate energy (90–110 kcal/kg), consideration of protein dose (3–4 g/kg), rate of infusion of carbohydrate for euglycemia (4–15 mg/kg/min), and sufficient fat to meet essential fatty acid requirements.
- Micronutrients including electrolytes, macrominerals, trace elements, and vitamins are essential components of parenteral nutrition regimens for neonates.
- Product shortages, contaminants, and solution compatibilities are challenges.
- Enteral feeding is the preferred source of nutrition; the transition from parenteral to enteral nutrition is a critical time period and should be managed carefully to ensure maintenance of adequate intake.

INTRODUCTION

Parenteral nutrition (PN) is a common therapy for preterm, very low birthweight (VLBW; birthweight <1500 g), and other high-risk newborns. PN is required for the period when enteral nutrition is either contraindicated or inadequate. PN is expensive and complicated; nutritional composition, administration of the solution, and monitoring of the therapy requires a multidisciplinary team that includes a neonatal dietitian.[1] Two critical timepoints in administration are the first week of life and during the transition from PN to enteral nutrition.

Key overarching themes include the following:

- PN is life saving for infants born with significant congenital gastrointestinal anomalies and there is general agreement that PN is required for extremely low birth weight (ELBW; birthweight <1000 g) infants.[2] Significant weight loss and nutritional deficits of energy and protein are common in infants less than 30 weeks'

[a] Nutrition and Pediatrics, Case Western Reserve University at MetroHealth Medical Center, 2500 MetroHealth Drive, C.G72, Cleveland, OH 44109-1998, USA; [b] Neonatal Dietitian, Department of Pediatrics, MetroHealth Medical Center, 2500 MetroHealth Drive, C.G72, Cleveland, OH 44109-1998, USA
* Corresponding author.
E-mail address: smerlino@metrohealth.org

Clin Perinatol 49 (2022) 355–379
https://doi.org/10.1016/j.clp.2022.02.002
0095-5108/22/© 2022 Elsevier Inc. All rights reserved.

gestation.[3] Complete and well-balanced PN during the first week of life optimizes nutritional intake, limits excessive early weight loss, improves growth, and decreases the accumulation of nutrient deficits.[4,5]

- Use of concentrated PN solutions when fluid restriction is required and continuation of PN until full, or near full, fluids are achieved decreases the time to regain birth weight and improves nutritional intake.[6,7] Early, optimal PN has the potential to decrease the incidence of bronchopulmonary dysplasia, necrotizing enterocolitis, sepsis, and retinopathy of prematurity.[8]
- The risk-benefit ratio of PN is less clear for larger, more mature infants. In a retrospective analysis, neonates greater than or equal to 32 weeks' gestation without major comorbidities seem unlikely to significantly benefit from PN supplementation.[9]

The initial PN solution for VLBW infants is usually a starter solution. These solutions may be called vanilla PN because they do not contain the multivitamin that gives PN the yellow color. Starter solutions contain glucose, amino acids, calcium, and, occasionally, phosphorus; are infused at 50 to 80 mL/kg/day; and provide maintenance carbohydrate and sufficient amino acids to prevent negative nitrogen balance. They generally run for the first 12 to 36 hours of life.[10–12]

Starter PN solutions are followed by PN solutions that provide protein to support positive nitrogen balance, fat to provide essential fatty acids, sufficient energy from carbohydrate and fat to support growth, and all essential micronutrients. Unit-specific, evidence-based PN guidelines are recommended.[1] The National Institute for Health and Care Excellence has published detailed PN guideline algorithms for preterm and term neonates.[13]

FLUID AND MACRONUTRIENTS

Premature infants have unique requirements that require specialized PN compositions. **Table 1** provides an overview of fluid, energy, carbohydrate, protein, and fat requirements and describes the progression from acute-phase requirements to goal PN requirements. Meeting these proposed requirements is challenging in smaller, sicker infants who are unable to maintain euglycemia and have electrolyte instability requiring frequent changing of fluids. With this clinical picture in mind, it is perhaps unsurprising that administration of lower energy and higher fluid in the first week of life is associated with higher rates of moderate-severe bronchopulmonary dysplasia in premature infants.[14] Similarly, increased protein and energy intake has been associated with higher Mental Developmental Index scores and improved growth at 18 months.[15] However, because of nutrition's critical role in lung and somatic growth, the inability to provide adequate nutrition and the development of severe/chronic illness should not simply be attributed to early life acuity; rather, this vicious cycle makes providing appropriate nutrition early and consistently, a true nutrition emergency in the preterm infant population.

Fluid

Fluid requirements increase as gestational age decreases because of higher rates of insensible water loss, immature renal function, and elevated energy needs. Extracellular fluid volume also increases with degree of prematurity, resulting in greater expected weight loss after birth.[16,17] Management of these elevated requirements is a challenging yet critical component of early life neonatal care because of the infant's expected fluid losses and rapidly changing serum electrolytes. A gradual increase of fluid administration is recommended for all infants and is described in **Table 1**.[18]

Table 1
Overview of fluid, energy, and macronutrient requirements based on major recommendations

		Day of Life 1	Advancing PN	Goal PN
Fluid (mL/kg/d)				
ESPGHAN[18]	Term	40–60	60–100	100–140
	Preterm	80–100	100–140	140–180
NICE[13]	Term	Use concentrated parenteral nutrition to meet energy		
	Preterm	goals within fluid requirements		
ASPEN[,23]	Term	—	—	—
	Preterm	—	—	—
Energy (kcal/kg/d)				
ESPGHAN[107]	Term	45–50	—	75–85
	Preterm	45–55	—	90–120
NICE[13]	Term	Nonnitrogen energy provided by 60%–75% carbohydrate,		
	Preterm	25%–40% fat		
		20–30 kcal nonnitrogen energy per gram of amino acid		
ASPEN[23]	Term	—	—	—
	Preterm	—	—	—
Carbohydrate (mg/kg/min)				
ESPGHAN[108]	Term	2.5–5	Advance	5–10 (max 12)
	Preterm	4–8	over 2–3 d	8–10 (max 12)
NICE[13]	Term	4–6.25	—	6.25–11.1
	Preterm		—	
ASPEN[23]	Term	6–8	7–10	10–14 (max 14–18)
	Preterm	6–8	7–10	10–14 (max 14–18)
Protein (g/k/d)				
ESPGHAN[24,]	Term	1.5	—	1.5–3
	Preterm	1.5	—	2.5–3.5
NICE[13]	Term	1–2	—	2.5–3
	Preterm	1.5–2	—	3–4
ASPEN[23]	Term	2.5–3	—	2.5–3
	Preterm	1–3	—	3–4
Fat (g/kg)				
ESPGHAN[109]	Term	—	—	4 (*max dose*)
	Preterm	Start no later than Day 2 of life	—	
NICE[13]	Term	1–2	—	3–4
	Preterm			
ASPEN[23]	Term	0.5–1	1–2	3
	Preterm	0.5–1	1–2	2.5–3

Abbreviations: ASPEN, American Society for Parenteral and Enteral Nutrition; ESPGHAN, European Society for Pediatric Gastroenterology Hepatology and Nutrition; NICE, National Institute for Health and Care Excellence.

Energy

Energy requirements of preterm infants on PN are determined by basal metabolic rate, growth requirements, and severity of illness. Meeting energy goals in the first week of life is associated with improved growth and neurodevelopment in preterm infants,[2,15,19] and may decrease the risk of adverse outcomes from critical illness in ELBW infants.[20]

Table 2 provides an overview of the macronutrients in PN and their energy contributions. Providing a balance of nonprotein energy from fat (25%–40%) and carbohydrate (60%–75%) with protein (23–34 total energy per gram amino acid) is suggested to meet requirements without exceeding an infant's metabolic capacity of administered macronutrients.[13] Excess carbohydrate administration can lead to hyperglycemia, which is associated with an increased risk of worse neurologic outcomes,[21] increased respiratory support requirements,[22] and increased mortality[21] in preterm infants. Excess protein administration may result in oxidation of amino acids and use of amino acids for energy, rather than tissue generation. This potential for excess nutrient administration highlights that more nutrition is not necessarily good nutrition, even for premature infants with exceedingly high nutrition requirements.

Protein

The early initiation of amino acids in PN is a practice strongly supported by the published literature and all major PN guidelines (see **Table 1** for specific protein recommendations).[13,23,24] Preterm infants have unique conditionally essential amino acids because of their relative biochemical immaturity[25,26]; conditionally essential amino acids are outlined in **Tables 3** and **4**. There are specialized amino acid solutions intended to meet preterm infants' unique requirements using cord blood or human milk amino acid profiles as templates (**Table 5** for a comparison of neonatal and adult amino acid solutions). However, the optimum amino acid formulation for parenteral administration is unknown and current products may not fully meet the amino acid requirements in very preterm infants.[27]

Early administration of amino acids is well tolerated,[28–30] particularly when combined with early lipid administration because of the promotion of albumin synthesis.[31] Serum urea nitrogen is not recommended as a biochemical marker of protein tolerance in early life, because it has not been correlated with amino acid intake in the first days of life of preterm infants.[32,33] There may be an increased risk of metabolic acidosis with earlier and higher intravenous amino acid administration.[34]

Evidence supports that early and higher doses amino acid administration may be beneficial in promoting growth, support bone growth, and preventing growth failure in preterm infants[35–38]; however, the heterogeneity of published studies makes this a low-quality recommendation. The influence of high amino acid doses on neurodevelopmental outcomes has been inconclusive.[39,40] Infusion of amino acids may be beneficial for management and prevention of hyperglycemia because of individual amino acids' role in stimulating insulin secretion.[41,42]

Table 2
Overview of macronutrients in parenteral nutrition

Macronutrient	Parenteral Nutrition Form	Calories per Gram	Example Products
Carbohydrate	Dextrose	3.4	—
Protein	Crystalline amino acid solution	4	Trophamine (B. Braun Medical Inc); Aminosyn-PF (ICU Medical Inc); Premasol (Baxter)
Fat	Intravenous fat emulsions	10* *9 kcal/g from fat 1 kcal/g from glycerol	Intralipid (Baxter); SMOFlipid (Fresenius Kabi)

Table 3
Essential, nonessential, and conditionally essential amino acids[24,25]

Essential	Nonessential	Semi-Essential
Histidine	Alanine	Arginine
Isoleucine	Aspartic acid	Glycine
Leucine	Asparagine	Proline
Lysine	Glutamic acid	Tyrosine
Methionine	Serine	Cysteine
Phenylalanine		Glutamine
Threonine		
Tryptophan		
Valine		

Carbohydrate

Carbohydrates are administered parenterally as dextrose (D-glucose), which provides 3.4 cal/g. Dextrose should be provided at a level to meet energy requirements, while preventing excess in administration and hyperglycemia. Glucose infusion rate (GIR) is a measure of the amount of carbohydrates an individual receives, expressed as milligrams (of dextrose) per kilograms (of body weight) per minute. **Box 1** provides an explanation on how to calculate GIR and other PN calculations. Minimum GIRs have been estimated to ensure organs that preferentially use glucose for energy, most importantly the brain, are able to receive a sufficient supply of carbohydrates (see **Table 1**). Advancement of GIR requires caution in the first week of life because of a reduction in glucose tolerance and insulin sensitivity. A more detailed discussion of glucose homeostasis is found in Cynthia L. Blanco and Jennifer Kim's article, "Glucose Homeostasis," in this issue.

Table 4
Discussion of conditionally essential amino acids in the premature infant[24,25]

Amino Acid	Why is It Conditionally Essential?	What is It Used for?
Arginine	High turnover in growing infants	Ammonia detoxification in the urea cycle Precursor for nitric oxide
Cysteine	Low/absent activity of cystathionase in preterm infants	Metabolic precursor for taurine and glutathione
Glycine	Increased requirements during critical illness or when receiving supplemental oxygen because of potential for oxidative injury	Inhibitory neurotransmitter Ammonia donor in the liver Precursor for glutathione synthesis
Proline	Preterm infants unable to synthesize proline from glutamate, have higher protein turnover and tissue accretion	Precursor for collagen Important in joint and tendon function and tissue repair
Taurine	Cysteine sulfinic acid decarboxylase may have lower activity in preterm infants	Fetal neurodevelopment Fat absorption, bile acid secretion, retinal function, and hepatic function
Tyrosine	Impaired hydroxylation of phenylalanine to tyrosine in preterm infants	Essential for neurotransmitter production, hormone creation and regulation, among other functions

Table 5
Comparison of neonatal and adult amino acid solutions

	Neonatal 10% Amino Acid Solution	Adult 10% Amino Acid Solution
Essential amino acids		
Histidine	0.31–0.48	0.30–0.48
Isoleucine	0.76–0.82	0.60–0.66
Leucine	1.20–1.40	0.73–1.00
Lysine	0.68–0.82	0.58–1.05
Methionine	0.18–0.34	0.17–0.4
Phenylalanine	0.43–0.48	0.30–0.56
Threonine	0.42–0.51	0.40–0.42
Tryptophan	0.18–0.20	0.18–0.20
Valine	0.67–0.78	0.50–0.58
Semi-essential amino acids		
Arginine	1.20–1.23	1.02–1.15
Cysteine	0*	0
Glycine	0.36–0.39	0.50–1.03
Proline	0.68–0.81	0.68–0.72
Tyrosine	0.24–0.44	0.27–0.40
Nonessential amino acids		
Alanine	0.54–0.70	0.99–2.07
Aspartic acid	0.32–0.53	0–0.7
Glutamic acid	0.50–0.82	0–0.74
Serine	0.38–0.50	0.5–0.53
Taurine	0.03–0.07	0
Other properties		
pH adjusted with glacial acetic acid USP	5.5 (5.0–6.0)	6.0 (5.0–7.0)
Calc. osmolarity (mOsm/L)	788–875	840–998
Total amino acids (g/L)	100	100
Total nitrogen (g/L)	15.2–15.5	15.3–16.5
Example products	Trophamine (B. Braun Medical Inc); Aminosyn-PF (ICU Medical Inc); Premasol (Baxter)	Travasol (Baxter); Aminosyn II (ICU Medical Inc)

Fat

Fat is provided in PN as intravenous fat emulsions (IVFEs), which provide energy, essential fatty acids, and aid in the delivery of lipid-soluble vitamins. An overview of recommended fat dosages is found in **Table 1**. The early initiation of IVFEs within the first 2 days of life is tolerated and may improve the nitrogen balance and improve growth in preterm infants.[43,44] Early lipid administration may also support greater cerebellar volume by term-equivalent age in very preterm infants.[45] Responding to hypertriglyceridemia by reducing the administered dose of IVFE in the first 10 days of life does not seem to negatively impact growth or neurodevelopment,[46] and this practice may improve respiratory outcomes.[47]

Box 1
Calculating glucose infusion rate

GIR is calculated as follows:

$$GIR = \frac{IV\ rate\left(\frac{mL}{hr}\right) \times\ dextrose\ concentration\left(\frac{g}{dL}\right) \times 1000\frac{mg}{g}}{weight\ (kg) \times 60\frac{min}{hr} \times 100\frac{mL}{dL}}$$

Example: 1.25-kg infant receiving parenteral nutrition at 7.5 mL/h with 12% dextrose.

$$GIR = \frac{7.5\frac{mL}{hr} \times 12\frac{g}{dL} \times 1000\frac{mg}{g}}{1.25\ kg \times 60\frac{min}{hr} \times 100\frac{mL}{dL}} = \frac{90,000\frac{mL*mg}{hr*dL}}{7,500\frac{kg*min*mL}{hr*dL}} = 12.0\ mg\Big/kg\Big/min$$

A shorter equation to solve for GIR is as follows:

$$GIR = \frac{IV\ rate\left(\frac{mL}{hr}\right) \times dextrose\ concentration\left(\frac{g}{dL}\right)}{weight(kg)} \times 0.167$$

Using the previous example, this 1.25-kg infant is receiving parenteral nutrition at a rate of 7.5 mL/h with a 12 g/dL dextrose concentration.

$$GIR = \left(\frac{7.5\frac{mL}{hr} \times 12\frac{g}{dL}}{1.25kg}\right) \times 0.167 = 12.0\ mg\Big/kg\Big/min$$

Carnitine, a derivative of the amino acid lysine, is a critical cofactor in beta-oxidation; carnitine facilitates the transport of long-chain fatty acids as acyl carnitines into the inner mitochondrial matrix. Premature infants have limited carnitine reserves, and thus it is a necessary component of PN to ensure normalized serum carnitine levels and improved fatty acid oxidation.[48,49] An ideal dose of parenteral carnitine has not been identified, but infants on an exclusive human milk diet are estimated to consume 2 to 5 mg/kg/d daily.

IVFEs are available in a variety of compositions internationally but, only a comparatively select products are clinically available in the United States. The growing number of IVFE products raises the important question of: what is the ideal fatty acid composition for a premature infant? It has not been determined that any single product is superior in promoting growth[50] or neurodevelopment[51] in the preterm infant population. Composite IVFEs that contain fish oil may be beneficial in preventing PN-associated cholestasis (PNAC).[52] A more detailed discussion on fatty acids and lipid metabolism is found in Kristin Santoro and Camilia R. Martin' article, "Lipids and Long Chain Polyunsaturated Fatty Acids in Preterm Infants," in this issue.

It is of critical importance to recognize the different dosage requirements to meet essential fatty acid requirements for different IVFE products. Biochemical essential fatty acid deficiency has been observed in premature infants receiving inadequately dosed IVFEs.[53,54] Differences in composition in available IVFE products are found in **Table 6** and an example calculation estimating dosage to meet essential fatty acid requirements is found in **Box 2**.

MICRONUTRIENTS
Electrolytes

Electrolytes are the category of micronutrients that are most often individualized in PN solutions. This is especially true in the first few days of life when fluids are highly

Table 6
Composition of intravenous fat emulsion products clinically available in the United States

| | Oil (%) | | | | EFA Content (%) | | Gram fat per 250 mL IVFE | % EFA per 250 mL IVFE |
| | | | | | LA (Omega-6) | ALA (Omega-3) | | |
Product	Soy	MCT	Olive	Fish				
Intralipid 20%	100%	—	—	—	44–62[a]	4–11[a]	50	48–73[a]
SMOFlipid 20%[b]	30%	30%	25%	15%	17.5	2.25	50	19.75

Abbreviations: ALA, α-linolenic acid; EFA, essential fatty acid; LA, linoleic acid; MCT, medium chain triglyceride.

[a] Fresenius Kabi provides the ranges of percent composition from LA and ALA for Intralipid. Please note that the midpoint of this range does not represent the average value of LA and ALA in Intralipid and could result in overestimating EFA intake.

[b] SMOFlipid is not approved for use in preterm infants in the United States, but is used frequently off-label in this population.

variable, and the newborn is adjusting to extrauterine life. Close monitoring for electrolyte imbalance, iatrogenic metabolic acidosis, and nonoliguric hyperkalemia is mandatory especially in the first week of life.[18] Acetate and chloride sources of sodium and potassium are chosen carefully based on acid-base balance.[23] Hyponatremia following discontinuation of PN may inhibit growth in preterm infants and 5 to 7 mEq/kg sodium may be required.[12,55] **Table 7** lists estimated sodium, potassium, and chloride requirements for initial PN solutions, stable neonates, and infants older than 1 month of age. VLBW infants tend to have electrolyte needs in the upper end of the ranges compared with preterm infants greater than 1500 g.[18]

Macrominerals

Calcium, phosphorus, and magnesium are essential micronutrients for muscle function, energy production, and bone health.[56] Magnesium requirements are available from several published sources.[23,57] Following some fluctuation during the first few

Box 2
Calculating IVFE dosage to meet essential fatty acid requirements in soy and composite IVFE products

A 1.0-kg infant receiving 100 kcal/kg/d from parenteral nutrition requires an estimated 3% of calories (or 3 kcal/kg, and in this case, 3 kcal) from linoleic acid (LA) to meet essential fatty acid requirements.
1. First, the total number of calories needed from LA is calculated: Calories needed from LA (kcal) = (grams of fat × 9 kcal/g) × % LA in IVFE
2. Then, determine the number of calories from LA in Intralipid. Fat has 9 kcal/g and approximately 50% of the fat in Intralipid is LA. Therefore: 1 g Intralipid = 9 kcal from fat = 4.5 kcal from LA
3. Next, determine the minimum dose of Intralipid to meet the patient's essential fatty acid requirements.
   3 kcal = X grams of fat × 4.5 kcal/g from LA
   X = 0.7 g Intralipid = 0.7 g/kg Intralipid for a 1-kg infant
4. Then, calculate the number of calories from LA in SMOFlipid; because fat has 9 kcal/g and 17.5% of the fat in SMOFlipid from LA. Therefore:
   1 g SMOFlipid = 9 kcal from fat = 1.6 kcal from LA
5. Finally, determine the minimum dose of SMOFlipid to meet the same patient's essential fatty acid requirements.
   3 kcal = X grams of fat × 1.6 kcal/g from LA acid
   X = 1.9 g SMOFlipid = 1.9 g/kg SMOFlipid for a 1-kg infant

Table 7
Recommended daily doses of parenteral electrolytes[18,58]

Usual Pediatric Range	Neonates Day of Life 1–2	Neonates	Infants 1– 12 mo
Sodium (mEq/kg)	0–2	2–5	2–3
Potassium (mEq/kg)	0–3	1–5	1–3
Chloride:			
mEq/kg	0–3	2–5	2–4
% anions	25–50	25	

days of extrauterine life, magnesium status is generally not a concern. Magnesium sulfate is the usual source of the mineral and, unlike calcium and phosphorus, does not present compatibility and solubility concerns.

Calcium and phosphorus are more complicated but there are several key points.

- Fetal accretion of calcium and phosphorus is enormous with about 80% of the total endowment occurring in the last trimester of pregnancy.[58]
- **Table 8** lists recommended daily parenteral doses for calcium, phosphorus, and magnesium; recommendations vary somewhat between sources.[23,57]
- Providing known calcium and phosphorus requirements within the solubility of PN solutions is a significant challenge; published solubility curves are available and should be used when ordering PN.[59]
- Solubility is driven by multiple factors (**Box 3**).
- Solubility is affected by the volume of solution with smaller volumes allowing less mineral; evaluate compatibility when PN provides less than 50 mL/kg/d.
- Calcium is generally provided as calcium gluconate, but calcium chloride is an alternative. Phosphorus is provided as either the potassium or sodium salt.[12,60]
- Inclusion of phosphorus within the first 24 to 48 hours should be considered especially if protein is provided at recommended levels and especially for ELBW infants and infants who have experienced intrauterine growth restriction. Early provision of phosphorus can prevent hypokalemia, hypophosphatemia,

Table 8
Recommended daily doses of parenteral calcium, phosphorus, and magnesium[23,57]

Usual Pediatric Range	Neonates Day of Life 1–2>	Neonates	Infants 1–12 mo
Calcium			
mEq/kg (mmol/kg)	0.8–2	1.6–3.5	0.5–1.5
mg/kg	32–80	100–140	20–60
Phosphorus			
mmol/kg	1–2	1.6–3.5	0.5–1.3
mg/kg	31–62	77–108	15–40
Calcium/phosphorus ratio			
mmol:mmol	0.8–1:1	1.3:1	
Magnesium			
mEq/kg	ESPGHAN: 0.1–0.2 ASPEN: 0.3–0.5	ESPGHAN: 0.2–0.3 ASPEN: 0.3–0.5	ESPGHAN: 0.1–0.2

> **Box 3**
> **Factors that increase calcium and phosphorus solubility in parenteral nutrition solutions for infants[12]**
>
> - Very acidic pH
> - Higher concentrations of dextrose and amino acids
> - Cysteine hydrochloride additive
> - Cooler temperature
> - Calcium and phosphorus in appropriate concentration and ratio
> - Addition of phosphorus before calcium during preparation
> - Fat emulsion by intravenous piggyback (rather than incorporated with dextrose and amino acids)

and hypercalcemia and avoid "neonatal refeeding syndrome," also called "placental incompletely restored feeding syndrome" (**Figs. 1** and **2**).[57,61–63]

- Attention to the ratio of calcium to phosphorus is required to maximize mineral retention (strong consensus for early ratio of 0.8–1:1 mmol).[57]
- Monitoring of calcium and phosphorus status is routine and screening for metabolic bone disease (MBD) recommended if PN extends beyond 2 weeks.
- The challenge of providing calcium and phosphorus parenterally is an important reason to transition to enteral nutrition as soon as possible.

Trace Elements

Eight trace elements are commonly mentioned for infants on PN: chromium, copper, iodine, iron, manganese, molybdenum, selenium, and zinc. Trace elements are cofactors and functional components of enzymes important to a wide variety of physiologic processes. Commercial multitrace element packages are generally not well designed; an individualized approach to trace element dosing in PN solutions for infants is recommended.[64] An excellent summary of typical symptoms observed in trace element deficiency states along with recommended tests for assessing and monitoring trace element status in infants on PN is available.[65]

Key issues for each of these important micronutrients include the following:

- Chromium: present as a contaminant in PN solutions; the need for additional dosing is not universally recommended.[23,66,67]
- Copper: a critically important trace element; monitor plasma copper and ceruloplasmin in patients on long-term PN, especially if PNAC/liver disease develops (consider decreased dose) or if high gastrointestinal fluid losses occur (consider increased dose).[66,68]
- Iodine: a critically important trace element. Iodine deficiency is prevalent among pregnant women; therefore, newborns are at risk of iodine deficiency especially because iodine-containing skin antiseptics are no longer commonly used and because sources of parenteral iodine are limited. Normal thyroid tests are considered surrogate makers of adequate iodine status.[66,69,70]
- Iron: parenteral iron is not required for short-term PN; enteral nutrition is the preferred source of iron; if PN is required long term, a daily dose is added to the solution or is given intermittently as a separate infusion. Iron status should be monitored regularly in patients on long-term PN therapy with assessment of serum ferritin and hemoglobin levels.[66]

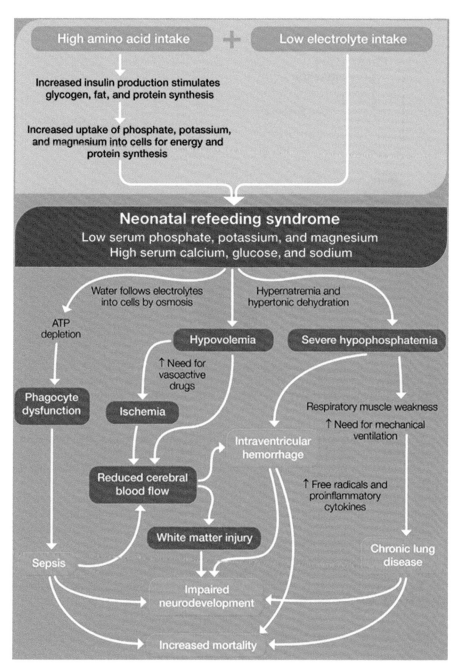

Fig. 1. Proposed mechanisms for neonatal refeeding syndrome and effects on clinical outcomes. (*From* Cormack BE, Jiang Y, Harding JE, Crowther CA, Bloomfield FH, Group ftPT. Neonatal Refeeding Syndrome and Clinical Outcome in Extremely Low-Birth-Weight Babies: Secondary Cohort Analysis From the ProVIDe Trial. Journal of Parenteral and Enteral Nutrition. 2021;45(1):65 to 78).

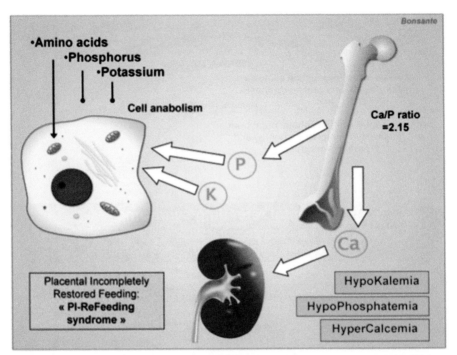

Fig. 2. Placental incompletely restored feeding syndrome. (*From* Bonsante F, Iacobelli S, La-torre G, Rigo J, De Felice C, Robillard PY, et al. Initial amino acid intake influences phos-phorus and calcium homeostasis in preterm infants–it is time to change the composition of the early parenteral nutrition. PLoS One. 2013;8(8):e72880).

- Manganese: present as a contaminant in PN solutions; the need for inclusion in infant PN solutions, especially in short-term PN, is questionable. Serum manga-nese concentrations should be monitored in patients on long-term PN, especially if PNAC/liver disease develops (consider decreased dose).[66,67]
- Molybdenum: generally added to PN solutions only in long-term situations.[66]
- Selenium: a critically important trace element related to antioxidant defense; monitor plasma selenium in long-term PN and consider a decreased dose in pa-tients with renal failure/oliguria; the dose recommended for preterm neonates varies from 2 to 7 μg/kg/d.[23,66]
- Zinc: a critically important trace element; zinc deficiency is expected when inad-equate zinc is provided, especially in the situation of high gastrointestinal and/or urinary losses.[65,66,71] **Fig. 3** provides a depiction of zinc deficiency in a premature infant.

Table 9 lists recommended daily parenteral doses for these eight essential trace elements.

Vitamins

Vitamins function as important coenzymes and cofactors required for the metabolism of macronutrients and must be supplied by the diet. An excellent summary of typical symptoms observed in vitamin deficiency states along with recommended tests for assessing and monitoring vitamin status in infants on PN is available.[65]

Key issues for essential fat- and water-soluble vitamins include the following:

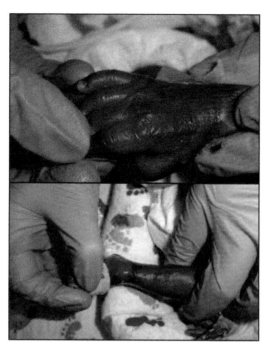

Fig. 3. Zinc deficiency in extremely premature infants after a nationwide shortage of injectable zinc. (*From* Notes from the field: Zinc deficiency dermatitis in cholestatic extremely premature infants after a nationwide shortage of injectable zinc - Washington, DC, December 2012. MMWR Morb Mortal Wkly Rep. 2013;62(7):136 to 7).

- Newborns, preterm and term, should receive daily vitamins when PN is initiated.[65,72]
- Vitamin requirements for infants on PN are not well established but preterm infants are assumed to have decreased stores of fat-soluble vitamins because of a shortened in-utero accretion time and excessive losses of water-soluble

Table 9
Recommended daily doses of parenteral trace elements[23,66]

Usual Pediatric Range	Preterm Infant <37 Week Gestation	Infant <12 Month Old (3–10 kg)	Maximum Dose per Day
Chromium µg/kg	0.05–0.3[a]	0.2[a]	5 µg
Copper µg/kg	40	20	0.5 mg
Iodine µg/kg	1–10	1	—
Iron µg/kg	200–250	50–100	5 mg
Manganese µg/kg	≤1	≤1	50 µg
Molybdenum µg/kg	1	0.25	5 µg
Selenium µg/kg	7	2–3	100 µg
Zinc µg/kg	400–500	100–250	5 mg

[a] ASPEN 2019.[23]

vitamins may occur after birth because of renal immaturity and increased urinary excretion.

- Substantial losses of vitamin A to adsorption into plastic bags and tubing are known to occur.[72]
- Vitamins A, E, and thiamin are particularly vulnerable to degradation by light.[72] Protection of the PN from light minimizes oxidation and has been shown to reduce mortality in preterm infants.[73]
- The total dose of vitamin E, from a multivitamin infusion and any vitamin provided by an IVFE, should not exceed 11 mg/d.
- Routine monitoring of vitamin concentrations, apart from vitamin D, is not usually recommended unless PN becomes long term.
- Current multivitamin preparations supply higher vitamin K amounts without apparent adverse clinical effects.[72]
- Thiamin plays an important role in glucose metabolism[74] and should be replaced with a single parenteral vitamin if a multivitamin product is not available.
- **Table 10** has a summary of recommended vitamin intakes in PN along with the composition of the multivitamin infusion products available in the United States.

MONITORING
Growth

A thorough review of growth assessment in newborns is available from Fenton and colleagues' article, "Neonatal and Preterm Infant Growth Assessment" in this issue. The first week of life is a critical time. Nutrient deficits can occur if careful attention to PN regimens is neglected.[3–5] In preterm infants, a weight loss of up to 0.8 z score is expected.[75] Weight gain velocity using the average method is calculated from the nadir, approximately 7 days of life, rather than the birth weight with an expected

Table 10
Recommended daily doses of parenteral vitamins[65,72]

Usual Pediatric Range	Preterm Infant <37 Week Gestation	Infant <12 Month Old	Composition of Pediatric Parenteral Multivitamin (1.5–5 mL[a])
Vitamin A: IU/kg	700–1500	500–1000	690–2300
Vitamin D: IU/d (IU/kg)	200–1000 (80–400)	400 (40–150)	120–400
Vitamin E: mg/kg	2.8–3.5		2.1–7
Vitamin K: μg/kg	10		60–200
Vitamin C: mg/kg	15–25		24–80
Thiamine B_1: mg/kg	0.35–0.5		0.36–1.2
Riboflavin: mg/kg	0.15–0.2		0.45–1.4
Niacin: mg/kg	4–6.8		5.1–17
Pyridoxine B_6: mg/kg	0.15–0.2		0.3–1
Pantothenic acid: mg/kg	2.5		1.5–5
Biotin: μg/kg	5–8		6–20
Vitamin B_{12}: μg/kg	0.3		0.3–1
Folic acid: μg/kg	56		42–140

[a] Recommended dose: 1.5 mL/d (<1 kg); 3.25 mL/d (1–3 kg); 5 mL/d (>3 kg) (Infuvite PEDiatric, Baxter; M.V.I. Pediatric, Hospira).

velocity at the intrauterine gain of 15 to 20 g/kg/d until 36 weeks. After that time, a weight gain of 20 to 40 g/d (like term newborns) is expected until about 2 months of age.[76]

Biochemical

Monitoring laboratory values balances the need for the information against the loss of blood to the baby and the cost of the test. Some general principles include the following:

- Glucose, electrolyte, and acid/base (blood gas) levels are essential for newborns on PN. Daily assessment, especially in ELBW infants, is recommended during the first week followed by one to two times per week for newborns who have stable electrolytes and normal acid-base status. Monitoring can then decrease to several times per month for infants with normal and stable levels.[12]
- Fat tolerance may be assessed with triglyceride levels at initiation and during dose increases; triene-tetraene ratios may be considered if adequacy of essential fatty acids is questionable.
- Phosphorus levels are important to monitor during in the first week to avoid "neonatal refeeding syndrome" (see **Figs. 1** and **2**); and are a sensitive screen for MBD if PN continues longer than a few weeks.
- Liver function tests: the direct bilirubin level is an important screen for PNAC; baseline levels should be obtained within the first few weeks after the infant is stable and then monitored several times a month if PN continues longer than a few weeks.
- Alkaline phosphatase: the alkaline phosphatase is elevated because of PNAC or, if the direct bilirubin is within normal limits, levels greater than 500 IU/L suggest bone demineralization and is a screen for MBD[77]; baseline levels should be obtained within the first few weeks after the infant is stable and then monitored several times a month if PN continues longer than a few weeks.
- Complete blood cell count: baseline levels should be obtained within the first few weeks after the infant is stable and then monitored several times a month if PN continues longer than a few weeks.
- Trace element and vitamin status: generally, "as indicated" with greatest suspicion for zinc, followed by copper, iodine, and selenium deficiency. If PN is exclusive of all enteral nutrition and continues into months, rather than weeks, a more complete micronutrient assessment should be considered.[12]

Nutrition-Focused Physical Examination

Micronutrient deficiencies can lead to cutaneous abnormalities involving the skin, hair, and nails. The micronutrients that most commonly present with cutaneous findings include the B vitamins riboflavin, niacin, pyridoxine, biotin, and vitamin B_{12}; vitamin C; the fat-soluble vitamins A, E, and K; the minerals zinc, iron, copper, and selenium; and essential fatty acids. A thorough review is available.[78] Infants are at risk if they have inadequate intake or increased losses. Of the micronutrients listed previously, deficiencies of zinc or essential fatty acids are the ones most likely to present in the newborn period.

COMPLICATIONS AND CONCERNS
Nutrition-Related Complications

Nutrition-related complications of prolonged PN use in the preterm infant population are most typically MBD and PNAC.

PN's role in MBD is briefly summarized in these key points:

- Approximately 80% of mineral accretion occurs in the third trimester, with 60 mg/d accretion at 25 weeks' gestation and rapidly increasing to more than 300 mg/d by 35 to 38 weeks' gestation.[79,80]
- PN cannot meet these exceedingly high calcium and phosphorus requirements because of the limitations to prevent precipitate formation in the parenteral solution.[81] **Box 3** describes factors that increase calcium and phosphorus solubility.
- Prolonged PN use and use of diuretics and glucocorticoids are risk factors for MBD development, and often seen in infants with sepsis, necrotizing enterocolitis, and chronic lung disease. This group of high-risk infants, and any infant on PN exceeding 2 weeks in time should be monitored for MBD development.
- Biochemical and radiographic evaluation of infants is used to monitor and diagnose MBD.[79,82] Serum phosphorus values less than 5.6 mg/dL and alkaline phosphatase levels greater than 500 IU/L are suggestive of poor bone mineralization and MBD.[79] Serum calcium is not a reliable biochemical marker for MBD, because this value remains stable in the setting of bone calcium depletion. Urinary calcium and phosphorus levels may also be considered in assessing for MBD.

PN's role in PNAC is briefly summarized in these key points:

- PNAC is multifactorial in origin; in infants with intestinal resection, the term "intestinal failure–associated liver disease" is used to reflect the critical role that gut atrophy plays in this disease etiology and progression.
- The high omega-6 fatty acid and phytosterol concentrations paired with the low bioavailability of vitamin E found in soy-based lipid emulsions have been hypothesized to contribute to PNAC development. Prolonged exposure to IVFEs is consistently correlated with the development of PNAC.[83]
- Provision of excessive intravenous dextrose parenterally may contribute to the development of PNAC.[84]
- Use of mixed oil lipid emulsions, which provide omega-3 fatty acids and more vitamin E and a lower amount of omega-6 fatty acids and phytosterol, has not been consistently shown to prevent PNAC.[85]
- Fish oil–based lipid emulsions have been successfully used to treat PNAC and intestinal failure–associated liver disease in infants,[86] but there are limited data available on the feasibility of long-term use of this product and meeting essential fatty acid requirements in the very preterm population.
- Transitioning from parenteral to enteral nutrition is the best method of resolving PNAC, when clinically feasible.

Compatibilities

Compatibilities of medications with PN solutions should be determined and monitored by the pharmacy team. Individual compatibilities may differ by

- Having a two-in-one versus a three-in-one PN solution
- The inclusion of IVFEs
- The type of IVFE; of note, there may be limited compatibility information on more novel IVFEs in the United States
- Line availability
- Solubility in solution (eg, calcium and phosphorus)

Contaminants

Trace element contaminants within PN bring potential for toxicity for the preterm infant. Aluminum, chromium, and manganese are the most well-documented and concerning contaminants and should be accounted for when purchasing PN admixtures and determining dosage.[67,87]

Aluminum

- Excess aluminum exposure through PN may have detrimental effects on neurodevelopment and bone mineralization in preterm infants and may play a role in the development of PNAC.[88–90]
- Aluminum is present as a contaminant in all PN ingredients, but is most concentrated in calcium gluconate, cysteine hydrochloride, and inorganic phosphates.[91–94]
- Calcium gluconate (in plastic vials), sodium phosphate, and sodium glycerophosphate are potential methods to minimize aluminum exposure in the premature infant, although product availability is subject to manufacturing and regulation restrictions.[92,94]

Manganese

- Multitrace element neonatal/pediatric solutions provide potentially toxic amounts of manganese.[95,96]
- Manganese has the potential to be neurotoxic, and deposits in the basal ganglia have been shown via MRI.[97]
- Given manganese's presence as a contaminant and a lack of evidence of potential for deficiency, it is likely not necessary to include manganese in standard PN administration for premature infants.[98]

Chromium

- Multitrace element neonatal/pediatric solutions provide potentially toxic amounts of chromium.[95,96] Preterm infants are at an increased risk for chromium toxicity.[64]
- Although the American Society for Parenteral and Enteral Nutrition recommends a reduced dose to be provided in PN (see **Table 9**), the European Society for Pediatric Gastroenterology Hepatology and Nutrition recommends that the presence of chromium as a contaminate in PN is sufficient to meet requirements.[23,66]
- Preterm infants with renal failure should not be supplemented with chromium.[64]

PRODUCT SHORTAGES

Unfortunately, because of a limited number of manufacturers the potential for shortages of critical PN components is occurring with greater frequency. The potential for deficiencies is greatest in the preterm infant population (see **Fig. 3** for an example), and thus it is critical to ensure a plan is in place to handle shortages. The following steps are recommended:

- Stay informed of product shortages with the American Society for Parenteral and Enteral Nutrition (http://www.nutritioncare.org/public-policy/product-shortages/)
- Limit use of products with a shortage to the most vulnerable populations
- Search for alternate suppliers and products
- Transition to enteral nutrition and enteral supplementation as is clinically feasible

Table 11
Published recommendations of maximum osmolarity of peripheral parenteral nutrition solutions

Source	Recommendation	Level of Evidence
ESPGHAN/ESPEN/ESPR/CSPEN Guidelines on Pediatric Parenteral Nutrition[101]	900 mOsm/L	conditional recommendation
ASPEN[87]	900 mOsm/L	Weak
NICE[13]	No recommendation	NA

- Be aware of increased risk for errors with alternate procedures and product usage
- Monitor patients for applicable clinical deficiencies
- Implement strategies early

OSMOLARITY

Osmolarity, the measure of osmotically active particles in solute per liter of solution, is most significantly influenced by dextrose and amino acid concentrations in PN. When considering the composition of a peripheral PN solution, it is critical to assess osmolarity because of the potential of thrombophlebitis and neonates. Published literature on osmolarity content of peripheral PN has ranged from low (400 mOsm/L) to high (1700 mOsm/L), with limited descriptions of the rate of infusion, and differing definitions of a "tolerable" rate of thrombophlebitis.[99,100] Major recommendations on maximum osmolarity have either been made with a noted weak level of evidence[87,101] or have opted to not make a recommendation because of the limitations in the literature (**Table 11**).[13]

TRANSITION TO ENTERAL NUTRITION

Meeting estimated nutrient (and in particular, protein) requirements when transitioning from PN to enteral nutrition is a challenging, yet essential consideration in developing neonatal intensive care unit nutrition guidelines. Optimizing and standardizing PN in this transition phase to ensure adequate protein intake leads to better growth and body composition development in preterm infants.[102–104]

Strategies to ensure appropriate nutrition in this transition phase include the following:

- Creating a guideline to ensure minimum nutrient requirements are met
- Using concentrated PN, rather than quickly transitioning to dextrose and electrolyte-only containing solutions
- Earlier initiation of human milk fortification

SUMMARY

PN is a life-saving therapy for high-risk newborns, but it carries risk. Unlike human milk, and commercial infant formulas that are designed to mimic it, PN is artificial; dependent of the expertise of the ordering health care professionals for balance and completeness; and bypasses the gate-keeping function of the gastrointestinal track, which protects against toxicity and adjusts absorption in the face of inadequate intake. An experienced, multidisciplinary team mitigates risk. The team, as a minimum, should include a physician, nurse, pharmacist, and dietitian.[105] Dietitians "...ensure that early, intense nutritional support is initiated and individualized to the infant, facilitate the smooth transition from parenteral to enteral nutrition, closely monitor growth on growth charts, and suggest adjustments to nutritional support aimed at maintaining steady growth."[106]

CLINICS CARE POINTS

A bulleted list of evidence-based pearls and pitfalls related to PN and relevant to the care of high-risks newborns.

- Starter PN: provide as first fluid for VLBW infants; consider need for phosphorus to prevent "neonatal refeeding syndrome"
- Balance: ensure physiologic macronutrient distribution to maximize high-quality weight gain (protein/calorie ratio) and normal metabolism (energy from fat and carbohydrate)
- Source of intravenous fat: consider components of fat emulsion regarding metabolism, nutrient adequacy, and contribution to long-term outcomes
- Electrolytes: monitor and individualize
- Bone health: maximize calcium and phosphorus within the safe limits of the solution; heed the calcium/phosphorus ratio
- Trace elements: focus on zinc, copper, selenium, and iodine
- Vitamins: remember that intravenous requirements are not well-defined; anticipate deficiency if your patient requires unusual fluid volumes, components, or treatments
- Complications: monitor for cholestasis and MBD if PN extends beyond 2 weeks
- Parenteral to enteral: transition as soon as possible
- Team: assemble a dedicated and experienced group

DISCLOSURE

S. Groh-Wargo is a consultant for Baxter. S.M. Barr has nothing to disclose.

REFERENCES

1. Embleton ND, Simmer K. In: Koletzko B, Poindexter B, Uauy R, editors. Practice of parenteral nutrition in VLBW and ELBW infants. Basel: Karger; 2014.
2. Moyses HE, Johnson MJ, Leaf AA, et al. Early parenteral nutrition and growth outcomes in preterm infants: a systematic review and meta-analysis. Am J Clin Nutr 2013;97(4):816–26.
3. Embleton NE, Pang N, Cooke RJ. Postnatal malnutrition and growth retardation: an inevitable consequence of current recommendations in preterm infants? Pediatrics 2001;107(2):270–3.
4. Senterre T, Rigo J. Optimizing early nutritional support based on recent recommendations in VLBW infants and postnatal growth restriction. J Pediatr Gastroenterol Nutr 2011;53(5):536–42.
5. Senterre T, Rigo J. Reduction in postnatal cumulative nutritional deficit and improvement of growth in extremely preterm infants. Acta Paediatr 2012; 101(2):e64–70.
6. Perrem L, Semberova J, O'Sullivan A, et al. Effect of early parenteral nutrition discontinuation on time to regain birth weight in very low birth weight infants: a randomized controlled trial. JPEN J Parenter Enteral Nutr 2019;43(7):883–90.

7. Späth C, Zamir I, Sjöström ES, et al. Use of concentrated parenteral nutrition solutions is associated with improved nutrient intakes and postnatal growth in very low-birth-weight infants. JPEN J Parenter Enteral Nutr 2020;44(2):327–36.

8. Hsiao CC, Tsai ML, Chen CC, et al. Early optimal nutrition improves neurodevelopmental outcomes for very preterm infants. Nutr Rev 2014;72(8):532–40.

9. Prusakov P, Speaks S, Magers JS. Parenteral nutrition in moderately preterm, otherwise healthy neonates is not associated with improved short-term growth outcomes. J Parenter Enteral Nutr 2020;44(8):1519–24.

10. Denne SC, Poindexter BB. Evidence supporting early nutritional support with parenteral amino acid infusion. Semin Perinatol 2007;31(2):56–60.

11. Patel P, Bhatia J. Total parenteral nutrition for the very low birth weight infant. Semin Fetal Neonatal Med 2017;22(1):2–7.

12. Carlson S, Kavars AM. Parenteral nutrition. In: Groh Wargo S, Thompson M, Cox J, editors. Academy of Nutrition and Dietetics pocket guide to neonatal nutrition. 2nd edition. Chicago: Academy of Nutrition and Dietetics; 2016. p. 32–76.

13. Excellence NIfHaC. Neonatal parenteral nutrition. 2020. Available at: https://www.nice.org.uk/guidance/indevelopment/gid-ng10037. Accessed December 7, 2021.

14. Al-Jebawi Y, Argawal N, Groh Wargo S, et al. Low caloric intake and high fluid intake during the first week of life are associated with the severity of bronchopulmonary dysplasia in extremely low birth weight infants. J Neonatal Perinatal Med 2020;13(2):207–14.

15. Stephens BE, Walden RV, Gargus RA, et al. First-week protein and energy intakes are associated with 18-month developmental outcomes in extremely low birth weight infants. Pediatrics 2009;123(5):1337–43.

16. Hartnoll G, Betremieux P, Modi N. Body water content of extremely preterm infants at birth. Arch Dis Child Fetal Neonatal Ed 2000;83(1):F56–9.

17. O'Brien F, Walker IA. Fluid homeostasis in the neonate. Paediatr Anaesth 2014; 24(1):49–59.

18. Jochum F, Moltu SJ, Senterre T, et al. ESPGHAN/ESPEN/ESPR/CSPEN guidelines on pediatric parenteral nutrition: fluid and electrolytes. Clin Nutr 2018; 37(6 Pt B):2344–53.

19. Martin CR, Brown YF, Ehrenkranz RA, et al. Nutritional practices and growth velocity in the first month of life in extremely premature infants. Pediatrics 2009; 124(2):649–57.

20. Ehrenkranz RA, Das A, Wrage LA, et al. Early nutrition mediates the influence of severity of illness on extremely LBW infants. Pediatr Res 2011;69(6):522–9.

21. van der Lugt NM, Smits-Wintjens VE, van Zwieten PH, et al. Short and long term outcome of neonatal hyperglycemia in very preterm infants: a retrospective follow-up study. BMC Pediatr 2010;10:52.

22. Talpers SS, Romberger DJ, Bunce SB, et al. Nutritionally associated increased carbon dioxide production. Excess total calories vs high proportion of carbohydrate calories. Chest 1992;102(2):551–5.

23. Crill CM, Gura KM. Parenteral nutrition support. In: Corkins MR, editor. The ASPEN pediatric nutrition support core curriculum. 2nd edition. Silver Spring, MD: ASPEN; 2015. p. 593–614.

24. van Goudoever JB, Carnielli V, Darmaun D, et al. ESPGHAN/ESPEN/ESPR/CSPEN guidelines on pediatric parenteral nutrition: amino acids. Clin Nutr 2018;37(6 Pt B):2315–23.

25. te Braake FW, van den Akker CH, Riedijk MA, et al. Parenteral amino acid and energy administration to premature infants in early life. Semin Fetal Neonatal Med 2007;12(1):11–8.

26. 3. Amino acids. J Pediatr Gastroenterol Nutr 2005;41:S12–8.

27. Morgan C, Burgess L. High protein intake does not prevent low plasma levels of conditionally essential amino acids in very preterm infants receiving parenteral nutrition. JPEN J Parenter Enteral Nutr 2017;41(3):455–62.

28. Valentine CJ, Fernandez S, Rogers LK, et al. Early amino-acid administration improves preterm infant weight. J Perinatol 2009;29(6):428–32.

29. Loui A, Bührer C. Growth of very low birth weight infants after increased amino acid and protein administration. J Perinat Med 2013;41(6):735–41.

30. Trintis J, Donohue P, Aucott S. Outcomes of early parenteral nutrition for premature infants. J Perinatol 2010;30(6):403–7.

31. Vlaardingerbroek H, Schierbeek H, Rook D, et al. Albumin synthesis in very low birth weight infants is enhanced by early parenteral lipid and high-dose amino acid administration. Clin Nutr 2016;35(2):344–50.

32. Ridout E, Melara D, Rottinghaus S, et al. Blood urea nitrogen concentration as a marker of amino-acid intolerance in neonates with birthweight less than 1250 g. J Perinatol 2005;25(2):130–3.

33. Roggero P, Giannì ML, Morlacchi L, et al. Blood urea nitrogen concentrations in low-birth-weight preterm infants during parenteral and enteral nutrition. J Pediatr Gastroenterol Nutr 2010;51(2):213–5.

34. Bonsante F, Gouyon JB, Robillard PY, et al. Early optimal parenteral nutrition and metabolic acidosis in very preterm infants. PLoS One 2017;12(11):e0186936.

35. Roelants JA, Vlaardingerbroek H, van den Akker CHP, et al. Two-year follow-up of a randomized controlled nutrition intervention trial in very low-birth-weight infants. JPEN J Parenter Enteral Nutr 2018;42(1):122–31.

36. Morgan C, McGowan P, Herwitker S, et al. Postnatal head growth in preterm infants: a randomized controlled parenteral nutrition study. Pediatrics 2014; 133(1):e120–8.

37. Osborn DA, Schindler T, Jones LJ, et al. Higher versus lower amino acid intake in parenteral nutrition for newborn infants. Cochrane Database Syst Rev 2018;3: Cd005949.

38. Scattolin S, Gaio P, Betto M, et al. Parenteral amino acid intakes: possible influences of higher intakes on growth and bone status in preterm infants. J Perinatol 2013;33(1):33–9.

39. Bellagamba MP, Carmenati E, D'Ascenzo R, et al. One extra gram of protein to preterm infants from birth to 1800 g: a single-blinded randomized clinical trial. J Pediatr Gastroenterol Nutr 2016;62(6):879–84.

40. Balakrishnan M, Jennings A, Przystac L, et al. Growth and neurodevelopmental outcomes of early, high-dose parenteral amino acid intake in very low birth weight infants: a randomized controlled trial. JPEN J Parenter Enteral Nutr 2018;42(3):597–606.

41. Yang S, Lee BS, Park HW, et al. Effect of high vs standard early parenteral amino acid supplementation on the growth outcomes in very low birth weight infants. JPEN J Parenter Enteral Nutr 2013;37(3):327–34.

42. Tottman AC, Bloomfield FH, Cormack BE, et al. Relationships between early nutrition and blood glucose concentrations in very preterm infants. J Pediatr Gastroenterol Nutr 2018;66(6):960–6.

43. Vlaardingerbroek H, Vermeulen MJ, Rook D, et al. Safety and efficacy of early parenteral lipid and high-dose amino acid administration to very low birth weight infants. J Pediatr 2013;163(3):638–44.e1-5.

44. Kim K, Kim NJ, Kim SY. Safety and efficacy of early high parenteral lipid supplementation in preterm infants: a systematic review and meta-analysis. Nutrients 2021;13(5):1535.

45. Ottolini KM, Andescavage N, Kapse K, et al. Early lipid intake improves cerebellar growth in very low-birth-weight preterm infants. JPEN J Parenter Enteral Nutr 2021;45(3):587–95.

46. Correani A, Giretti I, Antognoli L, et al. Hypertriglyceridemia and intravenous lipid titration during routine parenteral nutrition in small preterm infants. J Pediatr Gastroenterol Nutr 2019;69(5):619–25.

47. Boscarino G, Conti MG, De Luca F, et al. Intravenous lipid emulsions affect respiratory outcome in preterm newborn: a case-control study. Nutrients 2021; 13(4):1243.

48. Winther B, Jackson D, Mulroy C, et al. Evaluation of serum carnitine levels for pediatric patients receiving carnitine-free and carnitine-supplemented parenteral nutrition. Hosp Pharm 2014;49(6):549–53.

49. Crill CM, Storm MC, Christensen ML, et al. Carnitine supplementation in premature neonates: effect on plasma and red blood cell total carnitine concentrations, nutrition parameters and morbidity. Clin Nutr 2006;25(6):886–96.

50. Biagetti C, Correani A, D'Ascenzo R, et al. Does intravenous fish oil affect the growth of extremely low birth weight preterm infants on parenteral nutrition? Clin Nutr 2019;38(5):2319–24.

51. Biagetti C, Correani A, D'Ascenzo R, et al. Is intravenous fish oil associated with the neurodevelopment of extremely low birth weight preterm infants on parenteral nutrition? Clin Nutr 2021;40(5):2845–50.

52. Kasirer Y, Bin-Nun A, Raveh A, et al. SMOFlipid protects preterm neonates against perinatal nutrition-associated cholestasis. Am J Perinatol 2019;36(13): 1382–6.

53. Memon N, Hussein K, Hegyi T, et al. Essential fatty acid deficiency with SMOFlipid reduction in an infant with intestinal failure-associated liver disease. JPEN J Parenter Enteral Nutr 2019;43(3):438–41.

54. Carey AN, Rudie C, Mitchell PD, et al. Essential fatty acid status in surgical infants receiving parenteral nutrition with a composite lipid emulsion: a case series. JPEN J Parenter Enteral Nutr 2019;43(2):305–10.

55. Isemann B, Mueller EW, Narendran V, et al. Impact of early sodium supplementation on hyponatremia and growth in premature infants: a randomized controlled trial. JPEN J Parenter Enteral Nutr 2016;40(3):342–9.

56. Kleinman RE, Greer FR, editors. Pediatric nutrition. 8th edition. Itasca (Illinois): American Academy of Pediatrics; 2019. p. 1688.

57. Mihatsch W, Fewtrell M, Goulet O, et al. ESPGHAN/ESPEN/ESPR/CSPEN guidelines on pediatric parenteral nutrition: calcium, phosphorus and magnesium. Clin Nutr 2018;37(6 Pt B):2360–5.

58. Mimouni F, Mandel D, Lubetzky R, et al. In: Koletzko B, Poindexter BB, Uauy R, editors. Nutritional care of preterm infants: scientific basis and practical guidelines, 110. Basel: Karger; 2014. p. 140–51.

59. MacKay MW, Fitzgerald KA, Jackson D. The solubility of calcium and phosphate in two specialty amino acid solutions. JPEN J Parenter Enteral Nutr 1996; 20(1):63–6.

60. Huston RK, Christensen JM, Alshahrani SM, et al. Calcium chloride and calcium gluconate in neonatal parenteral nutrition solutions with added cysteine: compatibility studies using laser light obscuration methodology. JPEN J Parenter Enteral Nutr 2019;43(3):426–33.

61. Bonsante F, Iacobelli S, Latorre G, et al. Initial amino acid intake influences phosphorus and calcium homeostasis in preterm infants: it is time to change the composition of the early parenteral nutrition. PLoS One 2013;8(8):e72880.

62. Hair AB, Chetta KE, Bruno AM, et al. Delayed introduction of parenteral phosphorus is associated with hypercalcemia in extremely preterm infants. J Nutr 2016;146(6):1212–6.

03. Cormack BE, Jiang Y, Harding JE, et al. Neonatal refeeding syndrome and clinical outcome in extremely low-birth-weight babies: secondary cohort analysis from the ProVIDe trial. J Parenter Enteral Nutr 2021;45(1):65–78.

64. Zemrani B, McCallum Z, Bines JE. Trace element provision in parenteral nutrition in children: one size does not fit all. Nutrients 2018;10(11).

65. Hardy G, Wong T, Morrissey H, et al. Parenteral provision of micronutrients to pediatric patients: an international expert consensus paper. JPEN J Parenter Enteral Nutr 2020;44(Suppl 2):S5–23.

66. Domellof M, Szitanyi P, Simchowitz V, et al. ESPGHAN/ESPEN/ESPR/CSPEN guidelines on pediatric parenteral nutrition: iron and trace minerals. Clin Nutr 2018;37(6 Pt B):2354–9.

67. Olson LM, Wieruszewski PM, Jannetto PJ, et al. Quantitative assessment of trace-element contamination in parenteral nutrition components. JPEN J Parenter Enteral Nutr 2019;43(8):970–6.

68. Altarelli M, Ben-Hamouda N, Schneider A, et al. Copper deficiency: causes, manifestations, and treatment. Nutr Clin Pract 2019;34(4):504–13.

69. Kanike N, Groh-Wargo S, Thomas M, et al. Risk of iodine deficiency in extremely low gestational age newborns on parenteral nutrition. Nutrients 2020;12(6).

70. Zimmermann MB, Andersson M. Prevalence of iodine deficiency in Europe in 2010. Ann Endocrinol (Paris) 2011;72(2):164–6.

71. Notes from the field: zinc deficiency dermatitis in cholestatic extremely premature infants after a nationwide shortage of injectable zinc - Washington, DC, December 2012. MMWR Morb Mortal Wkly Rep 2013;62(7):136–7.

72. Bronsky J, Campoy C, Braegger C. ESPGHAN/ESPEN/ESPR/CSPEN guidelines on pediatric parenteral nutrition: vitamins. Clin Nutr 2018;37(6 Pt B):2366–78.

73. Chessex P, Laborie S, Nasef N, et al. Shielding parenteral nutrition from light improves survival rate in premature infants. JPEN J Parenter Enteral Nutr 2017; 41(3):378–83.

74. Polegato BF, Pereira AG, Azevedo PS, et al. Role of thiamin in health and disease. Nutr Clin Pract 2019;34(4):558–64.

75. Rochow N, Raja P, Liu K, et al. Physiological adjustment to postnatal growth trajectories in healthy preterm infants. Pediatr Res 2016;79(6):870–9.

76. Fenton TR, Anderson D, Groh-Wargo S, et al. An attempt to standardize the calculation of growth velocity of preterm infants: evaluation of practical bedside methods. J Pediatr 2018;196:77–83.

77. Abdallah EAA, Said RN, Mosallam DS, et al. Serial serum alkaline phosphatase as an early biomarker for osteopenia of prematurity. Medicine (Baltimore) 2016; 95(37):e4837.

78. DiBaise M, Tarleton SM. Hair, nails, and skin: differentiating cutaneous manifestations of micronutrient deficiency. Nutr Clin Pract 2019;34(4):490–503.

79. Faienza MF, D'Amato E, Natale MP, et al. Metabolic bone disease of prematurity: diagnosis and management. Front Pediatr 2019;7:143.

80. Kovacs CS. Bone development and mineral homeostasis in the fetus and neonate: roles of the calciotropic and phosphotropic hormones. Physiol Rev 2014;94(4):1143–218.

81. Fitzgerald KA, MacKay MW. Calcium and phosphate solubility in neonatal parenteral nutrient solutions containing TrophAmine. Am J Hosp Pharm 1986; 43(1):88–93.

82. Kavurt S, Demirel N, Yücel H, et al. Evaluation of radiologic evidence of metabolic bone disease in very low birth weight infants at fourth week of life. J Perinatol 2021;1–6.

83. Nayrouz MM, Amin SB. Cumulative amount of intravenous lipid intake and parenteral nutrition-associated cholestasis in neonates with gastrointestinal surgical disorders. Am J Perinatol 2014;31(5):419–24.

84. Gupta K, Wang H, Amin SB. Parenteral nutrition-associated cholestasis in premature infants: role of macronutrients. JPEN J Parenter Enteral Nutr 2016; 40(3):335–41.

85. Kapoor V, Malviya MN, Soll R. Lipid emulsions for parenterally fed preterm infants. Cochrane Database Syst Rev 2019;6:Cd013163.

86. Premkumar MH, Carter BA, Hawthorne KM, et al. Fish oil-based lipid emulsions in the treatment of parenteral nutrition-associated liver disease: an ongoing positive experience. Adv Nutr 2014;5(1):65–70.

87. Boullata JI, Gilbert K, Sacks G, et al. A.S.P.E.N. clinical guidelines: parenteral nutrition ordering, order review, compounding, labeling, and dispensing. JPEN J Parenter Enteral Nutr 2014;38(3):334–77.

88. Corkins MR. Aluminum effects in infants and children. Pediatrics 2019;144(6): e20193148.

89. Appleman SS, Kalkwarf HJ, Dwivedi A, et al. Bone deficits in parenteral nutrition-dependent infants and children with intestinal failure are attenuated when accounting for slower growth. J Pediatr Gastroenterol Nutr 2013;57(1):124–30.

90. Hall AR, Le H, Arnold C, et al. Aluminum exposure from parenteral nutrition: early bile canaliculus changes of the hepatocyte. Nutrients 2018;10(6):723.

91. Hernández-Sánchez A, Tejada-González P, Arteta-Jiménez M. Aluminum in parenteral nutrition: a systematic review. Eur J Clin Nutr 2013;67(3):230–8.

92. Huston RK, Heisel CF, Vermillion BR, et al. Aluminum content of neonatal parenteral nutrition solutions: options for reducing aluminum exposure. Nutr Clin Pract 2017;32(2):266–70.

93. Hall AR, Arnold CJ, Miller GG, et al. Infant parenteral nutrition remains a significant source for aluminum toxicity. JPEN J Parenter Enteral Nutr 2017;41(7): 1228–33.

94. Lima-Rogel V, Romano-Moreno S, de Jesus Lopez-Lopez E, et al. Aluminum contamination in parenteral nutrition admixtures for low-birth-weight preterm infants in Mexico. JPEN J Parenter Enteral Nutr 2016;40(7):1014–20.

95. Vanek VW, Borum P, Buchman A, et al. A call to action to bring safer parenteral micronutrient products to the U.S. market. Nutr Clin Pract 2015;30(4):559–69.

96. Hak EB, Storm MC, Helms RA. Chromium and zinc contamination of parenteral nutrient solution components commonly used in infants and children. Am J Health Syst Pharm 1998;55(2):150–4.

97. Uchino A, Noguchi T, Nomiyama K, et al. Manganese accumulation in the brain: MR imaging. Neuroradiology 2007;49(9):715–20.

98. Hardy G. Manganese in parenteral nutrition: who, when, and why should we supplement? Gastroenterology 2009;137(5 Suppl):S29–35.
99. Cies JJ, Moore WS 2nd. Neonatal and pediatric peripheral parenteral nutrition: what is a safe osmolarity? Nutr Clin Pract 2014;29(1):118–24.
100. Dugan S, Le J, Jew RK. Maximum tolerated osmolarity for peripheral administration of parenteral nutrition in pediatric patients. JPEN J Parenter Enteral Nutr 2014;38(7):847–51.
101. Hartman C, Shamir R, Simchowitz V, et al. ESPGHAN/ESPEN/ESPR/CSPEN guidelines on pediatric parenteral nutrition: complications. Clin Nutr 2018;37(6 Pt B):2418–29.
102. Miller M, Donda K, Dhutada A, et al. Transitioning preterm infants from parenteral nutrition: a comparison of 2 protocols. JPEN J Parenter Enteral Nutr 2017;41(8):1371–9.
103. Brennan A-M, Kiely ME, Fenton S, et al. Standardized parenteral nutrition for the transition phase in preterm infants: a bag that fits. Nutrients 2018;10(2):170.
104. Liotto N, Amato O, Piemontese P, et al. Protein intakes during weaning from parenteral nutrition drive growth gain and body composition in very low birth weight preterm infants. Nutrients 2020;12(5).
105. Embleton ND, Simmer K. Practice of parenteral nutrition in VLBW and ELBW infants. World Rev Nutr Diet 2014;110:177–89.
106. Ehrenkranz RA. Nutrition, growth and clinical outcomes. In: Koletzko B, Poindexter B, Uauy R, editors. Nutritional care of preterm infants: scientific basis and practical guidelines. 110. Basel: Karger; 2014. p. 11–26.
107. Joosten K, Embleton N, Yan W, et al. ESPGHAN/ESPEN/ESPR/CSPEN guidelines on pediatric parenteral nutrition: energy. Clin Nutr 2018;37(6 Pt B):2309–14.
108. Mesotten D, Joosten K, van Kempen A, et al. ESPGHAN/ESPEN/ESPR/CSPEN guidelines on pediatric parenteral nutrition: carbohydrates. Clin Nutr 2018;37(6 Pt B):2337–43.
109. Lapillonne A, Fidler Mis N, Goulet O, et al. ESPGHAN/ESPEN/ESPR/CSPEN guidelines on pediatric parenteral nutrition: lipids. Clin Nutr 2018;37(6 Pt B):2324–36.

Lipids and Long Chain Polyunsaturated Fatty Acids in Preterm Infants

Kristin Santoro, MD[a,b], Camilia R. Martin, MD, MS[b,c],*

KEYWORDS

- Lipids • Fatty acids • Lipid emulsions • Lipid supplements

KEY POINTS

- Preterm infants acquire postnatal deficits in DHA and ARA due to the inadequacy of available nutritional products and strategies to prevents these deficits.
- Preterm infants require parenteral lipids to meet dietary recommendations in fats and total energy; however, there are no parenteral lipid emulsions that meet the unique requirements of the preterm infant.
- Omegaven is recommended for infants with PNAC.

INTRODUCTION

Lipids represent a diverse class of bioactive compounds that are critical for fetal and infant development. Much of their function is dictated by the fatty acid moieties that comprise their structure. Critical factors include (1) carbon length, (2) saturated versus unsaturated (no double bonds vs double bonds, respectively), and (3) omega class. The omega class of an unsaturated fatty acid is denoted by the carbon position of the first double bond from the terminal methyl group. The 3 main classes of polyunsaturated fatty acids (PUFAs) are omega-3, omega-6, and omega-9 fatty acids. Alpha linoleic acid (ALA), an omega-3 fatty acid, and linoleic acid (LA), an omega-6 fatty acid, are not made endogenously and must be acquired through dietary sources and are referred to as essential fatty acids (EFA), as humans lack the enzymes necessary for their in vivo synthesis. These 2 fatty acids are elongated and desaturated to form the downstream long-chain PUFAs (LCPUFAs) docosahexaenoic acid (DHA) and arachidonic acid (ARA), respectively. Although not considered "essential" by strict

[a] Division of Newborn Medicine, Department of Pediatrics, Boston Children's Hospital, 300 Longwood Avenue, Boston, MA 02115, USA; [b] Harvard Medical School, Boston, MA, USA; [c] Department of Neonatology, Beth Israel Deaconess Medical Center, 330 Brookline Avenue, Rose3, Boston, MA 02215, USA
* Corresponding author. Department of Neonatology, Beth Israel Deaconess Medical Center, 330 Brookline Avenue, Rose3, Boston, MA 02215, USA
E-mail address: cmartin1@bidmc.harvard.edu

Clin Perinatol 49 (2022) 381–391
https://doi.org/10.1016/j.clp.2022.02.007
0095-5108/22/© 2022 Elsevier Inc. All rights reserved.
perinatology.theclinics.com

definition, DHA and ARA provide invaluable functions in utero and in the preterm neonate and are subject to acquired postnatal deficits and thus are sometimes referred to as "conditionally essential".

Beyond nutrition and growth, lipids and their constituent fatty acids also are critical in cellular level processes that contribute to angiogenesis, organogenesis, immune response, and regulation of inflammation. Structurally, they incorporate into cellular membranes and participate in regulatory activities at every tissue level—brain, eye, lung, gut, bone, and others. Lipids and fatty acids are highly concentrated in the retina and neuronal gray matter and therefore are important in neurodevelopment, cognitive functioning, and visual acuity. LCPUFAs also serve as precursors to oxygenated downstream products called oxylipins that include eicosanoids and specialized proresolving mediators (SPMs) that execute their pleiotropic bioactive roles in human health and disease.

The long history and continuing work in lipids and fatty acids in the preterm population has informed the critical role of DHA and ARA in growth and development, the unique perinatal transitions and fatty acid requirements in this population, the role of altered fatty acid profiles in neonatal diseases processes, and the challenges that arise in determining and providing adequate supplementation in preterm infants. This review discusses these topics through research findings across the T1 to T4 translational science pipeline, highlighting recent large, randomized control clinical trials aimed to reduce neonatal morbidities through enteral fatty acid supplementation. Emerging studies investigating the role of LCPUFA downstream lipid mediators, such as specialized proresolving mediators (SPMs), in neonatal physiology and disease will be examined as potential future strategies. The authors conclude with clinical practice recommendations and future directions for research.

MATERNAL TO FETAL TRANSFER OF LIPIDS AND FATTY ACIDS

The developing fetus relies on the transfer of LCPUFAs across the placenta for growth and organogenesis. During the first two trimesters of pregnancy, the maternal body deposits large amounts of fat stores necessary for fetal growth. As these maternal fat stores develop, the fetus first experiences a slow period of anabolic fat deposition from 22 to 32 weeks of gestation, followed by a sharp increase in anabolic fetal fat storage; this is achieved through a shift in maternal lipid metabolism from an anabolic to catabolic state in the third trimester, resulting in large maternal transfers of DHA and ARA to the fetus, in concentrations greater than their essential fatty acid precursors.[1] Early stores of adipose tissue undergo lipolysis, coupled by an increased maternal hepatic production of triglycerides, decrease in lipoprotein lipase activity, and an increase in placental lipoprotein lipase to promote transfer of LCPUFAs across the placental membrane.[2] ARA and DHA are thought to have particular significance in this metabolic exchange. Studies have shown selective preference for these lipids at the placental membrane over other nonessential fatty acids[3,4] and increases in ARA and DHA in cord blood of neonates compared with maternal plasma.[5] This differential of maternal to fetal concentrations is often referred to as "biomagnification."

In addition to the transfer of LCPUFAs to the fetus, they are also metabolized by the placenta into their eicosanoid derivates to participate in important biological activities throughout pregnancy and at the time of delivery; this includes an upregulation in cyclooxygenase-2, which plays an important role in the synthesis of prostaglandins, including prostaglandin E2, a proangiogenic factor that stimulates vascular endothelial growth factor and is a derivative of ARA.[6] This neovascularization process occurs in the first trimester during trophoblast infiltration of the uterus and spiral artery modulation, promoting placental development and providing proper growth and maintenance of the embryo. DHA has proangiogenic properties during the first trimester, which is unique to pregnancy, as the opposite effect is observed in tumor cells, where DHA is found to decrease angiogenic growth factors.[7] In addition, the placenta itself contains enzymes necessary to use fatty acids for energy and participate in fatty acid oxidation.[2]

Factors Influencing Maternal to Fetal Long-Chain Polysaturated Fatty Acid Transfer

Maternal levels of LCPUFAs affect the amount that transfers across the placenta[8]; this is influenced by maternal diet and maternal metabolic state.[9] For example, metabolic changes that result from maternal obesity and diabetes alter placental lipid metabolism by affecting the placental transfer of nutrients. Women with elevated prepregnancy body mass index and gestational diabetes mellitus have changes in gene expression involved in fatty acid uptake.[10] Alterations in activity and gene expression also occur with placental insufficiency, for example, changes in placental lipoprotein lipase and decreased fetal levels of LCPUFAs have been described in pregnancies complicated by infant in-utero growth restriction[11]; this results in storage of LCPUFA as triglycerides as opposed to their free fatty acid form, which can lead to impaired transport to the fetus, accounting for the poor growth observed in utero.[12]

Postnatal Transitions in Systemic Fatty Acid Levels in the Preterm Infant

The acquisition of large stores of LCPUFAs through placental transfer, with specific preference for DHA and ARA, is interrupted in infants born preterm. This initiates several challenges regarding adequate delivery postnatally. Inadequate tissue stores in the muscle and fat of preterm neonates lead to higher demands for dietary macronutrients to supply energy and improve fetal growth. The ability to meet these demands is met by the challenges in the lack of parenteral lipid emulsions specific for the unique needs of the preterm infant and a delay in enteral feeding.

Intravenous Lipid Emulsions

All very-low-birth-weight (VLBW) infants require lipid supplementation with intravenous lipid emulsions (ILE) in the first days of life to prevent essential fatty acid deficiency (EFAD). Infants fed diets absent in essential fatty acids can develop EFAD within 2 to 3 days.[13] EFAD is marked by failure to thrive, pathologic dermatologic conditions including scaly dermatitis and alopecia, increased susceptibility to bacterial infection, and laboratory abnormalities including thrombocytopenia.[14] At the minimum, 0.25 to 0.5 g/kg/d of intralipid intravenous emulsion is necessary to prevent EFAD in the preterm neonate.[15] The European Society of Pediatric Gastroenterology, Hepatology and Nutrition recommends 0.1 g/kg/d and 0.25 g/kg/d of LA to prevent EFAD in term infants and preterm infants, respectively.[16]

Intralipid (Sigma-Aldrich, Inc., St. Louis, Missouri) is currently the only Food and Drug Administration (FDA)-approved parental lipid emulsion for neonates. Common clinical practice is to begin the infusion within the first 24 to 48 hours of birth at 0.5 to 1 g/kg/d and advance by 0.5 g/kg/d to 3 g/kg/d with a general goal to reach 3 to 4 g/kg/d. However, at these current doses, levels of DHA and ARA fail to reach the high level of accretion achieved in utero. Although Intralipid does provide large amounts of the EFA parent compounds, LA and ALA, by 1 week of life circulating levels of fatty acids in infants mirror that in the emulsion and have higher levels of LA and ALA over DHA and ARA[17]; this is in direct contradiction to what is observed for gestationally aged match neonates during the process of biomagnification. In addition, Intralipid is criticized for its phytosterol content. Phytosterol is a cholesterol-like molecule derived from plants, with the same nucleus as cholesterol but a different side chain. Phytosterol has low levels of enteral absorption due to specialized transporters that excrete sterols back into the intestinal lumen. However, with intravenous administration, this intestinal excretion process is bypassed, and these products are systemically absorbed into the circulation, can incorporate into lipid membranes, and lead to adverse effects.[18] Phytosterols are thought to be a major contributor to parental nutrition–associated cholestasis (PNAC) and intestinal fatty acid liver disease (IFALD). PNAC/IFALD is a multifactorial disease marked by elevated direct bilirubin levels greater than 2 mg/dL in the absence of other liver disease and is associated with prolonged use of parental nutrition (PN) and ILE.[19]

Over the last 80 years, substantial effort led to the development of additional ILE compositions, with modifications to address the concerns regarding the first-generation lipid emulsion, Intralipid. Fish oil containing ILEs, sometimes referred to as fourth generation, were produced with the goal to create a lower, more favorable omega-6 to omega-3 ratio increasing the concentration of omega-3 fatty acids, including DHA. SMOFlipid (Fresenius Kabi, Bad Homburg, Germany) is composed of soybean oil, MCTs, olive oil, and fish oil, with an omega-6 to omega-3 ratio of 2.5:1. Omegaven (Fresenius Kabi, Bad Homburg, Germany) is composed 100% of fish oil, thus containing high levels of omega-3 fatty acids including DHA; this contrasts with Intralipid, with an omega-6 to omega-3 ratio of 7:1.

Fish oil–containing lipid emulsions have not been universally adopted into routine care due to the lack of large, multicentered randomized control trials that confirm their safety and superiority over exclusive soybean-based ILEs for infants without PNAC/IFALD. Although several trials have supported use of Omegaven to improve PNAC/IFALD (in 2018, Omegaven was approved by the FDA as monotherapy for PNAC/IFALD associated disease in infants and children), a recent meta-analysis is unable to draw proven clinical benefit of these emulsions as routine maintenance lipids. In addition, concern has been raised regarding the preterm infant's induced fatty acid profiles after exposure.[20,21] Although DHA levels are increased compared with soybean oil–based emulsions, the postnatal decline or acquired deficit in DHA is not prevented. In addition, clinical significance of the concomitant decreased levels of ARA and elevations in EPA is of potential concern.[22] Multicomponent emulsions such as SMOFlipid and fish oil–based emulsions have lower levels of ALA/LA, and it has been reported in the literature that its use confers a higher risk of EFAD when provided in doses less than approximately 2.0 g/k/d.[23] However, a randomized control trial that administered doses of Omegaven at 1 g/k/d did not report EFAD in late preterm infants older than 2 weeks.[24]

Enteral Feeding

Enteral feeding is the optimal source of fatty acid accruement in VLBW infants; however, breast milk concentration of DHA and ARA is highly variable. In general, the amount of lipids in breast milk can vary from start to end of a single feed and can vary in concentration 5-fold among different women.[25] On average, the amount of DHA in breast milk is about 20 mg/kg/d; however, the amount of DHA varies widely in breast milk and is reflective of maternal diet.[26] In the neonatal intensive care unit (NICU), a large population of infants receive pasteurized donor breast milk, which has been shown to have lower levels of DHA compared with mother's own milk.[27] Although studies have confirmed that both maternal and direct supplementation of DHA effectively increases DHA levels in preterm infants,[28] DHA-centric strategies further exacerbate deficits in ARA.[29] The appropriate amount of DHA/ARA is still unknown for the preterm population.

Ultimately, challenges in parenteral and enteral fatty acid delivery in preterm infants lead to a shift in blood fatty acid levels and ratios from what is found in utero, with a rapid decline in DHA and ARA levels and a concomitant increase in LA by 1 week postnatal age. Our group measured these levels in preterm neonates born less than 30 weeks gestational age and found an association with decreased levels of DHA with an increased odds ratio of bronchopulmonary dysplasia (BPD) and decreased levels of ARA with increased odds of late-onset sepsis.[17] These results from this study demonstrate the potential implications of DHA and ARA deficits and risk for increased morbidity. Over the last several decades, extensive evidence in both preclinical and clinical trials have demonstrated the importance of DHA and ARA in both developmental and disease processes in the brain, retina, lungs, gut, and bone of preterm infants.[30-35]

REVIEW OF RECENT CLINICAL TRIALS IN ENTERAL LIPID SUPPLEMENTATION

The heterogeneity of many early clinical trials on the beneficial effects of supplementation of LCPUFAs for preterm infants was secondary to limitations of study design, low subject numbers, late or inadequate LCPUFA dosing not meeting levels of fetal accretion in utero,[36] and failure to include very immature and critically ill preterm infants. Over the last 10 years, several large multicenter randomized control trials with sufficient power and broadened patient populations have investigated the effect of high-dose DHA with or without ARA supplementation (maternal or neonatal) on neurodevelopment, visual acuity, BPD, and retinopathy of prematurity (ROP) in preterm infants.

The DINO Trial

The DHA for the Improvement of Neurodevelopmental Outcome in preterm infants (DINO) trial was a multicenter randomized controlled trial conducted in 5 tertiary hospitals in Australia. The goal of the study was to determine the effect of maternal high-dose DHA supplementation (3000 mg/d) on neurodevelopmental outcomes of predominately breastfed preterm infants born before 33 weeks of gestational age. In this trial, the infants in the treatment group were exposed to levels of DHA equivalent to 1% total fatty acids, compared with infants receiving standard formula or breast milk from moms receiving placebo at 0.35% total fatty acids. The levels of ARA were the same in both groups at 0.6%. Maternal supplementation was successful in altering the infant's fatty acid profiles to reflect the effects of the DHA supplementation. Neurodevelopmental scores at 18 months were measured using the Mental Development Index (MDI) and The Psychomotor Development Index of the Bayley Scales of Infant Development, Second Edition. At 7 years of age general intellectual ability was assessed using the Full-Scale IQ of the Wechsler Abbreviated Scale of Intelligence. At 18 months of age, there was no difference in MDI scores between the DHA supplemented group and controls. However, on subgroup analysis, there was an increase in MDI score in girls on the high-dose DHA group versus controls.[36] This effect did not persist at the 7-year follow-up, as there was no benefit of DHA supplementation on IQ, visual-spatial perceptual skills, executive function, attention, educational process, or quality of life.[37] At both timepoints, parents reported decreased executive function and increased conduct problems in girls who received the high-dose DHA supplementation. Although it is difficult to make conclusions based on parental report, ultimately both studies provided strong evidence that high-dose DHA supplementation did not have any benefit on short- and long-term neurodevelopmental outcomes in preterm infants.

N3RO Trial

The n-3 Fatty Acids for Improvement in Respiratory Outcomes (N3RO) trial was a large multicenter randomized control trial with the primary aim to investigate the effect of enteral supplementation of DHA in preterm infants versus a soy emulsion on the outcome of BPD or death. In this trial, preterm infants born at less than 29 weeks gestational age tolerating full enteral feeds were randomized to receive enteral DHA supplementation at 60 mg/kg/d versus supplementation with soy placebo until 36 weeks corrected gestational age. The primary outcome was the development of BPD, defined physiologically by oxygen saturations at 36 weeks corrected gestation. The composite outcome of BPD or death was increased in the DHA supplemental group. There were no differences between groups in secondary outcomes, including time to reach enteral feeds, length of hospitalization, and odds ratio of other neonatal morbidities including ROP, necrotizing enterocolitis (NEC), sepsis, and intraventricular hemorrhage (IVH).[38]

MOBYDIck Trial

The Maternal Omega-3 Supplementation to Reduce Bronchopulmonary Dysplasia in Very Preterm Infants (MOBYDIck) was a multicenter, randomized placebo-controlled trial across 16 different NICUs in Canada. The primary outcome was to determine if maternal DHA supplementation decreased BPD-free survival in preterm infants born less than 29 weeks of gestation. BPD was defined based on a standard supplemental oxygen reduction test. This study had several additional secondary outcomes, including death, BPD, BPD severity, duration of respiratory therapy (supplemental oxygen, positive pressure ventilation), growth measurement data, and incidence of neonatal morbidities including IVH, sepsis, NEC, cholestasis, ROP, periventricular leukomalacia, patent ductus arteriosus (PDA), and maternal bleeding.

After reaching 50% of subject enrollment, an efficacy interim analysis revealed the intervention was potentially leading to harm. Although not statistically significant, there was an increased incidence of BPD in the intervention group versus control; and therefore, at that time, the data and safety monitoring board requested that the study stop recruiting patients. On final analysis of the data, the primary outcome of BPD-free survival was not statistically significant between the 2 groups, at 54.9% for the DHA group and 61.6% for controls. The incidence of BPD and severe BPD, however, was significantly decreased in the control group versus DHA group.[39] Regarding secondary outcomes, the incidence of grade 3 to 4 IVH was increased in the placebo group (16.1%) versus DHA (7.7%). The investigators attributed this finding to chance, as the occurrence of IVH was likely to occur before the infants achieved full enteral feeds and saw the effects of the intervention. Ultimately, this study was limited by the need for early termination; however, it supports the findings of the N3RO trial against the benefit of DHA supplementation of preterm neonates, particularly for the prevention of BPD.

The N3RO and MOBYDIck trials reinforce that DHA-centric enteral supplementation for preterm infants do not demonstrate clinical benefits, may lead to potential harm, and should be avoided.

Mega Donna Mega Trial

The Mega Donna Mega trial was a randomized clinical trial to investigate the frequency of severe ROP with or without supplementation of ARA and DHA. This trial was conducted in infants born less than 28 weeks gestation at 3 different NICUs in Sweden. Within 72 hours, infants were supplemented with an enteral lipid emulsion containing ARA and DHA daily until 40 weeks postmenstrual age (PMA). This emulsion contained 100 mg/kg/d of ARA and 50 mm/kg/d of DHA to match a 2:1 ARA:DHA ratio and recommended fetal accretion rates. Infants receiving the enteral lipid supplementation demonstrated decreased rates of severe ROP by 50% for infants less than 27 weeks gestational age. This effect was greatest in the most immature infants.

In infants less than 27 weeks' gestation, serum ARA levels were higher in the supplemented versus control group, and this remained true throughout the study. DHA levels were not significantly increased compared with controls until 34 weeks PMA. The infants born between 27 and 28 weeks' gestation had no appreciable differences in serum levels of the ratio of ARA to DHA compared with controls.

Additional secondary outcomes included neonatal morbidities, BPD, IVH, PDA, NEC, death, and growth. Overall, there were no differences between the treatment and nontreatment groups in any of these secondary outcomes. When stratified based on gestational age, there was a trend for the supplemented group to have a high relative risk of BPD, PDA, and death. However, sample size for this stratification was small, and this observation was not statistically significant. Overall, the investigators of the paper concluded that supplementation of both ARA and DHA in VLBW infants may help prevent severe-stage ROP.[40]

DERIVATIVES OF LONG-CHAIN POLYSATURATED FATTY ACIDS

Investigation of the downstream mediators of both DHA and ARA, known as oxylipins, and their alterations in different pathologic processes have provided new insights for understanding alterations in lipid metabolism during diseases states as well as new potential targets for therapeutic management. Downstream mediators of DHA and ARA that have important roles in the resolution phase of inflammation are known as specialized proresolving mediators (SPMs), which are characterized into 3 biological families: resolvins (resolution phase interaction products), maresins (macrophage mediators in resolving inflammation), and protectins.[41] These downstream mediators have both pro- and antiinflammatory activities that mediate different disease processes. Currently, active investigations are ongoing to determine the importance of these mediators as neuroprotective in certain adult neuroinflammatory diseases and psychiatric disorders and their potential as therapeutic targets in proinflammatory diseases such as inflammatory bowel disease, asthma, certain cancers, or postischemic brain injury in animal models.[42–44]

The downstream metabolites of arachidonic acid, called eicosanoids, have an important role in mediation and regulation of inflammation. The major classes of eicosanoids include prostaglandins, thromboxanes, leukotrienes, lipoxins, and eoxins. Although it is generally perceived that ARA is a proinflammatory agent, its eicosanoid mediators can be pro- and antiinflammatory and have more complex, tissue-specific roles and actions. For example, lipoxins have been found to have antiinflammatory effects in states of allergic anaphylaxis, whereas eoxins are more commonly proinflammatory.

Although the involvement of these mediators in neonatal development and different neonatal disease states is yet to be fully elucidated, recent effort is underway to quantify the levels of these mediators circulating in the preterm infant and in maternal breast milk, with the goal to understand how alterations in these levels might contribute to risk of disease and inform supplemental practices. A prospective clinical cohort study found alterations in oxylipin signatures in umbilical cord blood correlated with increased risk of BPD.[45] More specifically, increases in COX-derived prostaglandins and linolenic acid–derived hydroxy acids and ketones were correlated with an increase in BPD severity. These oxylipins are associated with increased levels of inflammation, apoptosis, and vasoconstriction through downstream G protein–coupled receptor activities.[45] Increased levels of another oxidation product of ARA, 9-HETE, was associated with development of pulmonary hypertension associated with BPD.[45] Animal models have shown that supplementation with proresolving mediators might lead to improved outcomes. In an animal model of BPD, Resolvin D1 and Lipoxin A4 were administered to neonatal mouse pups during exposure to hyperoxia, and the degree of hyperoxia lung injury was reduced with metrics approaching that of room air controls. Specifically, administration of these 2 SPMs attenuated inflammation induced by hyperoxia, reducing septal wall thickness, and Lipoxin A4 improved alveolarization of the lung.[46]

It is well established that DHA and ARA content is variable in human milk with decreases in content over time and in pasteurized donor milk compared with mother's own milk. In contrast, oxylipin levels remains consistent over the 1-month collection period.[47] Mothers taking DHA supplementation had correlating increases in breast milk DHA levels, although the supplementation did not increase oxylipin levels. There were no associations between levels of oxylipins and BPD, time to reach enteral feedings, incidence of NEC, or sepsis.[47] Larger multicenter cohort studies are necessary to further elucidate the role of breast milk oxylipins in neonatal development and disease.

KNOWLEDGE GAPS AND FUTURE RESEARCH DIRECTIONS

- Infants require early parenteral lipids for nutrition; however, none of the current lipid emulsions meet the unique needs of preterm infants. Correcting the fatty acid balance is just one unmet need. There are other critical complex lipids that need to be considered to support optimal development.
- It is likely an enteral lipid supplement enriched in DHA and ARA will be necessary to account for delayed enteral feedings, variable content in human milk, and increased needs. It remains to be determined the optimal dose to achieve the expected clinical benefits.
- Fatty acids are the building blocks of many simple and complex lipids; however, other lipids need further study in their role in infant development and the optimal delivery to support nutrition and growth. Examples include cholesterol, sphingolipids, endocannabinoids, and ceramides.

CLINICS CARE POINTS

- Given the induced fatty acid profiles of fish oil–containing lipid emulsions that include an exacerbated deficit in ARA and an excess of EPA, we recommend that Intralipid remain the first line maintenance parenteral lipid emulsion in preterm infants.
- If PNAC (or IFALD) develops, Omegaven should be instituted.
- It remains unclear whether SMOFlipid offers an advantage for infants at risk for PNAC/IFALD.
- Advance enteral nutrition and discontinue parenteral lipids as fast as possible.
- Enteral lipid supplementation remains undefined and is not routinely recommended at this time.
- Maternal DHA supplementation of 1.2 gm/d or greater should be avoided in mothers of preterm infants.

DISCLOSURE

KLS received funding support from the grant T32 HD 098061 for completion of this review..

REFERENCES

1. Cetin I, Alvino G, Cardellicchio M. Long chain fatty acids and dietary fats in fetal nutrition. J Physiol 2009;587(Pt 14):3441–51.
2. Duttaroy AK, Basak S. Maternal dietary fatty acids and their roles in human placental development. Prostaglandins Leukot Essent Fatty Acids 2020;155: 102080.
3. Campbell FM, Gordon MJ, Dutta-Roy AK. Preferential uptake of long chain poly-unsaturated fatty acids by isolated human placental membranes. Mol Cell Biochem 1996;155(1):77–83.
4. Woodard V, Thoene M, Van Ormer M, et al. Intrauterine transfer of polyunsaturated fatty acids in mother-infant dyads as analyzed at time of delivery. Nutrients 2021;13(3).
5. Duttaroy AK. Transport of fatty acids across the human placenta: a review. Prog Lipid Res 2009;48(1):52–61.
6. Zhang Y, Daaka Y. PGE2 promotes angiogenesis through EP4 and PKA Cgamma pathway. Blood 2011;118(19):5355–64.
7. Johnsen GM, Basak S, Weedon-Fekjaer MS, et al. Docosahexaenoic acid stimulates tube formation in first trimester trophoblast cells, HTR8/SVneo. Placenta 2011;32(9):626–32.
8. Haggarty P, Ashton J, Joynson M, et al. Effect of maternal polyunsaturated fatty acid concentration on transport by the human placenta. Biol Neonate 1999;75(6): 350–9.
9. Neuringer M, Connor WE, Lin DS, et al. Biochemical and functional effects of pre-natal and postnatal omega 3 fatty acid deficiency on retina and brain in rhesus monkeys. Proc Natl Acad Sci U S A 1986;83(11):4021–5.
10. Segura MT, Demmelmair H, Krauss-Etschmann S, et al. Maternal BMI and gestational diabetes alter placental lipid transporters and fatty acid composition. Placenta 2017;57:144–51.
11. Tabano S, Alvino G, Antonazzo P, et al. Placental LPL gene expression is increased in severe intrauterine growth-restricted pregnancies. Pediatr Res 2006;59(2):250–3.
12. Chassen SS, Ferchaud-Roucher V, Gupta MB, et al. Alterations in placental long chain polyunsaturated fatty acid metabolism in human intrauterine growth restriction. Clin Sci (Lond) 2018;132(5):595–607.
13. Friedman Z, Danon A, Stahlman MT, et al. Rapid onset of essential fatty acid deficiency in the newborn. Pediatrics 1976;58(5):640–9.
14. de Meijer VE, Le HD, Meisel JA, et al. Parenteral fish oil as monotherapy prevents essential fatty acid deficiency in parenteral nutrition-dependent patients. J Pediatr Gastroenterol Nutr 2010;50(2):212–8.
15. Martin CR. Lipids and fatty acids in the preterm infant, part 1: basic mechanisms of delivery, hydrolysis, and bioavailability. NeoReviews 2015;16(3):e160–8.
16. Gramlich L, Ireton-Jones C, Miles JM, et al. Essential fatty acid requirements and intravenous lipid emulsions. JPEN J Parenter Enteral Nutr 2019;43(6):697–707.
17. Martin CR, Dasilva DA, Cluette-Brown JE, et al. Decreased postnatal docosahexaenoic and arachidonic acid blood levels in premature infants are associated with neonatal morbidities. J Pediatr 2011;159(5):743–9.e741-742..
18. Savini S, D'Ascenzo R, Biagetti C, et al. The effect of 5 intravenous lipid emulsions on plasma phytosterols in preterm infants receiving parenteral nutrition: a randomized clinical trial. Am J Clin Nutr 2013;98(2):312–8.

19. Calkins KL, Robinson DT. Intravenous lipid emulsions in the NICU. Neoreviews 2020;21(2):e109–19.

20. Finn KL, Chung M, Rothpletz-Puglia P, et al. Impact of Providing a combination lipid emulsion compared with a standard soybean oil lipid emulsion in children receiving parenteral nutrition: a systematic review and meta-analysis. JPEN J Parenter Enteral Nutr 2015;39(6):656–67.

21. Frazer LC, Martin CR. Parenteral lipid emulsions in the preterm infant: current issues and controversies. Arch Dis Child Fetal Neonatal Ed 2021;106(6):683–4.

22. Zhao Y, Wu Y, Pei J, et al. Safety and efficacy of parenteral fish oil-containing lipid emulsions in premature neonates. J Pediatr Gastroenterol Nutr 2015;60(6): 708–16.

23. Memon N, Hussein K, Hegyi T, et al. Essential fatty acid deficiency with SMOFlipid reduction in an infant with intestinal failure-associated liver disease. JPEN J Parenter Enteral Nutr 2019;43(3):438–41.

24. Lam HS, Tam YH, Poon TC, et al. A double-blind randomised controlled trial of fish oil-based versus soy-based lipid preparations in the treatment of infants with parenteral nutrition-associated cholestasis. Neonatology 2014;105(4):290–6.

25. Michaelsen KF, Skafte L, Badsberg JH, et al. Variation in macronutrients in human bank milk: influencing factors and implications for human milk banking. J Pediatr Gastroenterol Nutr 1990;11(2):229–39.

26. Brenna JT, Varamini B, Jensen RG, et al. Docosahexaenoic and arachidonic acid concentrations in human breast milk worldwide. Am J Clin Nutr 2007;85(6): 1457–64.

27. Akinsulire O, Perides G, Anez-Bustillos L, et al. Early enteral administration of a complex lipid emulsion supplement prevents postnatal deficits in docosahexaenoic and arachidonic acids and increases tissue accretion of lipophilic nutrients in preterm piglets. JPEN J Parenter Enteral Nutr 2020;44(1):69–79.

28. Collins CT, Sullivan TR, McPhee AJ, et al. A dose response randomised controlled trial of docosahexaenoic acid (DHA) in preterm infants. Prostaglandins Leukot Essent Fatty Acids 2015;99:1–6.

29. Innis SM. Dietary (n-3) fatty acids and brain development. J Nutr 2007;137(4): 855–9.

30. Mallick R, Basak S, Duttaroy AK. Docosahexaenoic acid,22:6n-3: its roles in the structure and function of the brain. Int J Dev Neurosci 2019;79:21–31.

31. Connor KM, SanGiovanni JP, Lofqvist C, et al. Increased dietary intake of omega-3-polyunsaturated fatty acids reduces pathological retinal angiogenesis. Nat Med 2007;13(7):868–73.

32. Rogers LK, Valentine CJ, Pennell M, et al. Maternal docosahexaenoic acid supplementation decreases lung inflammation in hyperoxia-exposed newborn mice. J Nutr 2011;141(2):214–22.

33. Carlson SE, Montalto MB, Ponder DL, et al. Lower incidence of necrotizing enterocolitis in infants fed a preterm formula with egg phospholipids. Pediatr Res 1998;44(4):491–8.

34. Lu J, Jilling T, Li D, et al. Polyunsaturated fatty acid supplementation alters proinflammatory gene expression and reduces the incidence of necrotizing enterocolitis in a neonatal rat model. Pediatr Res 2007;61(4):427–32.

35. Boyan BD, Sylvia VL, Dean DD, et al. Differential regulation of growth plate chondrocytes by 1alpha,25-(OH)2D3 and 24R,25-(OH)2D3 involves cell-maturation-specific membrane-receptor-activated phospholipid metabolism. Crit Rev Oral Biol Med 2002;13(2):143–54.

36. Makrides M, Gibson RA, McPhee AJ, et al. Neurodevelopmental outcomes of preterm infants fed high-dose docosahexaenoic acid: a randomized controlled trial. JAMA 2009;301(2):175–82.

37. Collins CT, Gibson RA, Anderson PJ, et al. Neurodevelopmental outcomes at 7 years' corrected age in preterm infants who were fed high-dose docosahexaenoic acid to term equivalent: a follow-up of a randomised controlled trial. BMJ Open 2015;5(3):e007314.

38. Collins CT, Makrides M, McPhee AJ, et al. Docosahexaenoic acid and bronchopulmonary dysplasia in preterm infants. N Engl J Med 2017;376(13):1245–55.

39. Marc I, Piedbocuf B, Lacaze-Masmonteil T, et al. Effect of maternal docosahexaenoic acid supplementation on bronchopulmonary dysplasia-free survival in breastfed preterm infants: a randomized clinical trial. JAMA 2020;324(2):157–67.

40. Hellstrom A, Nilsson AK, Wackernagel D, et al. Effect of enteral lipid supplement on severe retinopathy of prematurity: a randomized clinical trial. JAMA Pediatr 2021;175(4):359–67.

41. Serhan CN, Levy BD. Resolvins in inflammation: emergence of the pro-resolving superfamily of mediators. J Clin Invest 2018;128(7):2657–69.

42. Dyall SC. Long-chain omega-3 fatty acids and the brain: a review of the independent and shared effects of EPA, DPA and DHA. Front Aging Neurosci 2015;7:52.

43. Sun GY, Simonyi A, Fritsche KL, et al. Docosahexaenoic acid (DHA): an essential nutrient and a nutraceutical for brain health and diseases. Prostaglandins Leukot Essent Fatty Acids 2018;136:3–13.

44. Zuo G, Zhang D, Mu R, et al. Resolvin D2 protects against cerebral ischemia/reperfusion injury in rats. Mol Brain 2018;11(1):9.

45. La Frano MR, Fahrmann JF, Grapov D, et al. Umbilical cord blood metabolomics reveal distinct signatures of dyslipidemia prior to bronchopulmonary dysplasia and pulmonary hypertension. Am J Physiol Lung Cell Mol Physiol 2018;315(5): L870–81.

46. Martin CR, Zaman MM, Gilkey C, et al. Resolvin D1 and lipoxin A4 improve alveolarization and normalize septal wall thickness in a neonatal murine model of hyperoxia-induced lung injury. PLoS One 2014;9(6):e98773.

47. Robinson DT, Palac HL, Baillif V, et al. Long chain fatty acids and related pro-inflammatory, specialized pro-resolving lipid mediators and their intermediates in preterm human milk during the first month of lactation. Prostaglandins Leukot Essent Fatty Acids 2017;121:1–6.

Neonatal Glucose Homeostasis

Cynthia L. Blanco, MD[a,b,*], Jennifer Kim, MD[a]

KEYWORDS

- Glucose • Hypoglycemia • Hyperglycemia • Euglycemia • Neonate • Newborn

KEY POINTS

- With current evidence, a specific concentration or range of plasma glucose (PG) concentration in asymptomatic newborns cannot be universally defined to provide specific treatment.
- There is no evidence of outcome improvement if actions are taken at any operational low PG threshold value in asymptomatic newborns; one should consider treatment depending on extrinsic and intrinsic risk factors.
- Hyperglycemia of prematurity is common, and peripheral insulin resistance (IR) seems to be the primary pathophysiological source.
- A specific high PG threshold for long-term deleterious effects in preterm infants is still unknown; the ideal management options are closely titrated IV glucose and early advancement of enteral feeds.

EUGLYCEMIA IN THE NEONATAL PERIOD

As glycogen stores are limited in the fetus, glucose accounts for 80% of fetal energy consumption. Maternal glucose is the only source of glucose for the fetus, and fluctuations in maternal levels have parallel effects on fetal levels. Maternal insulin, however, does not cross the placenta and fetal insulin fluctuates in response to glucose control in utero. At birth, cord glucose levels of 90.46 mg/dL (mmol/L) ±20.73 are typical.[1] Glycogen stores are exhausted within 12 hours of delivery[2]; therefore, infants must rely on breastmilk/formula.

The range within which a neonate is considered "euglycemic" is the range whereby organs receive an appropriate amount of energy without having side effects (ie, catabolism if too low, glucotoxicity if too high). Given the complicated nature of glucose homeostasis, and multiple factors affecting glucose regulation (**Fig. 1**), the ideal target for

[a] Division of Neonatology, Department of Pediatrics, UT Health San Antonio, 7703 Floyd Curl, San Antonio, TX 78229, USA; [b] Neonatology Services, University Health System, 4502 Medical Dr, San Antonio, TX, 78229, USA
* Corresponding author: Pediatrics, UT Health San Antonio, 7703 Floyd Curl, San Antonio, TX 78229.
E-mail address: blanco@uthscsa.edu

Clin Perinatol 49 (2022) 393–404
https://doi.org/10.1016/j.clp.2022.02.003
0095-5108/22/© 2022 Elsevier Inc. All rights reserved.

Abbreviations	
PG	Plasma Glucose
NH	Neonatal Hypoglycemia
IDM	Infant of Diabetic Mother
IR	Insulin Resistance

plasma glucose (PG) concentration and the thresholds below which treatment should be initiated remains to be determined.

HYPOGLYCEMIA IN THE NEONATAL PERIOD
Definition

Neonatal hypoglycemia (NH) can be difficult to diagnose due to its nonspecific symptoms, frequent variabilities in PG, and lack of data on long-term neurologic sequelae. Barriers to definitively establishing a specific threshold include: (1) differing brain responses to hypoglycemia across a range of PG concentrations, (2) effects of the presence of ketones and other alternative fuels, and (3) artifacts/technical factors complicating the accurate interpretation of any single PG value.[3] The generally adopted PG concentrations that define NH (<47 mg/dL), severe hypoglycemia (<36 mg/dL [2 mmol/L]), and extreme hypoglycemia (<27 mg/dL [1.5 mmol/L]) derive from associations with adverse neurodevelopmental outcomes but lack rigorous scientific justification.[1] According to the Pediatric Endocrine Society (PES), however, PG should be > 50 mg/dL in high-risk neonates at less than 48 hours of life (hol) and greater than 60 in high-risk neonates at greater than 48 hol. These thresholds are derived from studies in the 1980s that had a small sample size and less rigorous measurements of PG (**Fig. 2**A). A recent, larger study (GLOW) showed that breastfed, term infants may have PG values as low as 40 mg/dL during the first 48 hol (**Fig. 2**B) and these values increase to about 60 mg/dL by 96 hol (see **Fig. 2**B).[4] A recent multicenter prospective clinical trial comparing glucose thresholds of 36 mg/dL versus 47 mg/dL as an indicator of treatment in healthy newborns with asymptomatic hypoglycemia found

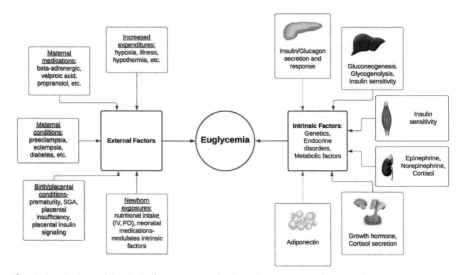

Fig. 1. Extrinsic and intrinsic factors modulating glucose control in newborns.

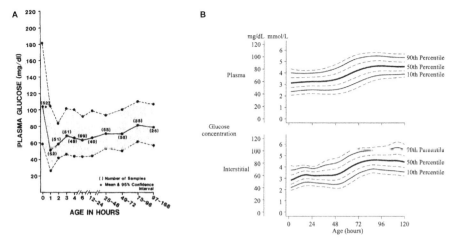

Fig. 2. Comparison of plasma glucose values in healthy newborns. (*A*). Plasma glucose values during the first week of life in 344 healthy term newborns published in 1986. (*B*). Plasma glucose values during the first week of life in 67 healthy newborns published in 2020. (*From* [*A*] Srinivasan G, Pildes S, Cattamanchi G, Voora S, Lilien D. Plasma glucose values in normal neonates: A new look. The Journal of Pediatrics. 1986;109(1):114-117; and [*B*] Harris DL, Weston PJ, Gamble GD, Harding JE. Glucose Profiles in Health Term Infants in the First 5 Days: The Glucose in Well Babies (GLOW) Study. The Journal of Pediatrics. 2020;223:34-41.)

no differences in the effects on psychomotor development at 18 months of age; a caveat was the mean PG was 57 and 61 mg/dL, respectively and therefore, further studies are needed.[5,6]

Given that none of the patients in the GLOW study met the hypoglycemia threshold of 25 mg/dL, and that a large percentage would have met the hypoglycemia threshold per PES's guideline (50 mg/dL) (**Fig. 3**), the proposed glucose range for further studies should be between 35 and 50 mg/dL in the first 48 hol.

Hypoglycemia Physiology

Healthy infants experience a drop in their PG concentrations after birth that reach a nadir at 30 to 90 minutes after birth before stabilizing by 12 to 48 hol.[2] PG concentrations previously reported as low as 30 mg/dL were found in healthy neonates 1 to 2 hours after birth; these low concentrations, seen in all mammalian newborns, are transient, asymptomatic, and a part of normal adaptation to postnatal life.[4]

Clinically significant NH, defined as PG concentrations low enough to impair brain function,[3] reflects an imbalance between supply and demand of glucose and alternative fuels. Infants are at risk of hypoglycemia due to one or more of the following underlying mechanisms: (1) insufficient glucose supply due to low glycogen/fat stores or impaired glucose production, (2) increased energy demands due to excessive insulin production or metabolic demands, or (3) pituitary/adrenal failure.[3] Screening at-risk infants for NH and institution of prophylactic measures to prevent prolonged NH is of utmost importance. The following conditions place newborns at highest risk.

Intrauterine Growth Restriction and Small for Gestational Age

Infants with intrauterine growth restriction (IUGR) or small for gestational age (SGA) are predisposed to NH due to inadequate glycogen and substrates for gluconeogenesis.[7] The risk of hypoglycemia may be as high as 72% in SGA infants. SGA infants also

Postnatal ages (h)	0–4	4–24	24–48	48–72	72–120
American Academy of Pediatrics[a]					
Plasma	0/64 (0)	2/67 (3)	1/67 (1)	1/67 (1)	0/67 (0)
Interstitial	0/60 (0)	6/55 (11)	3/57 (5)	1/56 (2)	0/47 (0)
British Association of Perinatal Medicine[b]					
Plasma	3/64 (5)	3/67 (4)	2/67 (3)	2/67 (3)	0/67 (0)
Interstitial	4/60 (7)	9/55 (16)	5/57 (9)	1/56 (2)	0/47 (0)
World Health Organisation[c]					
Plasma	12/64 (18)	16/67 (24)	9/67 (13)	7/67 (10)	1/67 (1)
Interstitial	23/60 (38)	35/55 (63)	19/57 (33)	17/56 (30)	4/47 (9)
Pediatric Endocrine Society[d]					
Plasma	16/64 (25)	27/67 (40)	15/67 (22)	31/67 (46)	4/67 (6)
Interstitial	30/60 (50)	40/55 (73)	33/57 (58)	41/56 (73)	26/47 (55)

Fig. 3. Comparison of glucose concentrations from GLOW study patients and various societies' threshold recommendations. Data are number (%). The American Academy of Pediatrics and Pediatric Endocrine Society guidelines refer to plasma glucose concentrations. The British Association of perinatal Medicine and world health organization guidelines refer to whole blood glucose concentrations. [a]<25 mg/dL [1.4 mmol/L] if 4 h, less than 35 mg/dL [1.9 mmol/L] if 4 to 24 h.[28] [b]< 36 mg/dL [2.0 mmol/L].[19] [c]< 47 mg/dL (2.6 mmol/L).[13] [d]50 mg/dL (2.8 mmol/L) in the first 48 h, ≤60 mg/dL (3.3 mmol/L)] after 48 h.[31] (*From* Harris DL, Weston PJ, Gamble GD, Harding JE. Glucose Profiles in Health Term Infants in the First 5 Days: The Glucose in Well Babies (GLOW) Study. The Journal of Pediatrics. 2020;223:34-41.)

showed a smaller increase in PG concentrations after dextrose gel administration compared with non-SGA infants.[8]

Infants of Diabetic Mothers

Newborn infants of diabetic mothers (IDM), whether type 1, 2, or gestational diabetes, are at higher risk for hypoglycemia (up to 40%) and associated adverse outcomes compared with infants born to nondiabetic mothers. As a result, the risk for short-term and long-term neurologic lesions is significantly higher among IDMs.[9] Hypoglycemia in IDMs is particularly severe in mothers with pre-existent, poorly controlled diabetes; it is thought to be due to fetal hyperinsulinism resulting from maternal hyperglycemia as glucose freely crosses the placenta. This hyperinsulinemia persists for ~4 to 7 days after birth, until the insulin production normalizes in the setting of appropriate glucose exposure.[9]

Prematurity

Many premature infants have abnormal glucose metabolism in the first weeks of life, and greater than 50% will develop hypoglycemia. Preterm infants are at greater risk for hypoglycemia because they are born with decreased glycogen stores in the liver and the proportion of glycogen concentration only increases after 36 weeks' gestation.[10] Studies in fetal and neonatal sheep have shown that enzymatic activities for glycogen incorporation in the liver are present in fetal life and decrease a few weeks after birth when compared with adults.[11] Consistent with this data, hepatic glycogen content increases with gestational age (GA) in preterm baboons but this is paired with impaired endogenous glucose production (EGP) due to the lack of enzymes involved in gluconeogenesis and hypoglucagonemia contributing to the risk of severe or prolonged low PG concentrations.[12,13]

Congenital Hyperinsulinemic Conditions

Hyperinsulinemic hypoglycemia (HH) is the most common cause of persistent hypoketotic hypoglycemia in neonates/infants and refers to a heterogeneous group of disorders associated with dysregulated insulin secretion. Patients with HH can present from asymptomatic to a medically unresponsive disease requiring near-total pancreatectomy.[14] While many risk factors contribute to the development of HH such as IDM, it can also be associated with congenital syndromes such as Beckwith–Wiedemann (BWS), Costello, and Soto. BWS is a multigenic disorder due to the dysregulation of growth regulatory genes within the chromosome 11p15 region.[15] Patients with this disorder present with macroglossia, anterior abdominal wall defects, organomegaly, hemihypertrophy, ear lobe creases, and helical pits and 5% experience persistent hypoglycemia.[16] Costello syndrome is a genetic disorder due to a mutation in the protooncogene HRAS.[17] Multiple congenital anomalies are associated with this syndrome, affecting the cardiac, musculoskeletal, and central nervous systems. Fasting hypoglycemia has been linked to growth hormone and cortisol deficiency and pancreatic hyperplasia and HH.[18] Soto syndrome is characterized by HH, learning difficulties, macrocephaly, and overgrowth with advanced bone age.[19]

Inborn Errors of Metabolism

Many inborn errors of metabolism can lead to hypoglycemia, among which maple syrup urine disease (MSUD) and fatty acid oxidation disorders (FAOD) are common.

MSUD is an inherited disorder caused by the inability to break down the branched-chain amino acids (leucine, valine, and isoleucine) and presents with nonspecific symptoms of neurologic dysfunction. The hypoglycemia associated with MSUD is thought to be secondary to preferential shunting of 3-carbon substrates from amino acids into glutamine, thus impairing gluconeogenesis by decreasing net oxaloacetate production.[20] FAODs lead to deficient energy production due to the disruption of FADH2 and NADH + for oxidative phosphorylation in the mitochondria and presents within the first few days after birth with profound cardiomyopathy, liver dysfunction, and hypoketotic hypoglycemia.[21] Other inborn errors of metabolism that are associated with NH include glycogen storage disease and hereditary fructose intolerance but tend to present after the neonatal period.

Consequences of Hypoglycemia

Neurologic dysfunction following hypoglycemia

Neurologic dysfunction is a major clinical pathology that can occur in infants with persistent hypoglycemia. Defining what constitutes clinically important NH, particularly regarding how it relates to brain injury, and that monitoring for, preventing, and treating NH remains largely empirical. However, repeated and prolonged very low PG concentrations (persistent hypoglycemia), particularly associated with conditions of excessive insulin secretion, have been associated with abnormal neurologic outcomes and should be investigated and treated.[22]

In the CHYLD study, hypoglycemia (PG <47 mg/dL), was treated with additional feeding, buccal dextrose gel (DexGel), and intravenous (IV) dextrose.[23] Follow-up at 4.5 years showed hypoglycemia was not associated with major neurologic deficits, but it was associated with a 2-fold to 3-fold increased risk of poor executive and visual motor performance.[23] Nevertheless, it should not be assumed that more aggressive intervention would necessarily improve outcomes. At 2 years, neurosensory impairment was associated with higher PG fluctuations in the first 48 hours, although still within the normal range. This association was strongest among hypoglycemic infants who received dextrose, raising concern that the rapid correction of hypoglycemia to higher glucose concentrations may lead to worse outcomes.[23] It remains to be determined whether glucose instability causes neuronal injury or is simply a marker of perinatal stress or severity of illness.

Methods for glucose measurement

There is no point-of-care method that is sufficiently reliable and accurate in the low range of BG to allow it to be used as the sole method for screening/treatment of NH. Newer glucose monitors have only been tested in few arterial neonatal samples during hypoglycemia (accuracy ±5–10 mg/dL, 94% samples), whereas venous/capillary samples have only been tested in adults. Laboratory determination by the glucose oxidase method is the most accurate method of measuring PG concentration, but one should not postpone the initiation of treatment of suspected NH while waiting for laboratory confirmation. Test-strip colorimetric methods are not accurate at low glucose concentrations (±10–20 mg/dL) and should not be used in neonate. Because of limitations with POC methods, any low PG concentration must be confirmed by the glucose oxidase method.

Continuous glucose monitoring

Given neonatal glucose instability and the invasiveness of heel lancing for serial glucose monitoring, continuous glucose monitoring (CGM) provides the possibility of adjusting treatment in real-time while reducing the number of BG measurements needed. A randomized trial involving preterm infants, glucose concentrations were measured either with the MiniMed Paradigm Real-Time System Sensor or the traditional intermittent arterial line glucose method revealing a strong correlation between the CGM and A-line measurements (r = 0.87).[24,25] Another randomized trial compared real-time CGM with intermittent BG monitoring in very low birth weight (VLBW; <1500 g) infants and found that CGM reduced the duration of hypoglycemic episodes by 50% and the number of capillary blood samples by 25%.[26] CGM does possess some drawbacks, such as the difficulty of keeping the probe in place, random errors, a drift component, and a time lag from glucose diffusion into the interstitial fluid from blood. Until these logistical issues are resolved, CGM remains under investigation but has promising clinical use.

Treatment

Screening. According to 2011 American Academy of Pediatrics (AAP) recommendations, infants with glucose levels less than 40 mg/dL and symptoms of hypoglycemia such as jitteriness, apnea, cardiac arrest, cyanotic spells, hypothermia, lethargy, seizures, and/or irritability require immediate treatment with IV glucose. Patients at high risk, namely preterm babies, large for GA or SGA babies, IDM, and those with perinatal asphyxia should receive a glucose screening test regardless of the presence or absence of symptoms. A stat PG level is always warranted to verify the results of a bedside glucose meter reading when the value is < 40 mg/dL. Any symptomatic newborn with a PG measuring less than 40 mg/dL (2.22 mmol/L) should receive IV dextrose. A suggested algorithm for the treatment of NH is shown in **Fig. 4**. Due to new data from the GLOW study whereby 40 mg/dL represents the 5th percentile in healthy newborns, one must act with caution in asymptomatic at-risk infants if glucose is < 40 mg/dL and take into account, if dealing with hyperinsulinemia and/or decreased PO intake, when balancing the decision for IV dextrose and the separation of mother–infant dyad.

Infant feeding. Feeding type, as well as time of feeding, impacts neonatal euglycemia. Breastfeeding has been associated with a reduced need for the treatment of hypoglycemia. In a study of the prevention of NH, the change in PG concentration after breastfeeding was similar to the use of formula or DexGel. However, breastfeeding was associated with a reduced need for a second treatment, independent of the initial BG concentration. Certain populations may benefit the most. IDMs who were breastfed within the first 30 minutes had higher PG concentrations than IDMs who were not fed or received infant formula, and those breastfed for >20 minutes soon after birth had less NH in the following 8 hours. These findings suggest that breastfeeding may have a slower but more sustained effect on PG concentrations than either infant formula or DexGel.[8]

Glucose. If an infant is deemed to be treated with IV glucose, the initial treatment consists of 200 mg/kg (2 mL/kg) of 10% dextrose in water administered over 1 minute. Recent data suggest steeper rise in PG may be associated with adverse long term outcomes,[23] and therefore, avoiding boluses while providing a continuious infusion in asymptomatic neonates might be preferred. As it is uncertain if this is due to glucose variability versus severity of illness, there is limited guidance on when and if glucose boluses should be avoided. A continuous glucose infusion should be administered at 6 to 8 mg/kg/min and titrated up by 1 to 2 mg/kg/min every 4 to 6 hours until

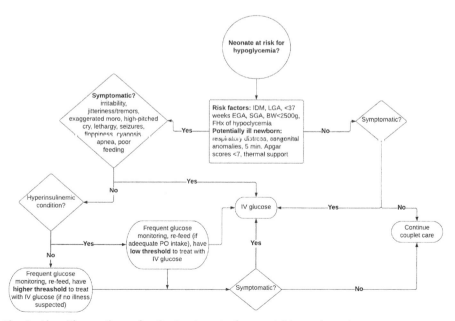

Fig. 4. Algorithm pathway for the treatment of neonatal hypoglycemia.

euglycemia is achieved, after which titration down can occur.[28] Other interventions may be necessary if the glucose infusion rate exceeds 12 to 14 mg/kg/min.

Other pharmacologic interventions

There are numerous other treatment options for NH beyond feeding and IV glucose. Hydrocortisone reduces the peripheral utilization of glucose while enhancing the effects of glucagon and gluconeogenesis and it can be given as a stress dose. If hyperinsulinemia is suspected, diazoxide 10 to 15 mg/kg/d divided TID is the drug of choice as it works by suppressing insulin release through the activation of potassium channels in the pancreatic cells. Glucagon 20-30 mcg/kg IM/IV can be given as a single-dose therapy for moderate to severe hypoglycemia. A trial dose of epinephrine can be used if a patient is unresponsive to hydrocortisone and/or diazoxide; the usual trial dosage is 0.01 mL/kg SQ of 1:1000 concentration. Epinephrine works by promoting glycogenolysis, gluconeogenesis, adipose lipolysis, and glucagon secretion. Patients with anterior pituitary deficiency can benefit from growth hormone supplementation. Ocreotide can be used alone or in conjunction with glucagon therapy at a dosage of 0.2-1.04 mcg/kg/hr continuous SQ to suppress both insulin and glucagon output. An alternative to somatostatin is its analog, octreotide. In a particular subset of infants with adenomatous pancreatic hyperplasia, a partial pancreatectomy may be needed if persistent hypoglycemia.

Dextrose gel

In 2013, double-blind study in at-risk infants with a GA of 35 to 42 weeks was randomized to receive 200 mg 40% DexGel versus placebo for hypoglycemia prophylaxis. NICU admission rates for hypoglycemia decreased among infants who received DexGel relative to those who received placebo but they had a low incidence of maternal diabetes.[8] A similar study using 4 different doses of DexGel indicated that infants who received the gel still developed hypoglycemia; however, the onset was delayed by 1.4 hours compared with infants who were given the placebo.[29] In the US, a quasi-experimental study was performed with 236 asymptomatic, at-risk infants and showed that one dose of insta-glucose (77% dextrose) prophylactically did not result in differences in glucose concentrations nor NICU admissions. The incidence of maternal diabetes was higher and they speculated the DexGel may have caused a hyperinsulinemic response in some patients.[29] Given the inconsistent evidence, DexGel could be transiently used as prophylaxis if infant's intake is adequate and no high-risk conditions for persistent hypoglycemia are identified. Particularly worrisome is the use as a treatment in infants with hyperinsulinemia as it might trigger further insulin secretion due to glucose variability.

HYPERGLYCEMIA IN THE NEONATAL PERIOD
Prematurity

Preterm birth increases the risk for hyperglycemia, affecting up to 80% of VLBW infants. Hyperglycemia has been associated with increased risk of death and neonatal morbidities, including retinopathy of prematurity (ROP) and intraventricular hemorrhage.[30] Furthermore, insulin resistance (IR) and an increased incidence of type 2 diabetes are seen in preterm babies who survive to adulthood, possibly as a direct consequence of early alterations in glucose metabolism.[31]

Nature of the Problem

Hyperglycemia pathophysiology in VLBW infants has been studied in human and animal models. Previously, it was thought hyperglycemia was caused by increased catecholamine release due to perinatal stress. Now, we understand this condition stems from developmental differences due to immaturity such as peripheral IR, which has been demonstrated in adipose and muscle tissue of premature animals via decreased adiponectin production and insulin signaling in skeletal muscle. Skeletal muscle impairments are demonstrated by the significant decrease in Akt phosphorylation and glucose uptake in preterm animals relative to term animals. In addition, hepatic IR has been shown in preterm infants when measuring EGP using stable isotopes, suggesting persistent hepatic glucose production despite hyperglycemic conditions.[32] This hepatic IR seems to be due to developmental differences in hepatic gene expression of insulin signaling molecules and alterations in hepatic gluconeogenic molecules due to immaturity as demonstrated in fetal and neonatal baboons.[31] This hepatic and skeletal muscles IR lead to the higher plasma insulin levels and higher serum c-peptide levels during fasting found in preterm animals and humans studies.[33] Persistent hepatic insulin impairments, particularly decreased IRS-1 phosphorylation, could explain the emergence of diabetes earlier in life in surviving preterm infants.[34] Future therapies should aim to improve IR to enhance hepatic and muscle glucose uptake in premature infants with hyperglycemia instead of insulin treatment.

Adverse Effects

High PG can lead to glucotoxicity, particularly in the pulmonary, endocrine, and neurologic systems. Studies have linked increased risk of death and brain MRI abnormalities at term-equivalent age if hyperglycemia occurs in the first 24 hours after birth in preterm infants.[35] Similarly, our group identified associations of increased ROP in a predominantly Hispanic population of preterm infants.[30] The oxidative stress caused by hyperglycemia via the polyol pathway has been shown to disrupt gene expression during neural tube formation and apoptosis leading to the disruption of normal development. Exposures at critical periods of development such as prematurity have shown to disrupt normal kidney development via increased oxidative stress.[36] Premature infants have increased incidence of type 1 and 2 diabetes.[37,38] Of greatest concern is the vulnerability of pancreatic development as it continues to have pluripotential cells as late as the last third of gestation and the effect of early exposure to hyperglycemia on the long-term effects on the number of beta cells in the endocrine pancreas remains unknown.[27]

Approach and Therapeutic Options

Hyperglycemia usually occurs during the first 7 to 10 days of life in VLBW infants. Due to the relative IR in these infants, insulin infusions are not effective. Therefore, we are left with the uncomfortable situation of limiting glucose infusions during this period to achieve euglycemia. One should not think we are "starving" the infant as the glucose will not be able to enter into the cells that can use it for growth even if we provide it. The inability of the preterm skeletal muscle to maximize utilization is due to impairments in insulin signaling (decreased insulin receptor and phosphorylation of Akt) which in turn, causes peripheral IR.[12] It seems as these developmental impairments improve after the first week of life and therefore, careful titration of glucose infusions are necessary to avoid glucotoxicity to pancreatic, liver, muscle, retina, neurons, and other organs that could be affected at critical periods of development. The ideal scenario is to provide glucose via enteral feeds to promote growth, stimulate incretin and insulin secretion naturally; however, some infants are unable to tolerate rapid feeding advancements due to their gut immaturity/dysmotility.

If enteral feeds are not established, the current approach should estimate the necessary IV glucose infusion rate depending on GA and severity of illness to avoid hyperglycemia regardless of glucose infusion rate. This should be paired with IV amino acid and intralipids via parenteral nutrition to avoid hypotonic solutions. The ideal medication would be insulin signaling up-regulators such as AMPK activators, thiazolidinediones, and sulfonylureas. Unfortunately, they have not been tested in neonates and limited research has been conducted in animal models. For now, we should promote early enteral feeds and develop algorithms to achieve euglycemia in at-risk infants until their developmental stage allows them to tolerate higher glucose infusion rates to achieve caloric goals.

CLINICS CARE POINTS

- The thresholds for plasma glucose (PG) below which neonatal hypoglycemia (NH) is diagnosed is without rigorous scientific justification; many studies and scientific organizations suggest using a threshold as low as 35 or as high as 50 mg/dL between 4 and 48 hrs of life and 60 mg/dL if > 48 hrs of age in the neonatal period.
- Neurologic dysfunction is the most significant morbidity related to NH, although the exact threshold at which each neonate develops adverse outcomes remains uncertain.
- The clinician must consider the neonate's perinatal history and metabolic conditions that predispose them to hyperinsulinemic conditions when deciding to treat an asymptomatic neonate. Symptomatic hypoglycemia should be treated as a neonatal emergency.
- Hyperglycemia affects preterm infants and thresholds at which the risk of short and long-term morbidity increases remain unknown. Euglycemia that mimics fetal PG is suggested between 60-100 mg/dL. A threshold of 150 mg/dL is widely used in the literature without scientific justification.
- Elevated PG can affect multiple organ systems in fetal life, particularly the endocrine, renal and neurologic systems secondary to the disruption of normal development, apoptosis pathways, and neural tube formation. It is likely to have similar effects in premature neonates.
- Current treatment of neonatal hyperglycemia includes the limitation of IV glucose and early enteral feeding along with strict monitoring of PG, until developmental insulin resistance improves; insulin infusions should not be routinely used and are rarely effective.

DISCLOSURE

Dr C.L. Blanco has received federal and nonfederal funding for glucose metabolism studies. All data utilized in this review have been published and funding sources are detailed in each article referenced.

REFERENCES

1. Khan K, Saha AR. A study on the correlation between cord blood glucose level and the apgar score. J Clin Diagn Res 2013;7(2):308–11.
2. Srinivasan G, Pildes RS, Cattamanchi G, et al. Plasma glucose values in normal neonates: a new look. J Pediatr 1986;109(1):114–7.
3. Thornton PS, Stanley CA, De Leon DD, et al. Recommendations from the pediatric endocrine society for evaluation and management of persistent hypoglycemia in neonates, infants, and children. J Pediatr 2015;167(2):238–45.
4. Harris DL, Weston PJ, Gamble GD, et al. Glucose profiles in healthy term infants in the first 5 days: the glucose in well babies (GLOW) study. J Pediatr 2020;223: 34–41.

5. van Kempen AAMW, Eskes PF, Nuytemans DHGM, et al. Lower versus traditional treatment threshold for neonatal hypoglycemia. N Engl J Med 2020;382(6): 534–44.

6. Zhang J, Shi W, Chen C. Neonatal glycogen storage disease ia. Pediatr Neonatal 2015;56(1):66–7.

7. Thompson-Branch A, Havranek T. Neonatal hypoglycemia. Pediatr Rev 2017; 38(4):147–57.

8. Harris DL, Gamble GD, Weston PJ, et al. What happens to blood glucose concentrations after oral treatment for neonatal hypoglycemia? J Pediatr 2017;190: 136–41.

9. Stanescu A, Stoicescu SM. Neonatal hypoglycemia screening in newborns from diabetic mothers–arguments and controversies. J Med Life 2014;7(Spec Iss 3):51–2.

10. Shelley HJ. Carbohydrate reserves in the newborn infant. Br Med J 1964;1(5378): 273–5.

11. Ballard FJ, Oliver IT. Carbohydrate metabolism in liver from foetal and neonatal sheep. Biochem J 1965;95(1):191–200.

12. Blanco CL, McGill-Vargas LL, Gastaldelli A, et al. Peripheral insulin resistance and impaired insulin signaling contribute to abnormal glucose metabolism in preterm baboons. Endocrinology 2015;156(3):813–23.

13. McGill-Vargas L, Gastaldelli A, Liang H, et al. Hepatic insulin resistance and altered gluconeogenic pathway in premature baboons. Endocrinology 2017; 158(5):1140–51.

14. Pierro A, Nah SA. Surgical management of congenital hyperinsulinism of infancy. Semin Pediatr Surg 2011;20(1):50–3.

15. Gaston V, Le Bouc Y, Soupre V, et al. Analysis of the methylation status of the KCNQ1OT and H19 genes in leukocyte DNA for the diagnosis and prognosis of Beckwith-Wiedemann syndrome. Eur J Hum Genet 2001;9(6):409–18.

16. Suri M. Approach to the diagnosis of overgrowth syndromes. Indian J Pediatr 2016;83(10):1175–87.

17. Aoki Y, Niihori T, Kawame H, et al. Germline mutations in HRAS proto-oncogene cause Costello syndrome. Nat Genet 2005;37(10):1038–40.

18. Alexander S, Ramadan D, Alkhayyat H, et al. Costello syndrome and hyperinsulinemic hypoglycemia. Am J Med Genet A 2005;139(3):227–30.

19. Matsuo T, Ihara K, Ochiai M, et al. Hyperinsulinemic hypoglycemia of infancy in Sotos syndrome. Am J Med Genet A 2012;161(1):34–7.

20. Haymond MW, Karl IE, Feigin RD, et al. Hypoglycemia and maple syrup urine disease: defective gluconeogenesis. Pediatr Res 1973;7(5):500–8.

21. Merritt JL 2nd, Norris M, Kanungo S. Fatty acid oxidation disorders. Ann Transl Med 2018;6(24):473.

22. Hay WW Jr, Raju TN, Higgins RD, et al. Knowledge gaps and research needs for understanding and treating neonatal hypoglycemia: workshop report from eunice kennedy shriver national institute of child health and human development. J Pediatr 2009;155(5):612–7.

23. McKinlay CJD, Alsweiler JM, Anstice NS, et al. Association of neonatal glycemia with neurodevelopmental outcomes at 4.5 years. JAMA Pediatr 2017;171(10): 972–83.

24. Saw H-P, Yao N-W, Chiu C-D, et al. The value of real-time continuous glucose monitoring in premature infants of diabetic mothers. PLoS One 2017;12(10). https://doi.org/10.1371/journal.pone.0186486.

25. Phillip M, Battelino T, Atlas E, et al. Nocturnal glucose control with an artificial pancreas at a diabetes camp. N Engl J Med 2013;368(9):824–33.
26. Uettwiller F, Chemin A, Bonnemaison E, et al. Real-time continuous glucose monitoring reduces the duration of hypoglycemia episodes: a randomized trial in very low birth weight neonates. PLoS One 2015;10(1). https://doi.org/10.1371/journal.pone.0116255.
27. Quinn AR, Blanco CL, Perego C, et al. The ontogeny of the endocrine pancreas in the fetal/newborn baboon. J Endocrinol 2012;214(3):289–99.
28. Lilien LD, Pildes RS, Srinivasan G, et al. Treatment of neonatal hypoglycemia with minibolus and intraveous glucose infusion. J Pediatr 1980;97(2):295–8.
29. Hegarty JE, Harding JE, Gamble GD, et al. Prophylactic oral dextrose gel for newborn babies at risk of neonatal hypoglycaemia: a randomised controlled dose-finding trial (the Pre-hPOD Study). PLoS Med 2016;13(10):e1002155. Published 2016 Oct 25.
30. Blanco CL, Baillargeon JG, Morrison RL, et al. Hyperglycemia in extremely low birth weight infants in a predominantly Hispanic population and related morbidities. J Perinatol 2006;26(12):737–41.
31. McGill-Vargas LL, Johnson-Pais T, Johnson MC, et al. Developmental regulation of key gluconeogenic molecules in nonhuman primates. Physiol Rep 2014;2: e12243.
32. Sunehag AL, Haymond MW, Schanler RJ, et al. Gluconeogenesis in very low birth weight infants receiving total parenteral nutrition. Diabetes 1999;48(4):791–800.
33. Mitanchez-Mokhtari D, Lahlou N, Kieffer F, et al. Both relative insulin resistance and defective islet beta-cell processing of proinsulin are responsible for transient hyperglycemia in extremely preterm infants. Pediatrics 2004;113:537–41.
34. Kajantie E, Osmond C, Barker DJP, et al. Preterm birth−a risk factor for type 2 diabetes?: the Helsinki birth cohort study. Diabetes Care 2010;33:2623–5.
35. Alexandrou G, Skiöld B, Karlén J, et al. Early hyperglycemia is a risk factor for death and white matter reduction in preterm infants. Pediatrics 2010;125(3): e584–91.
36. Callaway DA, McGill-Vargas LL, Quinn A, et al. Prematurity disrupts glomeruli development, whereas prematurity and hyperglycemia lead to altered nephron maturation and increased oxidative stress in newborn baboons. Pediatr Res 2018;83(3):702–11.
37. Li S, Zhang M, Tian H, et al. Preterm birth and risk of type 1 and type 2 diabetes: systematic review and meta-analysis. Obes Rev 2014;15(10):804–11.
38. Zhang J, Shi W, Chen C. Neonatal glycogen storage disease la. Pediatr Neonatal 2015;56(1):66–7.

Cerebral Effects of Neonatal Dysglycemia

Megan E. Paulsen, MD[a,b,]*, Raghavendra B. Rao, MD[a,b]

KEYWORDS

- Neurodevelopment • Blood glucose • Perinatal • Hypoxic-ischemic encephalopathy
- Hypoglycemia • Hyperglycemia • Brain • Preterm

KEY POINTS

- Dysglycemia is one of the most common pathologies in the neonatal intensive care unit.
- Hypoglycemia and hyperglycemia are detrimental to the neonatal brain as glucose metabolism and homeostasis are essential to brain growth and development.
- Prolonged, or severe, perinatal dysglycemia causes neurologic injury resulting in worse neurodevelopmental outcomes during childhood and adolescence.
- Controversy over the definitions of hypoglycemia and hyperglycemia may have an impact on expert consensus of prevention and treatment strategies for neonatal dysglycemia.

INTRODUCTION

Glucose metabolism is essential to promote growth and brain development in the fetus and newborn. Dysglycemia, including both hypoglycemia and hyperglycemia, is a biochemical disorder representing an imbalance between available glucose concentration and glucose utilization in tissue.[1] Repeated or prolonged periods of dysglycemia during critical windows of neurodevelopment can cause lasting changes in brain morphology and function. Whereas the risk of permanent brain injury with neonatal hypoglycemia has been known since 1959, a similar risk of long-term neurodevelopmental impairment due to neonatal hyperglycemia has begun to be appreciated only recently.[2,3] In the following sections, we review perinatal glucose metabolism, including cerebral glucose metabolism, epidemiology of hypoglycemia and hyperglycemia, pathogenesis and sequelae of brain injury with both conditions as well as respective management considerations. Management of hyperglycemia due to neonatal diabetes will not be discussed; however, a recent review of this genetic condition is available elsewhere.[4]

[a] Department of Pediatrics, University of Minnesota Medical School, Academic Office Building, 2450 Riverside Avenue S AO-401, Minneapolis, MN 55454, USA; [b] Masonic Institute for the Developing Brain, 2025 East River Parkway, Minneapolis, MN 55414
* Corresponding author.
E-mail address: mgosslin@umn.edu

Clin Perinatol 49 (2022) 405–426
https://doi.org/10.1016/j.clp.2022.02.008
0095-5108/22/Published by Elsevier Inc.

perinatology.theclinics.com

Perinatal Glucose Metabolism

In utero, the fetus receives a continuous supply of glucose from the mother. Following the birth and cessation of maternal glucose supply, blood glucose levels decrease, reaching a nadir as low as 30 mg/dL (1.7 mmol/L) at 1 to 2 hours of age.[5] This transient decrease in blood glucose occurs in all mammals and is likely essential for postnatal metabolic programming. In most infants, transient low blood glucose is well tolerated without long-term sequelae. However, under certain conditions, it could lead to complications, including brain injury. Glucose levels increase over the first 18 hours, remain stable until 48 hours, and then increase to a new plateau by the fourth day of life.[6] The common causes of hypoglycemia are shown in **Box 1**. Inadequate energy stores and failure of metabolic adaptation are the common causes of hypoglycemia soon after birth; hyperinsulinism is the most common cause of persistent hypoglycemia beyond 12 to 24 hours.

Most of the causes of hyperglycemia in the neonatal period are a result of the infant's metabolic response to their environment rather than an underlying genetic cause (**Table 1**). There are 3 critical environments when perinatal hyperglycemia may occur: (1) *In utero,* (2) preterm birth, and (3) term birth. For example, *in utero* exposure to hyperglycemia is most likely related to increased fetal glucose exposure secondary to maternal–placental metabolism of glucose.[7] Alternatively, neonates born prematurely have decreased insulin secretion, decreased suppression of hepatic glucose production, and aberrant counter hormone regulation.[1,8–15] Therefore, preterm infants who are more likely to be exposed to stress, parenteral glucose infusion, intrauterine growth restriction (IUGR), sepsis, and certain drugs are at increased the

---

Box 1
Infants at risk for hypoglycemia in the newborn period

Failure of metabolic adaptation
  Maternal drugs (beta-blockers [eg, labetalol] and beta-agonists [eg, terbutaline])
  Perinatal hypoxia-ischemia

Poor energy reserves
  Prematurity (gestational age <37 weeks)
  Intrauterine growth restriction
  Small-for-gestation (birth weight <10th percentile)

Increased energy demand
  Seizures
  Hypoxic-ischemic encephalopathy
  Sepsis
  Heart failure
  Cold stress

Endocrine causes
  Hyperinsulinism (transient and persistent) (eg, large-for-gestation [birth weight >90th percentile], maternal diabetes, maternal obesity)
  Failure of counter-regulation (eg, hypopituitarism, congenital adrenal hyperplasia)

Inborn errors of metabolism
  Disorders of carbohydrate metabolism (eg, disorders of gluconeogenesis, glycogen storage disease, galactosemia)
  Disorders of fatty acid oxidation (eg, medium-chain acyl-CoA dehydrogenase deficiency, very long-chain acyl-CoA dehydrogenase deficiency, and CPT-1 deficiency)
  Disorders of amino acid metabolism (eg, maple syrup urine disease)

Syndromes associated with hypoglycemia (eg, Beckwith–Wiedemann Syndrome)

Table 1	
Infants at risk for hyperglycemia in the perinatal period	
Critical Window of Brain Development	**Risk Factor for Hyperglycemia**
In utero	Maternal obesity Maternal overnutrition Maternal diabetes Maternal drugs
Postnatal	Prematurity Parenteral glucose infusion Neonatal drugs
Perinatal (*in utero* + postnatal)	Perinatal stress Neonatal diabetes

risk of hyperglycemia compared with the term neonate facing similar exposures.[16] Additionally, term infants who have experienced neonatal encephalopathy are at risk for hyperglycemia related to ineffective glucose metabolism.[17–22] They are also at risk for hypoglycemia.[23] A rare cause of hyperglycemia in term infants is neonatal diabetes mellitus which is the result of a monogenic disorder affecting pancreatic beta-cell function rather than the environmentally induced causes discussed previously.[4]

Definition and Epidemiology of Dysglycemia

Hypoglycemia

There are controversies in how to define hypoglycemia during the neonatal period. A blood glucose concentration of less than 47 mg/dL (<2.6 mmol/L) has typically been used to define hypoglycemia in the last 40 years. This value represents the 10th percentile for expected neonatal blood glucose during the first 48 hours in full-term infants.[6] Additionally, there is physiologic relevance that neonatal glucose levels of less than 47 mg/dL (<2.6 mmol/L) are associated with a counter-regulatory hormonal response and electrophysiological changes.[24] However, other studies have not found similar associations[25,26] thereby contributing to controversy over defining clinically significant neonatal hypoglycemia. Likewise, while some studies have demonstrated an association between blood glucose of less than 47 mg/dL (<2.6 mmol/L) and neurodevelopmental impairments,[27] others have not.[28] A glucose concentration of less than 36 mg/dL (2.0 mmol/L) is typically considered severe hypoglycemia.[29,30]

The frequency of neonatal hypoglycemia depends on the clinical interpretation of hypoglycemia, frequency of evaluation for hypoglycemia, and risk factors associated with hypoglycemia. For example, a study of 2000 infants between 23- and 42-weeks' gestation reported 19% incidence of hypoglycemia (blood glucose <45 mg/dL, <2.5 mmol/L) during the first 3 hours after birth with 6% having severe (blood glucose <35 mg/dL, <1.9 mmol/L) hypoglycemia.[31] A recent study using a combination of continuous glucose monitoring and intermittent plasma glucose measurements found that 39% of healthy full-term infants have one or more episodes of hypoglycemia (blood glucose <47 mg/dL, <2.6 mmol/L) during the first 4 days after birth.[6]

The incidence of hypoglycemia is substantially higher in neonates at higher risk for hypoglycemia. Standardized glucose screening in 514 infants who were preterm infants, infants of diabetic mothers, and small- or large-for-gestation infants had an incidence of hypoglycemia (blood glucose <47 mg/dL, <2.6 mmol/L) of 51% during the first 48 hours after birth.[29] Severe hypoglycemia (blood glucose <36 mg/dL,

<2.0 mmol/L) was seen in 19% of high-risk neonates. There were no differences in incidence among the different risk groups. Most episodes (81%) occurred on day 1 of life. In 37% of neonates, hypoglycemia occurred after 3 normal blood glucose values and 6% had their first episode on day 2 which is typically past the duration of standard hypoglycemia screening in newborn nurseries and NICUs. In contrast, severe hypoglycemia was more likely to occur soon after birth with 74% having the episode within 6 hours. Recurrent hypoglycemia occurred in 19% of neonates with most of the hypoglycemia episodes (70%) occurring on the first day of life.[29]

Two timely considerations in neonatal hypoglycemia risk are maternal obesity and cesarean section (C-section) without labor. These pregnancy complications are increasingly more common, both affecting approximately one-third of pregnancies in the United States.[32–34] Evidence investigating the associations between maternal obesity, or maternal C-section, and neonatal hypoglycemia continues to emerge in the literature and may inform neonatal screening guidelines which generally do not consider these maternal indications as risk factors for neonatal hypoglycemia.

Hyperglycemia
The threshold which defines hyperglycemia also remains uncertain.[10,15] In current literature, hyperglycemia is most often defined as plasma glucose greater than 150 mg/dL (>8.3 mmol/L).[35–42] Most neonatologists, however, intervene when the plasma blood glucose concentration is greater than 180 mg/dL (>10.0 mmol/L).[42–44] Perinatal hyperglycemia is most often discussed in the context of the preterm infant rather than the term infant. However, the biochemical phenomenon of hyperglycemia occurs throughout the perinatal (*in utero* + neonatal) time period.

The prevalence of perinatal hyperglycemia depends on clinical surveillance for the biochemical disorder. The direct causal relationship between maternal hyperglycemia and fetal hyperglycemia remains unknown. Increased fetal glucose exposure as a result of maternal hyperglycemia has been increasingly recognized as a potential exposure that programs adverse neurodevelopment outcomes in the fetus apparent later in life.[45] This is an important consideration as approximately 17% of pregnancies are affected by hyperglycemia in pregnancy globally.[46] Following preterm birth, greater than 50% of very low birthweight infants, and up to 80% of extremely low birthweight infants, develop hyperglycemia during the first 2 weeks.[39,47–54] Term infants treated for hypoxic-ischemic encephalopathy develop hyperglycemia 43% to 54% of the time.[21,22]

NEUROLOGIC EFFECTS OF DYSGLYCEMIA
Glucose and the Perinatal Brain

As in other ages, glucose is the primary energy substrate for the newborn brain. The brain depends on a continuous supply of glucose from the blood and there is minimal storage in the form of brain glycogen. Under physiologic conditions, the blood-to-brain transfer of glucose is maintained at 3:1.[55] More than 90% of transported glucose is oxidatively metabolized through the tricarboxylic acid (TCA) cycle. Additionally, the newborn brain can use alternate energy substrates, such as ketone bodies, lactate, and amino acids for energy metabolism and synthetic function, especially when glucose supply is limited.[56,57] Enhanced substrate delivery through brain glycogenolysis, increased cerebral blood flow, and potential suppression of neuronal activity to conserve energy are additional adaptive mechanisms during hypoglycemia. Depletion of alternative energy substrates leads to energy failure and brain injury.[57] Associated comorbidities such as hypoxia-ischemia and glycemic variations worsen brain injury.[20,23,30,58,59]

Brain Injury in Hypoglycemia

Animal data

Animal models demonstrate that relative to the mature brain, the neonatal brain is resistant to injury during acute hypoglycemia, likely because of the ability to maintain cerebral energy production using alternative substrates.[57,60] Neuronal injury is primarily seen in brain regions important for emotion, attention, learning, and cognitive function.[60] Glycemic fluctuations worsen acute hypoglycemia-induced brain injury.[58] In newborn monkeys, prolonged (10-hour duration) hypoglycemia leads to impaired motivation and adaptability at 22 to 24 months of age.[61] Unlike acute hypoglycemia, recurrent hypoglycemia in the neonatal period negatively impacts neurodevelopment and causes increased anxiety, affective dysregulation and poor socialization in the juvenile period, and exaggerated stress response in adulthood.[62]

Human data

Numerous studies have since affirmed the risk of brain injury in neonatal hypoglycemia since the first report establishing this association was published in 1959.[2] There is strong evidence for brain injury with hypoglycemia in newborn infants with genetic disorders of hyperinsulinism.[63] Similarly, concurrent hypoglycemia worsens brain injury due to hypoxic-ischemic encephalopathy.[23]

Most hypoglycemia episodes in the neonatal period are asymptomatic. In a large study, 79% of infants with hypoglycemia did not have any symptoms.[29] Clinical signs of newborn hypoglycemia in approximate order of frequency are jitteriness or tremors, cyanotic episodes, convulsions, intermittent apneic spells or tachypnea, weak or high-pitched crying, limpness or lethargy, difficulties feeding, and eye-rolling.[64]

Early MRI after severe hypoglycemia (blood glucose $\sim$ 20 mg/dL, 1.2 mmol/L) demonstrates white matter injury and hemorrhage, cortical injury in the occipital and posterior parietal regions, restricted diffusion in the occipital lobes, and basal ganglia/thalamic lesions.[65–67] These MRI changes correlate with cognitive deficits in infancy.[65] The optimal time for MRI acquisition is 5 to 14 days after the episode of hypoglycemia.[66,67]

A meta-analysis involving 11 studies and 1657 infants demonstrated that neonatal hypoglycemia is not associated with neurodevelopmental impairment (NDI) in early childhood (2–5 years).[68] However, there was an increased risk of visual-motor impairment (odds ratio (OR) = 3.46, 95% confidence interval (CI): 1.13–10.57) and executive dysfunction (OR = 2.50, 95% CI: 1.20–5.22). Hypoglycemia did not increase the risk of epilepsy, cognitive impairment, emotional and behavioral difficulty, visual and hearing impairment, motor deficits, or cerebral palsy. Hypoglycemia was associated with statistically nonsignificant low language and literacy.

Assessment at mid-childhood (6–11 years) showed that children with a history of neonatal hypoglycemia had an increased risk of NDI (OR = 3.62, 95% CI: 1.05–12.42), low language/literacy (OR = 2.04, 95% CI: 1.20–3.47), low numeracy (OR = 2.04, 95% CI: 1.21–3.44), and a statistically nonsignificant risk of emotional-behavioral difficulty. Risk of motor, cognitive, visual and hearing impairments, and epilepsy were not altered. The authors noted that the quality of evidence for primary and secondary outcomes at early and mid-childhood was low or very low.[68] The risk of visuo-motor and executive function impairments seems to be greater with severe (blood glucose <36 mg/dL, <2.0 mmol/L) and recurrent (3 or more episodes) hypoglycemia.[30,59] These studies also demonstrated that risk of neurosensory impairment in early childhood is greater in infants exhibiting glycemic fluctuations in the first 48 hours after birth and a steep rise in blood glucose after dextrose administration for hypoglycemia.[30,59]

Brain Injury in Hyperglycemia

Animal data

Perinatal exposure to hyperglycemia is associated with morphologic changes impacting brain structure and function. The direct influence of hyperglycemia on brain development depends on its timing, severity, and duration.[69] Exposure to hyperglycemia during fetal life, such as with maternal gestational diabetes or following preterm birth, coincides with a period of rapid brain development.[45,70,71] In comparison to preterm infants, term infants have completed the development of microglia and have further developed synaptic organization and function. Hyperglycemia in the setting of neuroinflammation (ie, asphyxia, sepsis, and meningitis) may potentiate neurologic injury.[70]

Preclinical studies have been instrumental in developing a biologic and mechanistic understanding of how hyperglycemia causes neurologic impairment in the developing brain. The majority of studies have used rodent models of streptozotocin-induced hyperglycemia.[72–89] These studies demonstrate that perinatal hyperglycemia causes decreased brain size, depletion of neuroprogenitor cells, altered neuronal distribution, altered synapse structure and function, increased apoptosis, increased oxidative stress and neuroinflammation, and altered regulatory gene/protein expression in the developing brain.[74–79,81–83,85–98] Functionally, long-term outcomes following perinatal hyperglycemia demonstrate increased anxiety, lower inhibition, altered object-place preference, learning and and memory deficits, structural changes in MRI, and altered *in vivo* neurochemical profile.[77,83,85,86,90–92,95–98]

Human data

A review of neurologic effects of hyperglycemia in human studies is summarized in **Table 2**. Most of the studies have investigated the association between maternal diabetes and offspring neurodevelopment.[99–124] The limitation to these studies is that the fetal glucose concentration is unknown thereby limiting any direct conclusions regarding fetal hyperglycemia and neurodevelopment. Additionally, there are limited studies reporting the association of maternal diabetes and immediate neurologic effects on the infant. Infants of diabetic mothers are predisposed to congenital central nervous system malformations, birth trauma, perinatal asphyxia, electrolyte derangements, polycythemia, hyperbilirubinemia, and hypoglycemia that may result in early neurologic state changes and seizures.[124,125]

Exposure to early hyperglycemia in the preterm infant is associated with short-term neurologic effects such as intraventricular hemorrhage and white matter reduction on imaging.[52,53,126–128] Long-term neurodevelopmental assessment demonstrates conflicting results with some studies reporting worse neurodevelopment while others showing no difference compared with preterm infants without hyperglycemia.[35,36,38,39,52,129] Clinical studies reporting associations between early hyperglycemia and neurologic effects have several confounding aspects limiting the ability to inform clinical practice. For example, the studies have varied widely in the methodology of blood glucose measurement and neurodevelopmental assessment (**Box 2**). Further research addressing these limitations would potentially eliminate the inconsistency of neurodevelopmental outcomes between studies.

Role of Glycemic Variability in Brain Injury

Glucose variability, whereby the fetus or newborn is exposed to both high and low glucose concentrations, is an emerging consideration in the effects of glucose metabolism on the developing brain. Preclinical studies have shown that glucose variability worsens neuronal injury and microglial activation in the developing rat brain.[93,130] As mentioned, glycemic instability worsens neurosensory outcome in preterm and term

Table 2			
Neurologic effects of perinatal hyperglycemia			
Exposure	**Outcomes**	**Hyperglycemia**	**Neurologic Effects of Hyperglycemia**
Fetus	Perinatal (Birth)	History of maternal gestational diabetes, type 2 diabetes mellitus, type 1 diabetes mellitus	• Neurologic changes as complications of macrosomia, birth trauma, glucose/electrolyte abnormalities, polycythemia, and vascular sludging[123,124]
	Postnatal (6 mo-27 y)		• Delayed language development[99–101] • Delayed motor development[100–103] • Lower intelligence and achievement[104–107] • Altered working memory[104,108–111] • Altered visual-spatial performance[104] • Attention-deficit/hyperactivity[102,112–116] • Autism spectrum disorder[117–119] • Psychiatric disorders[120–122]
Preterm infant	Perinatal (3–10 d,[52,53,126,127] 39–41 wk CGA[128]) Postnatal (1–7 y)	BG > 150 mg/dL (>8.3 mmol/L)	• Intraventricular hemorrhage[52,53,126,127] • White matter reduction[128] • Small head circumference[36] • Increased cognitive development at 4 mo CGA[36] • Duration of ≥ 5 d of hyperglycemia was associated with decreased cognition, language, and motor development at 12 mo CGA[35] • Abnormal neurologic examination at 2 y CGA[52] • Abnormal executive function at 2 y CGA[52] • Decreased odds ratio of survival without neurodevelopment impairment at 2 y CGA[39] • No difference in neurodevelopmental outcomes at 12 mo CGA or 7 y of age[38,129]
Term infant with HIE	Perinatal (0–11 d)	BG > 144 mg/dL (>8.0 mmol/L)	• Reduced risk of severity of multiorgan dysfunction[a;22] • Increased basal ganglia or global injury pattern on MRI[a,b;18,20]

(continued on next page)

Table 2 (continued)			
Exposure	Outcomes	Hyperglycemia	Neurologic Effects of Hyperglycemia
	Postnatal (18 mo- 3 y)		• Worse visual evoked potentials[a;17] • Increased frequency of seizures [a;163] • Worse background and sleep–wake cycling on aEEG[a;163] • Worse gross motor outcome[b;19] • Increased moderate or severe cerebral palsy and/or microcephaly[b;20] • No difference in neurodevelopmental outcomes[c;21]

Abbreviations: aEEG, amplitude electroencephalogram; BG, blood glucose; CGA, corrected gestational age; ERP, e event-related potential; HIE, hypoxic-ischemic encephalopathy; MRI, magnetic resonance imaging.

[a] infants received therapeutic hypothermia.
[b] some infants received therapeutic hypothermia.
[c] no infants received therapeutic hypothermia.

infants at-risk for hypoglycemia.[30,59] The Hyperglycemia and Adverse Pregnancy Outcome (HAPO) study demonstrated that maternal hyperglycemia was associated with neonatal hypoglycemia in a stepwise, linear fashion.[131] A recent study reported that infants of diabetic mothers with neonatal hypoglycemia had decreased adaptability, but no differences in gross motor, fine motor, language, or social skill development at 2 years of age.[131,132] Preterm infants are especially vulnerable to glucose instability[133,134] which is associated with neurosensory impairment.[133,135] The rate of change in glucose concentration in preterm infants was associated with worse neurodevelopmental outcomes rather than the glucose variability itself.[133] In infants with neonatal encephalopathy, glucose lability was associated with an increased incidence of watershed, multifocal, and basal ganglia injury patterns on MRI.[18] Further research investigating the neurologic effects of glucose variability are necessary to better characterize its effect on neurodevelopment.

MANAGEMENT CONSIDERATIONS
Hypoglycemia

The primary goal of management is the prevention of brain injury. Current clinical practice, based solely on blood glucose levels, is focused on raising blood glucose concentrations above a certain level with the assumption that this strategy will prevent brain injury. However, this strategy is flawed because (1) a specific blood glucose value that accurately predicts the risk of brain injury is not known, (2) the strategy does not consider the duration of hypoglycemia, nor the role of alternative substrates, and (3) currently, there is no evidence that normalizing blood glucose above a certain level (typically, >45 mg/dL, >2.5 mmol/L) will ensure normal neurodevelopment.[31,136,137]

Box 2
Clinical methods used to study long-term neurodevelopment following early hyperglycemia

- Achenbach System of Empirically Based Assessment child behavior checklist[38]
- ADHD Rating Scale-IV[102]
- Amplitude EEG[163]
- Autism diagnostic interview[117,119]
- Autism diagnostic observation schedule[117,119]
- Bayley Scales of Infant Development[35,36,39,103,108–112,129]
- Beery-Buktenica Developmental Test of Visual Motor Outcomes[38]
- Behavior Assessment System for Children-2[102]
- Behavior Rating Inventory of Executive Function[38]
- Childhood autism rating scale[117]
- Child Behavior Checklist/2 to 3[52]
- Continuous glucose monitoring[17,163]
- Cranial ultrasound[52,53,126,127]
- Developmental Neuropsychological Assessment[102]
- Diagnostic and Statistical Manual of Mental Disorders-IV-R[117]
- Early Development Instrument[99]
- ERP[17,108–110,112]
- Griffith's scales of Mental Development[21,129]
- Gross Motor Function Classification Scale[19,38]
- McArthur Communicative Development Inventory[99]
- Movement Assessment Battery for Children (2nd Ed)[38]
- Mullen Scales of Early Learning[119]
- MRI brain[18,20,128]
- Peabody Picture Vocabulary Test[99]
- Purdue Pegboard Dexterity Test[104]
- Temperament Assessment Battery for Children[102]
- Test of Everyday Attention in Children[38]
- Vineland Adaptive Behavior Scales[119]
- Wechsler Intelligence Scale[38,102,104,164]

Nevertheless, in the absence of alternative evidence-based strategies, professional societies recommend a blood glucose-based screening and treatment strategy for neonatal hypoglycemia.[64,138–141] Screening of at-risk infants, and not universal screening, which risks overdiagnosis and treatment, is recommended.[138] Typical recommendation is to screen within 1 to 4 hours after birth, and then every 3 to 4 hours until sustained euglycemia is confirmed. Screening is typically performed using point-of-care, nonenzymatic methods. The method is convenient, but not sensitive at lower glucose levels and could be confounded by a variety of factors. Hence, laboratory confirmation using the enzymatic method is needed for hypoglycemia management.

Some organizations recommend different lengths of screening periods depending on the underlying risk factor for hypoglycemia.[64,138] However, as there are no differences in the incidence and severity of hypoglycemia among the risk groups,[29] a uniform duration of screening may be more appropriate and easier to implement.

Interventions for hypoglycemia should consider blood glucose concentration, presence or absence of symptoms and signs, and the infant's ability to feed. Infants exhibiting signs, particularly neurologic signs, require measures to rapidly raise their blood glucose. Typically, this is achieved using an intravenous bolus of 10% dextrose at a dose of 200 mg/kg (2 mL/kg given more than 5–15 minutes), followed by a continuous infusion of 80 to 100 mL/kg per day to provide a glucose infusion rate of 4 to 8 mg/kg per min.[138,141] Infusion rates are adjusted by frequent glucose checks (typically, every 30 min). The goal is to maintain a blood glucose concentration of 40 to 50 mg/dL (2.2–2.8 mmol/L) and avoid an excessive and steep rise in blood glucose.[30,59,138] Persistently high glucose infusion rates (GIR, >8 mg/kg per min) and inability to wean off dextrose infusion after 3 days indicates the possibility of hyperinsulinism.

Asymptomatic infants with blood glucose less than 25 mg/dL (<1.4 mmol/L) in the first 4 hours and less than 35 mg/dL (<1.9 mmol/L) between 4 and 24 hours, and who can feed are offered breastfeeding or formula feeding with follow-up blood glucose checks 1-hour later.[64,138] Persistent low blood glucose is treated using intravenous dextrose. Application of 40% dextrose gel at a dose of 0.5 mL/kg (200 mg/kg of glucose) to the buccal mucosa has emerged as an alternative to intravenous dextrose infusion.[64,142,143] Dextrose gel application is followed with breastfeeding or bottle feeding of expressed mother's milk or pasteurized donor breastmilk or formula. Dextrose gel application reduces the need for intravenous dextrose infusion and improves success with breastfeeding.[142,143] It does not improve neurosensory outcome at 2 years of age.[136,144] Preventive application of dextrose gel reduces the risk of hypoglycemia and potentially major neurologic disability at 2 years of age in at-risk infants.[145]

Hyperglycemia

While management, including prevention, of hyperglycemia is an essential consideration during fetal and early postnatal life, the preterm infant is at the most iatrogenic risk for chronic, severe exposure to hyperglycemia during a critical period of brain development. Additionally, the treatment of hyperglycemia is an area of controversy in neonatology. Therefore, the focus in this review will be the prevention and management of hyperglycemia in the preterm infant.

Early enhanced nutrition, typically using the parenteral route, is important to promote early growth and brain development.[146–151] Enhanced nutrition, however, is also associated with an increased risk of hyperglycemia.[152] Careful consideration of macronutrient balance in parenteral nutrition, as well as early initiation of enteral breastmilk feeds, can decrease the risk of hyperglycemia in the preterm infant. Initial energy goals of preterm infants should focus on preventing the catabolism of endogenous energy stores.

Initiation of small enteral breastmilk feeds in the first 24 hours of life in the stable preterm infant is associated with a decreased incidence of hyperglycemia.[153] Enteral feeding increases incretin hormone secretion, particularly GLP-1, which stimulates insulin secretion in the early postnatal period.[12] A GIR of 4 to 6 mg/kg/min in a preterm infant may be enough to meet early resting metabolic needs once hepatic glucose production has been established. Protein intake has the strongest association, compared with GIR reduction or lipid reduction, in decreasing hyperglycemia in preterm infants.[153] Amino acids enhance endogenous insulin secretion thereby reducing glucose concentrations. Lipids, the most calorically dense macronutrient, can help achieve nutrient requirements and lower glucose infusion rates.

Similar to the variation in definitions of hyperglycemia there is variation in management practices for hyperglycemia. Neonatologists differ in glucose thresholds for treatment, strategies implemented in treatment, and target glucose achieved with treatment.[10] The most widely practiced treatment strategy is GIR reduction which can prevent and treat hyperglycemia effectively.[154] A lower energy intake early in the NICU course, however, is associated with worse neurodevelopment.[8,36,38,39,149,153,155] Insulin, alternatively, lowers glucose concentration and improves weight gain.

Prophylactic Insulin, in the prevention of hyperglycemia, has shown to be associated with both increased mortality and worse neurologic outcomes.[49,154] Pharmacokinetics of infused insulin is not well understood in extremely preterm infants. Similarly, the physiologic implications and later health consequences of suppressing β-cell function in early developmental stages have not been thoroughly studied. Biologic concerns for insulin use in the preterm infant population include increased fat deposition and cellular dysfunction leading to lactic acidosis which may be associated with worse long-term metabolic outcomes such as obesity, fatty liver disease, and cardiovascular disease.[14,48] Alternatively, insulin may indirectly improve neurodevelopmental outcomes by allowing increased caloric intake and controlling hyperglycemia. Preclinical studies, however, have not demonstrated a direct benefit of insulin on neurodevelopment. Specifically, insulin does not promote brain glucose uptake or utilization enhance neuronal growth, or dendritic development.[14]

Hyperglycemia management may vary depending on the clinical scenario when targeting neurodevelopment and minimizing the potential metabolic risk for each preterm infant. For example, if hyperglycemia is transient, one may consider a stepwise reduction in GIR followed by limiting the intravenous lipid infusion to meet the resting energy needs of the preterm infant. A different approach to hyperglycemia management, however, may be required in the unstable preterm infant or when the preterm infant's NICU course is complicated by significant risk for postnatal growth failure.

It has been clearly established that adequate early calorie intake correlates with long-term neurodevelopment in preterm infants.[35,36,146,156] A GIR as low as 6 to 8 mg/kg/min can cause hyperglycemia, especially in the physiologic stressed and unstable preterm infant.[1,8] Further limiting the GIR, especially past a transient period of hyperglycemia, may contribute to insufficient caloric intake impacting the preterm infant's neurodevelopment. Additionally, prevention of postnatal growth failure requires higher dextrose concentrations to achieve target energy intake thus adding risk to limiting GIR.[157] These clinical scenarios, therefore, may prompt consideration for insulin. While providing an insulin infusion, a higher glucose target (150–180 mg/dL, 8.3–10.0 mmol/L) should be considered in an effort to avoid hypoglycemic episodes which also can be detrimental to neurodevelopment. Further research dedicated to understanding the role of insulin in treating neonatal hyperglycemia, and its effect on neurodevelopment, is necessary to understand the benefits and risks associated with insulin use.

Role of Continuous Glucose Monitoring

Intermittent blood glucose surveillance leads to selection bias toward sicker infants with a history of dysglycemia. Continuous glucose monitoring (CGM), which can be performed via a subcutaneous glucose sensor, may provide more accurate surveillance of glucose homeostasis and therefore an improved understanding of the association between glucose concentration and neurodevelopment. CGM detects more episodes of hypoglycemia than intermittent glucose checks.[6,158] CGM has been shown to strongly correlate with the point of care glucose measurements in preterm infants (R = 0.94).[159] Although CGM remains investigational, studies using CGM coupled with computer algorithm approaches are promising to standardize glucose and insulin dosing decision algorithms in the management and treatment of neonatal hyperglycemia.[160,161] Specifically, these studies have shown increased time spent in the euglycemia range, reduced glycemic variably, decreased duration of hyperglycemia, and fewer episodes of hypoglycemia during insulin infusion in preterm infants.[159–162]

SUMMARY

Dysglycemia, one of the most common pathologies in the neonatal intensive care unit, is detrimental to the perinatal brain as glucose metabolism is essential to brain growth and development. The definition of hypoglycemia and hyperglycemia are controversial as evidence examining the neurologic effects of dysglycemia has used different blood glucose thresholds, different methodologies, and has reported varying outcome measures at different timepoints. Both preclinical and clinical studies demonstrate that severe, prolonged hypoglycemia or unstable blood glucose causes neurologic injury which translates to later neurosensory impairment, worse executive function, and behavioral difficulty in children and adolescents. Long-term neurodevelopmental outcomes following early hyperglycemia in neonates are reported less; however, several studies have demonstrated short-term complications such as intraventricular hemorrhage and white matter reduction on imaging. Although short-term clinical outcomes are of importance and inform long-term outcomes, dysglycemia management strategies should be weighted toward optimizing long-term health outcomes.

CLINICS CARE POINTS

- Current management practices in the prevention and treatment of perinatal dysglycemia are limited by (1) controversies in the definition of hypoglycemia and hyperglycemia and (2) a paucity of large prospective studies using consistent neurodevelopmental outcome measures beyond early childhood.

- Strategies to promote optimal perinatal nutrition, while maintaining euglycemia, are foundational to improving long-term neurodevelopmental outcomes.

- Treatment of asymptomatic hypoglycemia by increasing glucose infusion rate, rather than dextrose bolus, may prevent worse neurologic injury in preterm infants.

- Continuous glucose monitoring may reduce the severity and duration of dysglycemia in high-risk infants thus improving long-term neurodevelopmental outcomes.

DISCLOSURE

Dr M.E. Paulsen was supported by the National Institute of Health Building Interdisciplinary Research Careers in Women's Health (BIRCWH) grant K12HD055887.

REFERENCES

1. Hay WW Jr. Nutritional support strategies for the preterm infant in the neonatal intensive care unit. Pediatr Gastroenterol Hepatol Nutr 2018;21(4):234–47.
2. Cornblath M, Odell GB, Levin EY. Symptomatic neonatal hypoglycemia associated with toxemia of pregnancy. J Pediatr 1959;55:545–62.

3. Paulsen M, Brown SJ, Satrom KM, et al. Long-term outcomes after early neonatal hyperglycemia in vlbw infants: a systematic review. Neonatology 2021;118(5):509–21.

4. Lemelman MB, Letourneau L, Greeley SAW. Neonatal diabetes mellitus: an update on diagnosis and management. Clin Perinatol 2018;45(1):41–59.

5. Srinivasan G, Pildes RS, Cattamanchi G, et al. Plasma glucose values in normal neonates: a new look. J Pediatr 1986;109(1):114–7.

6. Harris DL, Weston PJ, Gamble GD, et al. Glucose profiles in healthy term infants in the first 5 days: the glucose in well babies (GLOW) Study. J Pediatr 2020;223: 34–41.e34.

7. Rosario FJ, Kanai Y, Powell TL, et al. Increased placental nutrient transport in a novel mouse model of maternal obesity with fetal overgrowth. Obesity (Silver Spring) 2015;23(8):1663–70.

8. Hay WW Jr. Aggressive nutrition of the preterm infant. Curr Pediatr Rep 2013;1(4).

9. Mitanchez-Mokhtari D, Lahlou N, Kieffer F, et al. Both relative insulin resistance and defective islet beta-cell processing of proinsulin are responsible for transient hyperglycemia in extremely preterm infants. Pediatrics 2004;113(3 Pt 1): 537–41.

10. Morgan C. The potential risks and benefits of insulin treatment in hyperglycaemic preterm neonates. Early Hum Dev 2015;91(11):655–9.

11. Bonner-Weir S. Perspective: postnatal pancreatic beta cell growth. Endocrinology 2000;141(6):1926–9.

12. Shoji H, Watanabe A, Ikeda N, et al. Influence of gestational age on serum incretin levels in preterm infants. J Dev Orig Health Dis 2016;7(6):685–8.

13. Beardsall K, Vanhaesebrouck S, Frystyk J, et al. Relationship between insulin-like growth factor I levels, early insulin treatment, and clinical outcomes of very low birth weight infants. J Pediatr 2014;164(5):1038–1044 e1031.

14. Thureen PaH, William W. Nutritional requirements of the very-low-birthweight infant. In: Neu J, editor. Gastroenterology and nutrition: neonatology questions and controversies. 2nd edition. Philadelphia (PA): Elsevier/Saunders; 2012. p. 107–28.

15. Louik C, Mitchell AA, Epstein MF, et al. Risk factors for neonatal hyperglycemia associated with 10% dextrose infusion. Am J Dis Child 1985;139(8):783–6.

16. Ogilvy-Stuart AL, Beardsall K. Management of hyperglycaemia in the preterm infant. Arch Dis Child Fetal Neonatal Ed 2010;95(2):F126–31.

17. Kamino D, Almazrooei A, Pang EW, et al. Abnormalities in evoked potentials associated with abnormal glycemia and brain injury in neonatal hypoxic-ischemic encephalopathy. Clin Neurophysiol 2021;132(1):307–13.

18. Basu SK, Ottolini K, Govindan V, et al. Early glycemic profile is associated with brain injury patterns on magnetic resonance imaging in hypoxic ischemic encephalopathy. J Pediatr 2018;203:137–43.

19. Spies EE, Lababidi SL, McBride MC. Early hyperglycemia is associated with poor gross motor outcome in asphyxiated term newborns. Pediatr Neurol 2014;50(6):586–90.

20. Chouthai NS, Sobczak H, Khan R, et al. Hyperglycemia is associated with poor outcome in newborn infants undergoing therapeutic hypothermia for hypoxic ischemic encephalopathy. J Neonatal Perinatal Med 2015;8(2):125–31.

21. Nadeem M, Murray DM, Boylan GB, et al. Early blood glucose profile and neurodevelopmental outcome at two years in neonatal hypoxic-ischaemic encephalopathy. BMC Pediatr 2011;11:10.

22. Basu SK, Salemi JL, Gunn AJ, et al. Hyperglycaemia in infants with hypoxic-ischaemic encephalopathy is associated with improved outcomes after therapeutic hypothermia: a post hoc analysis of the CoolCap Study. Arch Dis Child Fetal Neonatal Ed 2017;102(4):F299–306.

23. Salhab WA, Wyckoff MH, Laptook AR, et al. Initial hypoglycemia and neonatal brain injury in term infants with severe fetal acidemia. Pediatrics 2004;114(2):361–6.

24. Koh TH, Aynsley-Green A, Tarbit M, et al. Neural dysfunction during hypoglycaemia. Arch Dis Child 1988;63(11):1353–8.

25. Cowett RM, Howard GM, Johnson J, et al. Brain stem auditory-evoked response in relation to neonatal glucose metabolism. Biol Neonate 1997;71(1):31–6.

26. Harris DL, Weston PJ, Williams CE, et al. Cot-side electroencephalography monitoring is not clinically useful in the detection of mild neonatal hypoglycemia. J Pediatr 2011;159(5):755–60.e751.

27. Lucas A, Morley R, Cole TJ. Adverse neurodevelopmental outcome of moderate neonatal hypoglycaemia. BMJ 1988;297(6659):1304–8.

28. Tin W, Brunskill G, Kelly T, et al. 15-year follow-up of recurrent "hypoglycemia" in preterm infants. Pediatrics 2012;130(6):e1497–503.

29. Harris DL, Weston PJ, Harding JE. Incidence of neonatal hypoglycemia in babies identified as at risk. J Pediatr 2012;161(5):787–91.

30. McKinlay CJ, Alsweiler JM, Ansell JM, et al. Neonatal glycemia and neurodevelopmental outcomes at 2 Years. N Engl J Med 2015;373(16):1507–18.

31. Kaiser JR, Bai S, Gibson N, et al. Association between transient newborn hypoglycemia and fourth-grade achievement test proficiency: a population-based study. JAMA Pediatr 2015;169(10):913–21.

32. Turner D, Monthe-Dreze C, Cherkerzian S, et al. Maternal obesity and cesarean section delivery: additional risk factors for neonatal hypoglycemia? J Perinatol 2019;39(8):1057–64.

33. Neumann K, Indorf I, Hartel C, et al. C-section prevalence among obese mothers and neonatal hypoglycemia: a cohort analysis of the department of gynecology and obstetrics of the University of Lubeck. Geburtshilfe Frauenheilkd 2017;77(5):487–94.

34. Suk D, Kwak T, Khawar N, et al. Increasing maternal body mass index during pregnancy increases neonatal intensive care unit admission in near and full-term infants. J Matern Fetal Neonatal Med 2016;29(20):3249–53.

35. Gonzalez Villamizar JH JL, Scheurer JM, Rao R, et al. Relationships between early nutrition, illness, and later outcomes among infants born preterm with hyperglycemia. J Pediatr 2020;1–5.

36. Ramel SE, Long JD, Gray H, et al. Neonatal hyperglycemia and diminished long-term growth in very low birth weight preterm infants. J Perinatol 2013;33(11):882–6.

37. Scheurer JM, Gray HL, Demerath EW, et al. Diminished growth and lower adiposity in hyperglycemic very low birth weight neonates at 4 months corrected age. J Perinatol 2016;36(2):145–50.

38. Tottman AC, Alsweiler JM, Bloomfield FH, et al. Long-term outcomes of hyperglycemic preterm infants randomized to tight glycemic control. J Pediatr 2018;193:68–75 e61.

39. Tottman AC, Alsweiler JM, Bloomfield FH, et al. Relationship between measures of neonatal glycemia, neonatal illness, and 2-year outcomes in very preterm infants. J Pediatr 2017;188:115–21.

40. Alsweiler JM, Harding JE, Bloomfield FH. Tight glycemic control with insulin in hyperglycemic preterm babies: a randomized controlled trial. Pediatrics 2012; 129(4):639–47.
41. Ramel S, Rao R. Hyperglycemia in extremely preterm infants. Neoreviews 2020; 21(2):e89–97.
42. Hay WW Jr, Rozance PJ. Neonatal hyperglycemia-causes, treatments, and cautions. J Pediatr 2018;200:6–8.
43. Alsweiler JM, Kuschel CA, Bloomfield FH. Survey of the management of neonatal hyperglycaemia in Australasia. J Paediatr Child Health 2007;43(9): 632–5.
44. Paize FMA, Morgan C. Effect of differences in parenteral nutrition policies on preterm macronutrient intake: a telephone survey of all UK level 3 neonatal services. Arch Dis Child 2012;97:A49–50.
45. Camprubi Robles M, Campoy C, Garcia Fernandez L, et al. Maternal diabetes and cognitive performance in the offspring: a systematic review and meta-analysis. PLoS One 2015;10(11):e0142583.
46. Guariguata L, Linnenkamp U, Beagley J, et al. Global estimates of the prevalence of hyperglycaemia in pregnancy. Diabetes Res Clin Pract 2014;103(2): 176–85.
47. Zamir I, Tornevi A, Abrahamsson T, et al. Hyperglycemia in extremely preterm infants-insulin treatment, mortality and nutrient intakes. J Pediatr 2018;200: 104–110 e101.
48. Beardsall K, Vanhaesebrouck S, Ogilvy-Stuart AL, et al. Prevalence and determinants of hyperglycemia in very low birth weight infants: cohort analyses of the NIRTURE study. J Pediatr 2010;157(5):715–9.e711-713.
49. Beardsall K, Vanhaesebrouck S, Ogilvy-Stuart AL, et al. Early insulin therapy in very-low-birth-weight infants. N Engl J Med 2008;359(18):1873–84.
50. Blanco CL, Baillargeon JG, Morrison RL, et al. Hyperglycemia in extremely low birth weight infants in a predominantly Hispanic population and related morbidities. J Perinatol 2006;26(12):737–41.
51. Yoon JY, Chung HR, Choi CW, et al. Blood glucose levels within 7 days after birth in preterm infants according to gestational age. Ann Pediatr Endocrinol Metab 2015;20(4):213–9.
52. van der Lugt NM, Smits-Wintjens VE, van Zwieten PH, et al. Short and long term outcome of neonatal hyperglycemia in very preterm infants: a retrospective follow-up study. BMC Pediatr 2010;10:52.
53. Hays SP, Smith EO, Sunehag AL. Hyperglycemia is a risk factor for early death and morbidity in extremely low birth-weight infants. Pediatrics 2006;118(5): 1811–8.
54. Szymonska I, Jagla M, Starzec K, et al. The incidence of hyperglycaemia in very low birth weight preterm newborns. results of a continuous glucose monitoring study–preliminary report. Dev Period Med 2015;19(3 Pt 1):305–12.
55. Pardridge WM. Brain metabolism: a perspective from the blood-brain barrier. Physiol Rev 1983;63(4):1481–535.
56. Nehlig A. Respective roles of glucose and ketone bodies as substrates for cerebral energy metabolism in the suckling rat. Dev Neurosci 1996;18(5–6): 426–33.
57. Rao R, Ennis K, Long JD, et al. Neurochemical changes in the developing rat hippocampus during prolonged hypoglycemia. J Neurochem 2010;114(3): 728–38.

58. Ennis K, Dotterman H, Stein A, et al. Hyperglycemia accentuates and ketonemia attenuates hypoglycemia-induced neuronal injury in the developing rat brain. Pediatr Res 2014;77(1–1):84–90.
59. McKinlay CJD, Alsweiler JM, Anstice NS, et al. Association of neonatal glycemia with neurodevelopmental outcomes at 4.5 years. JAMA Pediatr 2017;171(10): 972–83.
60. Ennis K, Tran PV, Seaquist ER, et al. Postnatal age influences hypoglycemia-induced neuronal injury in the rat brain. Brain Res 2008;1224:119–26.
61. Schrier AM, Wilhelm PB, Church RM, et al. Neonatal hypoglycemia in the Rhesus monkey: effect on development and behavior. Infant Behav Dev 1990; 1990(13):189–207.
62. Moore H, Craft TK, Grimaldi LM, et al. Moderate recurrent hypoglycemia during early development leads to persistent changes in affective behavior in the rat. Brain Behav Immun 2010;24(5):839–49.
63. Menni F, de Lonlay P, Sevin C, et al. Neurologic outcomes of 90 neonates and infants with persistent hyperinsulinemic hypoglycemia. Pediatrics 2001;107(3): 476–9.
64. Narvey MR, Marks SD. The screening and management of newborns at risk for low blood glucose. Paediatr Child Health 2019;24(8):536–54.
65. Burns CM, Rutherford MA, Boardman JP, et al. Patterns of cerebral injury and neurodevelopmental outcomes after symptomatic neonatal hypoglycemia. Pediatrics 2008;122(1):65–74.
66. Boardman JP, Wusthoff CJ, Cowan FM. Hypoglycaemia and neonatal brain injury. Arch Dis Child Educ Pract Ed 2013;98(1):2–6.
67. Tam EW, Widjaja E, Blaser SI, et al. Occipital lobe injury and cortical visual outcomes after neonatal hypoglycemia. Pediatrics 2008;122(3):507–12.
68. Shah R, Harding J, Brown J, et al. Neonatal glycaemia and neurodevelopmental outcomes: a systematic review and meta-analysis. Neonatology 2019;115(2): 116–26.
69. Kretchmer N, Beard JL, Carlson S. The role of nutrition in the development of normal cognition. Am J Clin Nutr 1996;63(6):997S–1001S.
70. Mottahedin A, Ardalan M, Chumak T, et al. Effect of neuroinflammation on synaptic organization and function in the developing brain: implications for neurodevelopmental and neurodegenerative disorders. Front Cell Neurosci 2017; 11:190.
71. Cusick SE, Georgieff MK. The role of nutrition in brain development: the golden opportunity of the "first 1000 days. J Pediatr 2016;175:16–21.
72. Yamano T, Shimada M, Fujizeki Y, et al. Quantitative synaptic changes on Purkinje cell dendritic spines of rats born from streptozotocin-induced diabetic mothers. Brain Dev 1986;8(3):269–73.
73. Ji S, Zhou W, Li X, et al. Maternal hyperglycemia disturbs neocortical neurogenesis via epigenetic regulation in C57BL/6J mice. Cell Death Dis 2019;10(3):211.
74. Jing YH, Song YF, Yao YM, et al. Retardation of fetal dendritic development induced by gestational hyperglycemia is associated with brain insulin/IGF-I signals. Int J Dev Neurosci 2014;37:15–20.
75. Plagemann A, Harder T, Rake A, et al. Hypothalamic insulin and neuropeptide Y in the offspring of gestational diabetic mother rats. Neuroreport 1998;9(18): 4069–73.
76. Franke K, Harder T, Aerts L, et al. 'Programming' of orexigenic and anorexigenic hypothalamic neurons in offspring of treated and untreated diabetic mother rats. Brain Res 2005;1031(2):276–83.

77. Steculorum SM, Bouret SG. Maternal diabetes compromises the organization of hypothalamic feeding circuits and impairs leptin sensitivity in offspring. Endocrinology 2011;152(11):4171–9.
78. Fu J, Tay SS, Ling EA, et al. High glucose alters the expression of genes involved in proliferation and cell-fate specification of embryonic neural stem cells. Diabetologia 2006;49(5):1027–38.
79. Plagemann A, Harder T, Lindner R, et al. Alterations of hypothalamic catecholamines in the newborn offspring of gestational diabetic mother rats. Brain Res Dev Brain Res 1998;109(2):201–9.
80. Razi EM, Ghafari S, Golalipour MJ. Effect of gestational diabetes on purkinje and granule cells distribution of the rat cerebellum in 21 and 28 days of postnatal life. Basic Clin Neurosci 2015;6(1):6–13.
81. Adam CL, Findlay PA, Chanet A, et al. Expression of energy balance regulatory genes in the developing ovine fetal hypothalamus at midgestation and the influence of hyperglycemia. Am J Physiol Regul Integr Comp Physiol 2008;294(6): R1895–900.
82. Hami J, Sadr-Nabavi A, Sankian M, et al. The effects of maternal diabetes on expression of insulin-like growth factor-1 and insulin receptors in male developing rat hippocampus. Brain Struct Funct 2013;218(1):73–84.
83. Singh BS, Westfall TC, Devaskar SU. Maternal diabetes-induced hyperglycemia and acute intracerebral hyperinsulinism suppress fetal brain neuropeptide Y concentrations. Endocrinology 1997;138(3):963–9.
84. Rosa AP, Jacques CE, de Souza LO, et al. Neonatal hyperglycemia induces oxidative stress in the rat brain: the role of pentose phosphate pathway enzymes and NADPH oxidase. Mol Cell Biochem 2015;403(1–2):159–67.
85. Satrom KM, Ennis K, Sweis BM, et al. Neonatal hyperglycemia induces CXCL10/CXCR3 signaling and microglial activation and impairs long-term synaptogenesis in the hippocampus and alters behavior in rats. J Neuroinflammation 2018; 15(1):82.
86. Rao R, Nashawaty M, Fatima S, et al. Neonatal hyperglycemia alters the neurochemical profile, dendritic arborization and gene expression in the developing rat hippocampus. NMR Biomed 2018;31(5):e3910.
87. Yang G, Cancino GI, Zahr SK, et al. A Glo1-methylglyoxal pathway that is perturbed in maternal diabetes regulates embryonic and adult neural stem cell pools in murine offspring. Cell Rep 2016;17(4):1022–36.
88. Liao DM, Ng YK, Tay SSW, et al. Altered gene expression with abnormal patterning of the telencephalon in embryos of diabetic Albino Swiss mice. Diabetologia 2004;47(3):523–31.
89. Shyamasundar S, Jadhav SP, Bay BH, et al. Analysis of epigenetic factors in mouse embryonic neural stem cells exposed to hyperglycemia. PLoS One 2013;8(6):e65945.
90. Aviel-Shekler K, Hamshawi Y, Sirhan W, et al. Gestational diabetes induces behavioral and brain gene transcription dysregulation in adult offspring. Transl Psychiatry 2020;10(1):412.
91. Vuong B, Odero G, Rozbacher S, et al. Exposure to gestational diabetes mellitus induces neuroinflammation, derangement of hippocampal neurons, and cognitive changes in rat offspring. J Neuroinflammation 2017;14(1):80.
92. Chandna AR, Kuhlmann N, Bryce CA, et al. Chronic maternal hyperglycemia induced during mid-pregnancy in rats increases RAGE expression, augments hippocampal excitability, and alters behavior of the offspring. Neuroscience 2015;303:241–60.

93. Gisslen T, Ennis K, Bhandari V, et al. Recurrent hypoinsulinemic hyperglycemia in neonatal rats increases PARP-1 and NF-kappaB expression and leads to microglial activation in the cerebral cortex. Pediatr Res 2015;78(5):513–9.

94. Tayman C, Yis U, Hirfanoglu I, et al. Effects of hyperglycemia on the developing brain in newborns. Pediatr Neurol 2014;51(2):239–45.

95. Lin B, Ginsberg MD, Busto R. Hyperglycemic exacerbation of neuronal damage following forebrain ischemia: microglial, astrocytic and endothelial alterations. Acta Neuropathol 1998;96(6):610–20.

96. Park WS, Chang YS, Lee M. Effects of hyperglycemia or hypoglycemia on brain cell membrane function and energy metabolism during the immediate reoxygenation-reperfusion period after acute transient global hypoxia-ischemia in the newborn piglet. Brain Res 2001;901(1–2):102–8.

97. Blomstrand S, Hrbek A, Karlsson K, et al. Does glucose administration affect the cerebral response to fetal asphyxia? Acta Obstet Gynecol Scand 1984;63(4):345–53.

98. Vannucci RC, Vasta F, Vannucci SJ. Cerebral metabolic responses of hyperglycemic immature rats to hypoxia-ischemia. Pediatr Res 1987;21(6):524–9.

99. Dionne G, Boivin M, Seguin JR, et al. Gestational diabetes hinders language development in offspring. Pediatrics 2008;122(5):e1073–9.

100. Ornoy A. Growth and neurodevelopmental outcome of children born to mothers with pregestational and gestational diabetes. Pediatr Endocrinol Rev 2005;3(2):104–13.

101. Ornoy A, Wolf A, Ratzon N, et al. Neurodevelopmental outcome at early school age of children born to mothers with gestational diabetes. Arch Dis Child Fetal Neonatal Ed 1999;81(1):F10–4.

102. Nomura Y, Marks DJ, Grossman B, et al. Exposure to gestational diabetes mellitus and low socioeconomic status: effects on neurocognitive development and risk of attention-deficit/hyperactivity disorder in offspring. Arch Pediatr Adolesc Med 2012;166(4):337–43.

103. He XJ, Dai RX, Tian CQ, et al. Neurodevelopmental outcome at 1 year in offspring of women with gestational diabetes mellitus. Gynecol Endocrinol 2021;37(1):88–92.

104. Bolanos L, Matute E, Ramirez-Duenas Mde L, et al. Neuropsychological impairment in school-aged children born to mothers with gestational diabetes. J Child Neurol 2015;30(12):1616–24.

105. Fraser A, Almqvist C, Larsson H, et al. Maternal diabetes in pregnancy and offspring cognitive ability: sibling study with 723,775 men from 579,857 families. Diabetologia 2014;57(1):102–9.

106. Fraser A, Nelson SM, Macdonald-Wallis C, et al. Associations of existing diabetes, gestational diabetes, and glycosuria with offspring IQ and educational attainment: the avon longitudinal study of parents and children. Exp Diabetes Res 2012;2012:963735.

107. Clausen TD, Mortensen EL, Schmidt L, et al. Cognitive function in adult offspring of women with Type 1 diabetes. Diabet Med 2011;28(7):838–44.

108. Deregnier RA, Nelson CA, Thomas KM, et al. Neurophysiologic evaluation of auditory recognition memory in healthy newborn infants and infants of diabetic mothers. J Pediatr 2000;137(6):777–84.

109. Nelson CA, Wewerka S, Thomas KM, et al. Neurocognitive sequelae of infants of diabetic mothers. Behav Neurosci 2000;114(5):950–6.

110. Nelson CA, Wewerka SS, Borscheid AJ, et al. Electrophysiologic evidence of impaired cross-modal recognition memory in 8-month-old infants of diabetic mothers. J Pediatr 2003;142(5):575–82.
111. DeBoer T, Wewerka S, Bauer PJ, et al. Explicit memory performance in infants of diabetic mothers at 1 year of age. Dev Med Child Neurol 2005;47(8):525–31.
112. Cai S, Qiu A, Broekman BF, et al. The influence of gestational diabetes on neurodevelopment of children in the first two years of life: a prospective study. PLoS One 2016;11(9):e0162113.
113. Xiang AH, Wang X, Martinez MP, et al. Maternal gestational diabetes mellitus, type 1 diabetes, and type 2 diabetes during pregnancy and risk of ADHD in offspring. Diabetes Care 2018;41(12):2502–8.
114. Ji J, Chen T, Sundquist J, et al. Type 1 diabetes in parents and risk of attention deficit/hyperactivity disorder in offspring: a population-based study in Sweden. Diabetes Care 2018;41(4):770–4.
115. Nielsen PR, Benros ME, Dalsgaard S. Associations between autoimmune diseases and attention-deficit/hyperactivity disorder: a nationwide study. J Am Acad Child Adolesc Psychiatry 2017;56(3):234–40.e231.
116. Instanes JT, Halmoy A, Engeland A, et al. Attention-deficit/hyperactivity disorder in offspring of mothers with inflammatory and immune system diseases. Biol Psychiatry 2017;81(5):452–9.
117. Xu G, Jing J, Bowers K, et al. Maternal diabetes and the risk of autism spectrum disorders in the offspring: a systematic review and meta-analysis. J Autism Dev Disord 2014;44(4):766–75.
118. Li M, Fallin MD, Riley A, et al. The association of maternal obesity and diabetes with autism and other developmental disabilities. Pediatrics 2016;137(2): e20152206.
119. Krakowiak P, Walker CK, Bremer AA, et al. Maternal metabolic conditions and risk for autism and other neurodevelopmental disorders. Pediatrics 2012; 129(5):e1121–8.
120. Cannon M, Jones PB, Murray RM. Obstetric complications and schizophrenia: historical and meta-analytic review. Am J Psychiatry 2002;159(7):1080–92.
121. Hultman CM, Sparen P, Takei N, et al. Prenatal and perinatal risk factors for schizophrenia, affective psychosis, and reactive psychosis of early onset: case-control study. BMJ 1999;318(7181):421–6.
122. Kong L, Norstedt G, Schalling M, et al. The risk of offspring psychiatric disorders in the setting of maternal obesity and diabetes. Pediatrics 2018;142(3).
123. Nold JL, Georgieff MK. Infants of diabetic mothers. Pediatr Clin North Am 2004; 51(3):619–37, viii.
124. Kalhan SCPP, Lindsay CA. Pregnancy complicated by diabetes mellitus. In: Fanaroff AAMR, editor. Neonatal-perinatal medicine: diseases of the fetus and infant. 7th edition. Philadelphia (PA): Mosby; 2002. p. 1357–62.
125. Georgieff MK. The effect of maternal diabetes during pregnancy on the neurodevelopment of offspring. Minn Med 2006;89(3):44–7.
126. Kao LS, Morris BH, Lally KP, et al. Hyperglycemia and morbidity and mortality in extremely low birth weight infants. J Perinatol 2006;26(12):730–6.
127. Bermick J, Dechert RE, Sarkar S. Does hyperglycemia in hypernatremic preterm infants increase the risk of intraventricular hemorrhage? J Perinatol 2016;36(9): 729–32.
128. Alexandrou G, Skiold B, Karlen J, et al. Early hyperglycemia is a risk factor for death and white matter reduction in preterm infants. Pediatrics 2010;125(3): e584–91.

129. Heald A, Abdel-Latif ME, Kent AL. Insulin infusion for hyperglycaemia in very preterm infants appears safe with no effect on morbidity, mortality and long-term neurodevelopmental outcome. J Matern Fetal Neonatal Med 2012; 25(11):2415–8.

130. Ennis K, Dotterman H, Stein A, et al. Hyperglycemia accentuates and ketonemia attenuates hypoglycemia-induced neuronal injury in the developing rat brain. Pediatr Res 2015;77(1–1):84–90.

131. Group HSCR, Metzger BE, Lowe LP, et al. Hyperglycemia and adverse pregnancy outcomes. N Engl J Med 2008;358(19):1991–2002.

132. Qiao LX, Wang J, Yan JH, et al. Follow-up study of neurodevelopment in 2-year-old infants who had suffered from neonatal hypoglycemia. BMC Pediatr 2019; 19(1):133.

133. Burakevych N, McKinlay CJD, Harris DL, et al. Factors influencing glycaemic stability after neonatal hypoglycaemia and relationship to neurodevelopmental outcome. Sci Rep 2019;9(1):8132.

134. Mola-Schenzle E, Staffler A, Klemme M, et al. Clinically stable very low birth-weight infants are at risk for recurrent tissue glucose fluctuations even after fully established enteral nutrition. Arch Dis Child Fetal Neonatal Ed 2015;100(2): F126–31.

135. Fendler W, Walenciak J, Mlynarski W, et al. Higher glycemic variability in very low birth weight newborns is associated with greater early neonatal mortality. J Matern Fetal Neonatal Med 2012;25(7):1122–6.

136. Harris DL, Alsweiler JM, Ansell JM, et al. Outcome at 2 years after dextrose gel treatment for neonatal hypoglycemia: follow-up of a randomized trial. J Pediatr 2016;170:54–9.e51-52.

137. Rasmussen AH, Wehberg S, Portner F, et al. Neurodevelopmental outcomes after moderate to severe neonatal hypoglycemia. Eur J Pediatr 2020;179(12): 1981–91.

138. Adamkin DH. Postnatal glucose homeostasis in late-preterm and term infants. Pediatrics 2011;127(3):575–9.

139. Thornton PS, Stanley CA, De Leon DD, et al. Recommendations from the Pediatric Endocrine Society for Evaluation and Management of Persistent Hypoglycemia in Neonates, Infants, and Children. J Pediatr 2015;167(2):238–45.

140. Wackernagel D, Gustafsson A, Edstedt Bonamy AK, et al. Swedish national guideline for prevention and treatment of neonatal hypoglycaemia in newborn infants with gestational age >/=35 weeks. Acta Paediatr 2020;109(1):31–44.

141. Levene I, Wilkinson D. Identification and management of neonatal hypoglycaemia in the full-term infant (British Association of Perinatal Medicine-Framework for Practice). Arch Dis Child Educ Pract Ed 2019;104(1):29–32.

142. Harris DL, Weston PJ, Signal M, et al. Dextrose gel for neonatal hypoglycaemia (the Sugar Babies Study): a randomised, double-blind, placebo-controlled trial. Lancet 2013;382(9910):2077–83.

143. Plummer EA, Ninkovic I, Rees A, et al. Neonatal hypoglycemia algorithms improve hospital outcomes. J Matern Fetal Neonatal Med 2020;1–8.

144. Weston PJ, Harris DL, Battin M, et al. Oral dextrose gel for the treatment of hypoglycaemia in newborn infants. Cochrane Database Syst Rev 2016;(5): CD011027.

145. Edwards T, Liu G, Hegarty JE, et al. Oral dextrose gel to prevent hypoglycaemia in at-risk neonates. Cochrane Database Syst Rev 2021;5:CD012152.

146. Ramel SE, Demerath EW, Gray HL, et al. The relationship of poor linear growth velocity with neonatal illness and two-year neurodevelopment in preterm infants. Neonatology 2012;102(1):19–24.

147. Ramel SE, Haapala J, Super J, et al. Nutrition, illness and body composition in very low birth weight preterm infants: implications for nutritional management and neurocognitive outcomes. Nutrients 2020;12(1):145.

148. Franz AR, Pohlandt F, Bode H, et al. Intrauterine, early neonatal, and postdischarge growth and neurodevelopmental outcome at 5.4 years in extremely preterm infants after intensive neonatal nutritional support. Pediatrics 2009;123(1): e101–9.

149. Stephens BE, Walden RV, Gargus RA, et al. First-week protein and energy intakes are associated with 18-month developmental outcomes in extremely low birth weight infants. Pediatrics 2009;123(5):1337–43.

150. Tottman AC, Alsweiler JM, Bloomfield FH, et al. Relationships between early neonatal nutrition and neurodevelopment at school age in children born very preterm. J Pediatr Gastroenterol Nutr 2020;70(1):72–8.

151. Tottman AC, Bloomfield FH, Cormack BE, et al. Sex-specific relationships between early nutrition and neurodevelopment in preterm infants. Pediatr Res 2020;87(5):872–8.

152. Stensvold HJ, Strommen K, Lang AM, et al. Early enhanced parenteral nutrition, hyperglycemia, and death among extremely-low-birth-weight infants. JAMA Pediatr 2015;169(11):1003–10.

153. Tottman AC, Bloomfield FH, Cormack BE, et al. Relationships between early nutrition and blood glucose concentrations in very preterm infants. J Pediatr Gastroenterol Nutr 2018;66(6):960–6.

154. Bottino M, Cowett RM, Sinclair JC. Interventions for treatment of neonatal hyperglycemia in very low birth weight infants. Cochrane Database Syst Rev 2011;(10):CD007453.

155. Ehrenkranz RA, Dusick AM, Vohr BR, et al. Growth in the neonatal intensive care unit influences neurodevelopmental and growth outcomes of extremely low birth weight infants. Pediatrics 2006;117(4):1253–61.

156. Ramel SE, Brown LD, Georgieff MK. The impact of neonatal illness on nutritional requirements-one size does not fit all. Curr Pediatr Rep 2014;2(4):248–54.

157. Morgan C, McGowan P, Herwitker S, et al. Postnatal head growth in preterm infants: a randomized controlled parenteral nutrition study. Pediatrics 2014; 133(1):e120–8.

158. Harris DL, Battin MR, Weston PJ, et al. Continuous glucose monitoring in newborn babies at risk of hypoglycemia. J Pediatr 2010;157(2):198–202.e191.

159. Beardsall K, Vanhaesebrouck S, Ogilvy-Stuart AL, et al. Validation of the continuous glucose monitoring sensor in preterm infants. Arch Dis Child Fetal Neonatal Ed 2013;98(2):F136–40.

160. Galderisi A, Facchinetti A, Steil GM, et al. Continuous glucose monitoring in very preterm infants: a randomized controlled trial. Pediatrics 2017;140(4): e20171162.

161. Le Compte AJ, Lynn AM, Lin J, et al. Pilot study of a model-based approach to blood glucose control in very-low-birthweight neonates. BMC Pediatr 2012; 12:117.

162. Karon BS, Meeusen JW, Bryant SC. Impact of glucose meter error on glycemic variability and time in target range during glycemic control after cardiovascular surgery. J Diabetes Sci Technol 2015;10(2):336–42.

163. Pinchefsky EF, Hahn CD, Kamino D, et al. Hyperglycemia and glucose variability are associated with worse brain function and seizures in neonatal encephalopathy: a Prospective Cohort Study. J Pediatr 2019;209:23–32.

164. Clausen TD, Mortensen EL, Schmidt L, et al. Cognitive function in adult offspring of women with gestational diabetes–the role of glucose and other factors. PLoS One 2013;8(6):e67107.

Enteral Nutrition

The Intricacies of Human Milk from the Immune System to the Microbiome

Jaclyn B. Wiggins, MD[a],*, Rachael Trotman, RD, CNSC[b],
Patti H. Perks, MS, RDN, CNSC[b], Jonathan R. Swanson, MD, MSc[a]

KEYWORDS

- Human milk • Pasteurized donor milk • Microbiome • Gut–brain axis
- Enteromammary pathway

KEY POINTS

- The protein content in human milk is highest in a mother's own milk after preterm delivery, and decreases steadily until it reaches a steady state around 6 months postpartum.
- The enteromammary pathway contributes to the presence of bacteria and secretory IgA found in breastmilk. Human milk oligosaccharides aid in host defense.
- Pasteurized donor human milk is safe and recommended for preterm infants when mom's milk is not available or of insufficient quantity.
- Fortifiers and modular additives are essential tools for meeting the nutritional needs of infants receiving human milk and should be selected according to specific nutritional goals for the infant.
- Evidence suggests that human milk plays an important role in microbial colonization of the preterm gut and lungs, which participate in bidirectional communication.

INTRODUCTION

Human milk is the preferred nutrition for premature infants. In 2012, the American Academy of Pediatrics revised its policy on breastfeeding. It stated that all preterm infant diets should consist of human milk, either their mother's own milk (MoM) or, if not available, pasteurized donor human milk (PDM).[1] The clinical reasons supporting this policy are many, including reducing infections (necrotizing enterocolitis [NEC], pneumonia, late-onset sepsis) and retinopathy of prematurity, decreased length of stay in the neonatal intensive care unit, and subsequent readmissions, as well as a decrease in mortality and improved neurodevelopmental outcomes.[2–7]

[a] Division of Neonatology, Department of Pediatrics, University of Virginia, Box 800386, Charlottesville, VA 22908, USA; [b] Neonatal Intensive Care Unit, PO Box 800673, Nutrition Services, Ground Floor, UVA Main Hospital, 1215 Lee Street, Charlottesville, VA 22908-0673, USA
* Corresponding author.
E-mail address: JY9NZ@hscmail.mcc.virginia.edu

Clin Perinatol 49 (2022) 427–445
https://doi.org/10.1016/j.clp.2022.02.009
0095-5108/22/© 2022 Elsevier Inc. All rights reserved.

This article focuses on human milk, its composition and bioactive factors, and how it affects the gut–brain axis through the microbiome. We focus on the role that various components of human milk have on the premature infant and subsequently evaluate the immunologic properties seen in human milk. Finally, we will also examine the differences between a MoM and PDM and how those differences may affect the premature infant.

BIOACTIVE PROPERTIES
Protein

More than 400 known proteins within human milk play various roles in nutrition, digestion, and immune defense.[8] The protein content in human milk is highest shortly after birth (14–16 g/L) and decreases as lactation continues when content is approximately 7 to 8 g/L by 6 months postpartum.[9] It has also been found that milk from mothers who delivered premature infants is higher in protein than mothers who delivered term infants.[10] Proteins within human milk are derived from 1 of 3 classes, namely, whey, casein, or mucins (known now as the milk fat globule membrane [MFGM]). The majority of the protein in human milk is synthesized by the maternal lactocyte, with less than 20% of the protein directly taken up from the maternal circulation.[8]

Whey protein makes up the majority of protein in human milk. Colostrum is approximately 90% whey, whereas more mature milk is 60% to 70% whey.[11,12] Whey protein, unlike casein, is found in liquid form, which is thought to be why human milk is easier to digest than commercial formulas, in which casein is the major protein component. Whey proteins may also be responsible for improving gastric emptying time. Alpha-lactalbumin, lactoferrin, secretory IgA, lysozyme, and osteopontin make up the majority of the whey proteins. Of these, alpha-lactalbumin makes up to 40% of whey protein in human milk, whereas in bovine milk, beta-lactalbumin is found in relative abundance and is not found in human milk. Alpha-lactalbumin is also an essential component in the complex involved in lactose synthase.[13] Lactoferrin, in conjunction with lysozyme, plays a significant role in aiding the newborn infant's immune system by degrading the outer wall of bacteria.[14] This protective mechanism contributes to the observed outcomes of decreased infection in those premature neonates fed human milk.

The casein component of human milk is composed of beta and kappa casein. Accounting for approximately 13% of total protein content in human milk, the lowest percentage known in any species, caseins form micelles, which are more difficult to digest.[8] They are also thought to aid in the development of increased fat mass in infants.[15] Kappa casein in particular aids against infection and increases micronutrient absorption and has also been found to prevent *Helicobacter pylori* adhesion to the surface of the gastric mucosa.[16]

The MFGM compose less than 5% of total protein in human milk; however, they potentially play a crucial part in infant nutrition. They are responsible for delivering one-half of the energy content of each feed by surrounding the milk fat vesicle.[17] MFGM proteins, of which there are more than 120, affect multiple systems within the body, playing a key role by interacting with various other components in the small and large intestine, the brain, and the metabolic system.[17]

Carbohydrates

The principal carbohydrate component of human milk is lactose, which increases in content through the first months of lactation. Lactose is a disaccharide composed of galactose and glucose and accounts for approximately 5% of human milk.[18] It is believed that lactose concentrations are correlated with milk volume and that concentrations may be decreased in preterm milk.[19–21] Lactose also plays a role in stool consistency and improved mineral absorption within the small intestine.

Lipids

The fat content in human milk is the most variable component compared with other macronutrients. It accounts for approximately 50% of the content volume over 24 hours of lactation and is integral in the development of the central nervous system.[11,22] Several studies have demonstrated that, as the breast empties, the lipid content increases, with one-half of the content found in the last one-quarter of milk expressed.[18] The fat content of human milk also increases over time, with higher concentrations found in human milk at 12 weeks compared with 1 to 3 days postpartum.[11,23] The majority of milk triglycerides, which contribute up to 98% of the lipid content, are found in the core of the MFGM.[24] Surrounding this core is a trilayer of phospholipids, in addition to membrane proteins and glycoproteins, as noted elsewhere in this article. Finally, surrounding the core are cholesterols, phosphatidylcholine, cerebrosides, and sphingomyelin.[25]

The most common saturated fatty acid in human milk is palmitic acid, which has specific properties that aid in absorbing calcium and magnesium.[26] Because of its unique position in the triglyceride and association with bile salt stimulated lipases in human milk, palmitic acid is converted to monoacylglycerol, which is absorbed easily. However, in infant formula, where palmitic acid is converted to free fatty acids, it binds calcium to form insoluble calcium soaps in the intestine.[27]

In addition to triglycerides, human milk also provides 2 essential fatty acids, namely, linoleic acid and alpha-linolenic acid.[11] These are converted into arachidonic acid and eicosapentaenoic acid. Eicosapentaenoic acid is ultimately converted into docosahexaenoic acid (DHA). DHA cannot be synthesized in the body, so lactating women need to eat a diet rich in omega-3 fatty acids or supplement with DHA. These components play an integral role in signal transduction, such as progression through the cell cycle, and development of the central nervous system and retina.[11]

IMMUNOLOGIC COMPONENTS OF HUMAN MILK

There are many bioactive properties to human milk, but there is also an abundance of immunologic properties. After birth, the neonate encounters a barrage of microorganisms from the environment they had previously been protected from in utero. Particularly for preterm neonates, the innate immune system is not fully developed, increasing sepsis-related morbidity and mortality.[28] Within the enteromammary immune system, there are immunoglobins, growth factors, hormones, and enzymes that interact with each other and the intestines to build the neonate's first defense against outside pathogens.[29]

The enteromammary pathway was first described in the 1970s when scientists discovered that the long-held notion that breastmilk was sterile was incorrect while looking to understand how similar bacterial species were found in maternal feces, neonatal feces, the neonatal oral cavity, and breast milk.[30] Scientists then realized that this same pathway was used to facilitate the presence of secretory IgA in breast milk.[30,31] Foreign antigens in the maternal distal ileum are transported through the intestinal epithelium through M cells in Peyer's Patches.[31] These antigens are then bound to IgM + B cells, which causes the conversion of these cells from IgM to IgA. These activated B cells then migrate through the intestinal lymphatic system to the mesenteric lymph nodes and eventually end up in the mammary gland (**Fig. 1**).

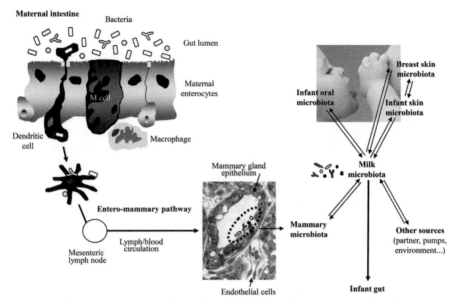

Fig. 1. How bacteria may be transferred from the maternal mammary gland to the neonatal gut. (*From* Rodríguez JM. The origin of human milk bacteria: is there a bacterial entero-mammary pathway during late pregnancy and lactation? Adv Nutr. 2014 Nov 14;5(6):779–84.)

Once in the mammary gland, the B cells become plasma cells that secrete an IgA dimer that is cleaved at the mammary epithelium to produce secretory IgA in the breast milk. Through this enteromammary pathway, the neonatal intestine acquires the first line of defense against foreign antigens.[30–32]

In addition to secretory IgA, which provides the neonatal gut with specific antigen-targeted protection, 2 other immunoglobulins are found in breast milk. IgM, the second most abundant immunoglobulin in breast milk, provides complement activation, and IgG provides some antimicrobial properties.[33] Fetal development of the immune system begins early in gestation, around 9 to 12 weeks; however, significant immunoglobulin synthesis does not typically begin until after birth at term gestation.[34] The majority of the IgG detected in the fetus at birth is acquired transplacentally from the maternal circulation. IgA levels do not increase significantly in neonates until 2 to 3 weeks after birth, once the neonate has established breastfeeding.[34] This phenomenon demonstrates the importance of initiating breast milk feeds in premature neonates as early as possible to protect and develop premature intestinal defenses. This factor may be one of the primary reasons why premature neonates exposed to maternal breast milk have significantly lower rates of NEC than those neonates exposed to formula.[35,36]

Another key immunologic component of breast milk is human milk oligosaccharides (HMOs).[37] This collection of indigestible complex sugars aids in host defense through several mechanisms, including antiadhesive actions, immune modulation, and impacting bacterial flora development.[38] For bacteria and viruses to proliferate and cause disease, they must first adhere to the epithelium. Any unbound pathogen gets excreted and therefore cannot cause disease. HMOs act as a fake binding site for pathogens and then block that pathogen from binding to the epithelium.[39,40]

They also modify the glycan-binding sites on the epithelium to make it increasingly difficult for pathogens to recognize the glycan-binding site and bind.[38] In addition, HMOs are also thought to modulate the immune response by promoting leukocyte extravasation and mucosal infiltration. During an inflammatory process, HMOs promote the expression of specific proteins on endothelial cells, which interact with leukocytes that respond to the source of inflammation.[38] Finally, HMOs aid in developing the unique neonatal microbiome that is predominantly occupied by *Bifidobacteria*. These *Bifidobacteria* ferment oligosaccharides, causing the pH in the intestine to decrease and become more acidic. This acidic environment is bacteriostatic to pathogenic bacteria.[38,41] There have been nearly 200 HMOs identified, and research continues to elucidate their role in infant immune function.[40,42]

Lactoferrin, a glycoprotein, also plays a vital role in the innate immune system. This protein binds iron, decreasing the available iron in the intestines for pathogenic bacteria to use.[43] The low iron environment is optimized for nonpathogenic bacteria such as *Lactobacillus* and *Bifidobacteria*, allowing them to proliferate.[44] Lactoferrin can also bind to the cell wall of bacteria and induce cell lysis. In addition to these properties, lactoferrin, like HMOs, can upregulate or downregulate the inflammatory response by affecting Toll-like receptors in the intestine.[45]

Another immunologic component of breast milk are growth factors that promote many organs' maturation, including the gastrointestinal tract. One of the most significant growth factors in intestine maturation is epidermal growth factor (EGF).[46] EGF can be found in both breast milk and amniotic fluid. However, the premature neonate must rely on breast milk alone to provide an adequate source of EGF.[47] A member of the EGF family, heparin-binding growth factor, is responsible for intestinal repair and can help to prevent damage from intestinal ischemia–reperfusion injury, NEC, and hemorrhagic shock.[48] Transforming growth factor-β is an important anti-inflammatory growth factor that also promotes the secretion of IgA. It is produced by lymphocytes, macrophages, and platelets. Its role is to decrease T lymphocyte activity ,allowing the neonate to tolerate breast milk in the intestine without significant inflammatory response to the foreign (maternal) components of breast milk.[49] It is also known to help decrease atopic sensitization, which is one theory why breastfed neonates have fewer allergies and a lower risk for eczema than formula-fed neonates.[10] Other growth factors found in breast milk include neuronal growth factors, which promote the development of the nervous system; insulin-like growth factors, which protect enterocytes after injury; and vascular endothelial growth factors, which mediate vascularization in all organ systems, including the eyes.[50]

In addition to growth factors that promote maturation of the intestinal tract, hormones in breast milk promote metabolism, which is essential for premature neonatal growth. Leptin is an anorexigenic hormone that downregulates the desire for energy consumption and increases energy expenditure.[51] Distinctive leptin levels can be found in the breast milk of small for gestational age, appropriate for gestational age, and large for gestational age neonates, with the greatest amount of leptin found in large for gestational age neonates.[52] Counteracting leptin is adiponectin, which increases energy consumption. It also has anti-inflammatory properties, which affect the vascular endothelium.[53] Calcitonin and somatostatin are also found in breast milk, and they help to promote the development of enteric neurons and regulate the growth of the gastric epithelium, respectively.[50]

Finally, anti-inflammatory or proinflammatory cytokines can be found in breast milk. In general, anti-inflammatory cytokines are in greater abundance than the proinflammatory cytokines in preterm and term breast milk. The most abundant anti-inflammatory cytokines are IL-7, which aids in thymus development, and IL-10.[50] IL-10 is less understood, but research has linked lower IL-10 levels in preterm infants to increased rates of NEC.[54] Proinflammatory cytokines include tumor necrosis factor-alpha, IL-1β, IL-6, IL-8, and interferon gamma. These proteins increase the immune response in several organ systems.[50]

PASTEURIZED DONOR MILK

The American Academy of Pediatrics supports the preferred use of human milk for all infants, term or preterm, with appropriate fortification to meet nutritional needs, particularly preterm infants less than 1.5 kg.[55] Moro and colleagues[56] recommend fortification of human milk for all infants less than 1.8 kg. In the absence of MoM despite adequate lactation support, preterm infants, especially those at born less than 1500 g (VLBW), should receive PDM. This recommendation is based on clinical evidence to support improved tolerance, faster attainment of full feeds, and reduced risk of NEC with feeds of human milk compared with cow's milk-based formula.[57–60] Direct sharing of unpasteurized human milk exposes the infant to risks of bacterial and viral transmission, including cytomegalovirus, hepatitis viruses, and HIV, as well as pesticides, mercury, medications, drugs, or herbs.[55,61] PDM is pooled from multiple screened donors, then collected, pasteurized, tested, and shipped to hospitals or individuals for consumption.[62]

In the United States, the first human milk bank opened in Boston, Massachusetts, in 1910, shortly after the first human milk bank opened in Vienna, Austria, in 1909.[62] Milk banks associated with the Human Milk Bank Association of North America (www. hmbana.org) are nonprofit operations that follow internationally recognized guidelines for PDM. There are currently 31 Human Milk Bank Association of North America milk banks. Typically, milk from 3 to 5 donors is pooled, and the Holder method of pasteurization is used along with strict, specified quality control measures.[60] At this time, there are 3 commercial sources for PBM and its derived products. Company websites provide specific information on their products and processes:

- Medolac, www.medolac.com (Boulder City, NV) https://www.medolac.com/products.
- NicQ, www.ni-q.com, (Wilsonville, Oregon) https://www.ni-q.com/about-us/
- Prolacta Bioscience, www.prolacta.com (Minerva, CA) https://www.prolacta.com/en/resource-library/technical-brief-pasteurization-and-processing/

Vat (batch) pasteurization, used by Prolacta Bioscience, is similar to Holder pasteurization, but a large volume of milk is heated to a set temperature and prescribed time. Retort sterilization is used by Medolac and Ni-Q and combines high temperature and high pressure.

Impact of Pasteurization on Biological and Nutritional Components

Human milk is a bioactive substance that contributes to the newborn's maturation of immune and digestive systems and is considered a species-specific dynamic system.[63] PDM and MoM are often treated similarly when discussing the benefits of human milk for an infant. Meier and colleagues[64] emphasize that the maternal-specific microbial content of MoM and its positive impact on the infant's microbiome cannot be replicated through pasteurized PDM. Meier and colleagues[64] posit that PDM itself may be less of a factor in the protection against NEC versus the earlier initiation of feeds if not waiting for mom's milk, and the avoidance of formula. Most studies showing the impact of the exclusive human milk diet do not define the amount of PDM received. The authors emphasize the importance of focusing resources on the provision of MoM.[64]

The more that is known about the impact of pasteurization and treatment processes on the components and properties of PDM, the better equipped clinicians are for discussing the benefits and limitations of PDM for preterm and term infants. The goal for pasteurization is the effective inactivation of pathogenic bacteria and viruses while maintaining important immunologic and nutrient components.[60] The impact of pasteurization processes on biological components is presented in **Table 1**. Note that reported changes to nutritional and biological components can vary greatly, reflecting specific processing methods and equipment, sample size, and assay methods.

Table 1
Pasteurization processes

Holder pasteurization or low temperature, long time
  62.5°C, 30 min
    Standard method for Human Milk Banking Association of North America milk banks

Benefits[60,64–67]	Limitations[60,65,66,68,69]
Removes bacteria and viruses	Spore-forming *Bacillus cereus*, if
Maintains bactericidal activity against	present, could survive; however,
Escherichia coli better than high	stringent testing before and after
temperature short time	pasteurization and strict procedures
IgA and sIgA reduced but present	for handling and storage minimize
Lysozyme diminished but retained—	this risk
wide range reported	IgM destroyed
Cytokine activity—largely retained	Lactoferrin reduced by 50%–85%
Many growth factors, IgG, hormones,	Glutathione decreased
and antioxidants reduced but	Lipases and alkaline phosphatase
present	inactivated
HMOs preserved	Destroys B- and T-cell lymphocytes,
Retains long-chain polyunsaturated	which diminishes bactericidal
fatty acids, including linoleic and	properties but also reduces risk of a
α-linolenic	graft-versus-host immune reaction
Retains free fatty acids and	Vitamin C and tocopherols (vitamin E)
monoglycerides which help destroy	likely largely destroyed
viruses and protozoans	Modest decrease in lysine
Vitamins A, D, E, and B_{12}, and folic acid	Lysozyme activity significantly
preserved	decreased
Protein and energy, iron, copper, zinc	
largely preserved; protein	
digestibility maintained	

High temperature short time
  72°C for 15 s
    Variations of temperature and time exist

Benefits[56,60]	Limitations[60,65,68]
Removes bacteria and viruses, except	Spore-forming *Bacillus cereus*, if
Hep A but considered at least	present, could survive; however,
equivalent to Holder pasteurization	stringent testing before and after
Retains IgA and IgG, similar or	pasteurization and strict procedures
potentially better than Holder	for handling and storage minimize
pasteurization	this risk
HMOs preserved	Bactericidal activity against *Escherichia*
Preserves majority of lysozyme,	*coli* decreased as compared with high
cytokines activity	temperature short time
Retains total protein, folic acid, vitamin	IgG decreased
B_{12}, and vitamin C	IgM destroyed

(*continued on next page*)

Table 1 (continued)	
Some retention of lactoferrin and antioxidant properties	Lipase and alkaline phosphatase destroyed (some tests show bile salt stimulated lipase retained to some degree)
May preserve bile salt stimulated lipase—results vary	Modest decrease in lysine
Antioxidant capacity generally preserved	
Lactoferrin reduced but less so than Holder pasteurization	

High pressure processing (HPP)
Nonthermal
High hydrostatic pressure for short time, 4°C or 37° C

Benefits[60,70]	Limitations[60]
Removes bacteria and viruses; efficacy depends on pressure and time	Limited destruction of spore-forming bacteria such as *Bacillus cereus*, requiring 37°C
Preserves more IgA, IgG, and IgM, dependent on pressure and temperature (exception: ↓IgM in 37° C HPP method)	Protein quality negatively impacted
Lysozyme, cytokine, lipase activity seems to be better retained that low temperature, long time and high temperature short time methods	Fatty acids—unclear if negative impact at higher pressures
Improved preservation of lactoferrin	Leukocytes destroyed
Antioxidants, vitamin C, and tocopherols (vitamin E) retained	More costly, less available method and equipment

Ultraviolet C irradiation
Short-wavelength ultraviolet radiation
Destroys DNA of microorganisms
Limited information; not yet used to pasteurize large volumes of milk

Retort sterilization (high temperature and high pressure) is not represented in **Table 1**. Evidence supports the effective elimination of all bacteria, but also shows decreased lysozyme and sIgA activity as compared with Holder processing.[66] An analysis of PDM processed by retort sterilization shows reduced protein and fat content and a decreased immune-modulating proteins, in addition to a decreased lysozyme and sIgA content.[71]

The degree of reduction of immunologic components and, in some cases, the macronutrient composition of PDM is impacted by the specific pasteurization or sterilization method. PDM treated by the Holder and vat methods retain many active biological components not found in infant formula, likely contributing to the demonstrated benefits and protective clinical outcomes.[63,72,73] The preservation of HMOs is likely partly responsible for the protective effect of PDM.[67] The specific HMO profile of PDM is lower in quantity and different in composition from MoM, attributed less to the pasteurization process itself and more to the impact of genetics, environmental factors, and stage of lactation on HMO composition.[74] Alternative pasteurization methods presented in **Table 1** offer the potential benefit of destroying microorganisms while retaining a higher percentage of immune-enhancing components and warrant further evaluation.[69,70,73]

An assessment of the nutrient content of PDM has produced conflicting results. Some reviews of published studies on the Holder method's impact on nutrient content conclude that energy and protein content are largely preserved.[63,69] The method of analysis impacts results, including measurements of amino acid profile and total lipid content. One hypothesis for decreased growth in infants receiving PDM is that the destruction of bile salt–stimulated lipase decreases the intestinal absorption of milk fat. However, clinical evidence has not supported this finding; lingual lipase remains available, and pasteurization increases the amount of free fatty acids, which are well-digested and likely beneficial.[60,63,65] Zinc, also essential for growth, is preserved in pasteurization; however, the potential impact on bioavailability requires further study.[60,63,75]

An analysis of the nutritional composition of PDM as compared with fresh MoM seem to be impacted more by the variability between donors and stage of lactation, the number of pooled donors, and the storage and delivery process, rather than by pasteurization itself, except for heat-labile vitamins deactivated by pasteurization. The maturity of the mammary gland (preterm MoM vs term milk), mature milk versus colostrum and transitional milk, and freeze–thaw cycles involved in the shipping, processing, and storage of PDM are key determinants of nutrient levels.[64] Freezing negatively impacts the fat and energy content of PDM[76] and further decreases lactoferrin content to nominal levels.[77] Human milk, frozen for more than 90 days, has decreased fat, protein, calories, and lactoferrin and increased acidity.[78] Further fat loss occurs through adherence to storage containers, whether glass, polyethylene, or polypropylene.[78]

Evidence Supporting the Use of Pasteurized Donor Human Milk and Related Research Opportunities

Despite the disparities between MoM and PDM, studies support the benefits of PDM as compared with formula[72,79]:

- reduction in NEC and feeding intolerance
- reduced risk of sepsis
- protection against bronchopulmonary dysplasia (BPD)
- protection against long-term complications, such as cardiovascular diseases

PDM retains the lipid and fatty acid composition necessary for central nervous system development.[63] Gastric emptying of unfortified PDM is generally faster and may be better digested than formula. However, the rapidity of gastric emptying may depend on the formula's characteristics, which is important to consider in infants with dysmotility, gastrointestinal anomalies, or surgery. Growth factors that remain following pasteurization include secretory IgA and HMOs to help support gut maturation and mitigate damage from pathogens in the infant GI tract.

Milk from mothers who deliver prematurely or early in lactation contains higher concentrations of HMOs, which may support providing preterm PDM for preterm infants and term PDM for term infants.[74] Research is needed on the impact of PDM on the gut microbiota and microbial diversity with implications for short-term and long-term health outcomes.[80]

Concerns often expressed regarding potential limitations of PDM for preterm or term infants with increased nutritional needs include slower growth and a decrease of MoM availability and use.

Achieving adequate growth has been demonstrated with the use of human milk–derived fortifiers[81,82] or cow's milk–based fortifiers.[55,75] Important clinical interventions that support optimal growth include initiation of enteral feeds as soon as clinically safe, early and aggressive parenteral nutrition, and adherence to standardized nutritional plans.[83]

Apprehension has been expressed that the availability of PDM could discourage or decrease the provision of MoM. Studies have shown the opposite impact.[61,75]

Kantorowska and colleagues[83] demonstrated that the availability of PDM for very low birth weight infants in a neonatal intensive care unit was associated with improved breast milk feeding rates at discharge and a decreased incidence of NEC.[84,85] Although the use of PDM has not been shown to decrease the availability of MoM to infants in the neonatal intensive care unit, the support of MoM production and education regarding the unique benefits therein remain essential.[55]

HUMAN MILK AND THE MICROBIOME

There is substantial evidence that the microbiome is connected to human health and various disease states. Although colonization of the gut continues until the age of 3, evidence shows that the first 1000 days of life are a critical window for microbial health.[86] Preterm infants are vulnerable to microbial dysbiosis for various reasons, such as antibiotic exposure, alternate delivery method, changes in feeding patterns, and stress.[87] Breast milk is a protective factor and plays a vital role in microbial colonization and symbiosis.

Human Milk Microbiome

Different methods have been used to analyze and study the human milk microbiome. The results of these analyses point to a complex and variable composition. Some of the contributing factors to its variation include the length of gestation, delivery mode, milk expression method, maternal diet, and geographic location (**Fig. 2**).[80] Data from the Canadian Healthy Infant Longitudinal Development (CHILD) study found an association between the mode of human milk feed and human milk microbiome features.[88] When compared with expressed breast milk, breastfeeding was associated with an increase in microbial diversity and the abundance of the beneficial bacteria, *Bifidobacterium*.[80] This research has led to a theory connecting the colonization of human milk with salivary backwash during breastfeeding. Additional research is needed to understand the intricacies of human milk microbiome. Refer to **Table 2** for a list of the most common microbes found in human milk.

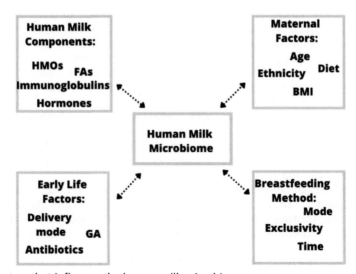

Fig. 2. Factors that influence the human milk microbiome.

Table 2
Common bacteria found in human milk

Human Milk Microbiome		
Staphylococcus aureus	Propionibacterium acnes	Streptococcus agalactiae
Staphylococcus epidermidis	Enterococcus faecalis	Escherichia coli
Streptococcus sanguinis	Bifidobacterium breve	Lactobacillus gasseri
Salmonella enterica		

Data from Beghetti I, Biagi E, Martini S, Brigidi P, Corvaglia L, Aceti A. Human Milk's Hidden Gift: Implications of the Milk Microbiome for Preterm Infants' Health. Nutrients. 2019; 11(12):2944.

Components of Human Milk

Breast milk is not only nutritive, but serves as the first functional food for neonates. Various components of human milk play a role in colonizing the microbiome, but one of the most studied is HMOs. Maternal factors influence the exact type and amount of HMOs.[87] Additionally, various fatty acids, hormones, immune cells, and antibodies found in human milk help to mold and shape the microbiome's composition.[80] Lactoferrin and sIgA play a role in changing the infant's microbiota after birth by decreasing the presence of Enterobacteriacae in the preterm gut (**Fig. 3**).[87]

Gut Respiratory Access

The presence of a microbial community in healthy lungs has emerged, and research is focusing on the correlation between the lung microbiome and various disease states, such as BPD. Increased microbial community turnover, changes in the abundance of proteobacteria and firmicutes, and decreased lactobacilli have been reported with BPD progression.[89] Clearly, there is evidence that the neonatal lung microbiome plays a role in BPD outcomes; however, the exact evolution and interactions are yet to be determined. One theory that has emerged links the gut microbiome with the lung microbiome. This placenta–gut–lung triangle represents the bidirectional impact of the microbial community from one system to the next (**Fig. 4**).[90] This theory aligns with research connecting human milk with respiratory development; the short chain fatty acids found in human milk may impact the intestinal lymphatic system and modulate lung immune balance.[90,91] Additionally, breastfeeding is associated with decreased wheezing and asthma in childhood.[90] Therefore, it is reasonable to suspect human milk to play a prominent role in establishing and regulating the lung and gut microbiomes.

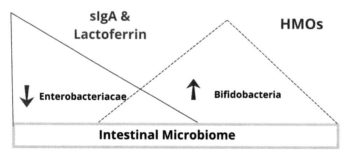

Fig. 3. Components of human milk.

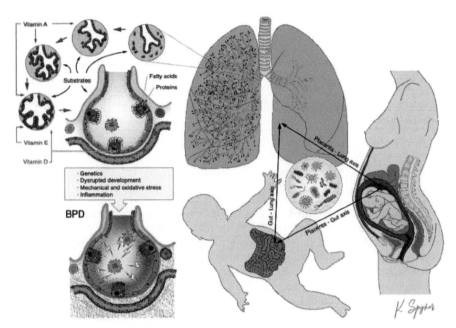

Fig. 4. Placenta–gut–lung triangle. (*From* Piersigilli F, Van Grambezen B, Hocq C, Danhaive O. Nutrients and Microbiota in Lung Diseases of Prematurity: The Placenta-Gut-Lung Triangle. Nutrients. 2020 Feb 13;12(2):469.)

Gut–Brain Access

The bidirectional relationship between the gut and brain, coined the gut–brain axis, represents the communication via the intestinal microbes and established psycho-neuroimmunologic pathways. Evidence suggests that the gut microbiome impacts cognition, mood, anxiety, and sociability. The neonatal microbiota most likely impacts early life neurocognitive and emotional development.[86] Research has shown improvements in IQ testing of breastfed infants.[92] Additionally, a longitudinal study for infants less than 30 weeks or less than 1250 g discovered an association between breast milk feeds with more extensive deep nuclear gray matter at term age, better performance, IQ, mathematics, working memory, and motor testing at 7 years of age.[93] Therefore, breast milk may be beneficial for the cognitive development of the preterm infant.

Maternal Factors Affecting Breast Milk

Maternal diet

As mentioned elsewhere in this article, variations in maternal diet may impact the human milk microbiome. However, there does not seem to be variation in the macronutrient content of breast milk among mothers, even among a malnourished population.[94] This finding supports the hypothesis that a buffer exists against variations in maternal dietary intake and human milk nutrition status. Following this trend, the micronutrient content of breast milk is not significantly correlated with maternal diet changes or supplementation.[94,95] However, there seems to be a link between human milk fatty acid content and maternal nutrition.[96] Some studies have shown significant improvement in fat-soluble vitamins and fat content of breast milk after maternal supplementation. Additionally, DHA supplementation among breastfeeding mothers may impact BPD rates.[90]

Drugs

Illicit drug use is a contraindication to breastfeeding, because illicit drugs are found in breast milk and are associated with long-term neurobehavioral outcomes. In the clinical setting, breastfeeding should be discouraged when a positive toxicology is confirmed.[97] The most common drug used during pregnancy and lactation is marijuana, which has been linked to long-term neurobehavioral effects.[98] It is discouraged to use marijuana while breastfeeding; however, the current evidence is insufficient to make its use a contraindication.[99] Nonetheless, the feasibility of tailored breastfeeding support for substance-exposed mothers and babies exists and should be implemented when clinically appropriate. Research has shown that breastfed infants with neonatal opioid withdrawal syndrome are less likely to require pharmacotherapy for neonatal withdrawal and have shorter lengths of stay.[97,100]

Neurodevelopmental outcomes

Current evidence shows that human milk is beneficial for preterm infants' cognitive development from infancy to adolescence. Among the research, a study showed improved Bayley scores in preterm infants fed fortified breast milk.[2] In another study, breastfed preterm infants with the greatest volume of human milk had greater motor maturity and range of state on the Brazelton examination at the time of discharge and higher Bayley scores at 6 months corrected age. Human milk feeds in preterm infants are associated with increases in the motor developmental index, psychomotor developmental index, and behavior rating scale percentiles at 12 months.[101] Additionally, breast milk is associated with higher IQs, an increase in total brain volume, and an increase in white matter among breastfed preterm infants into adolescence. Although additional research is needed, the current body of evidence for breastfed preterm infants is promising.

CLINICS CARE POINTS

- Lactose is the main carbohydrate in human milk, and its concentration in preterm milk may be decreased compared to term human milk.

- DHA cannot be synthesized in the body, so lactating women need to eat a diet rich in omega-3 fatty acids or supplement with DHA.

- HMOs, a collection of indigestible complex sugars, aid in host defense through several mechanisms, including anti-adhesive actions, immune modulation, and impacting bacterial flora development.

- Term infants likely benefit from PDM when mom's milk is unavailable; more research is needed to define what clinical scenarios and for what duration.Current research suggests the human milk diet impacts clinical outcomes during admission and early life neurocognitive and emotional development of preterm infants.

DISCLOSURE

Dr J.R. Swanson has received speaker's honoraria from Prolacta Bioscience, Inc.

REFERENCES

1. American Academy of Pediatrics Section on Breastfeeding. Breastfeeding and the use of human milk. Pediatrics 2012;129(3):e827–41.
2. Vohr BR, Poindexter BB, Dusick AM, et al, NICHD Neonatal Research Network. Beneficial effects of breast milk in the neonatal intensive care unit on the

developmental outcome of extremely low birth weight infants at 18 months of age. Pediatrics 2006;118(1):e115–23.

3. Vohr BR, Poindexter BB, Dusick AM, et al, National Institute of Child Health and Human Development National Research Network. Persistent beneficial effects of breast milk ingested in the neonatal intensive care unit on outcomes of extremely low birth weight infants at 30 months of age. Pediatrics 2007; 120(4):e953–9.

4. Sullivan S, Schanler RJ, Kim JH, et al. An exclusively human milk-based diet is associated with a lower rate of necrotizing enterocolitis than a diet of human milk and bovine milk-based products. J Pediatr 2010;156(4):562–7.

5. Ip S, Chung M, Raman G, et al. A summary of the Agency for Healthcare Research and Quality's evidence report on breastfeeding in developed countries. Breastfeed Med 2009;4(suppl 1):S17–30.

6. Delaney Manthe E, Perks PH, Swanson JR. Team-based implementation of an exclusive human milk diet. Adv Neonatal Care 2019;19(6):460–7.

7. Chetta KE, Schulz EV, Wagner CL. Outcomes improved with human milk intake in preterm and full-term infants. Semin Perinatol 2021;45(2):151384.

8. Andreas NJ, Kampmann B, Le-Doare KM. Human breast milk: a review on its composition and bioactivity. Early Hum Dev 2015;91:629–35.

9. Martin CR, Ling PR, Blackburn GL. Review of infant feeding: key features of breast milk and infant formula. Nutrients 2016;8:279.

10. Ballard O, Morrow AL. Human milk composition: nutrients and bioactive factors. Pediatr Clin North Am 2013;60(1):49–74.

11. Kim SY, Yi DY. Components of human breast milk: from macronutrient to microbiome and microRNA. Clin Exp Pediatr 2020;63(8):301–9.

12. Donovan SM. Human milk proteins: composition and physiological significance. In: Donovan SM, German JB, Lonnerdal B, et al, editors. Human milk: composition, clinical benefits and future opportunities. Nestle nutrition workshop series. Basel Switzerland: Nutrition Institute/Karger AG; 2019.

13. Monaco MH, Kim J, Donovan SM. Human milk: composition and nutritional value. In: Caballero B, Finglas P, Toldra F, editors. Encyclopedia of food and health. Elsevier; 2016.

14. Thai JD, Gregory KE. Bioactive factors in human breast milk attenuate intestinal inflammation during early life. Nutrients 2020;12(2):E581.

15. Gridneva Z, Tie WJ, Rea A, et al. Human milk casein and whey protein and infant body composition over the first 12 months of lactation. Nutrients 2018;10:1332.

16. Stromqvist M, Falk P, Bergström S, et al. Human milk kappa-casein and inhibition of Helicobacter pylori adhesion to human gastric mucosa. J Pediatr Gastroenterol Nutr 1995;21:288–96.

17. Brink LR, Lonnerdal B. Milk fat globule membrane: the role of its various components in infant health and development. J Nutr Biochem 2020;85:108465.

18. Dror DK, Allen LH. Overview of nutrients in human milk. Adv Nutr 2018;9: 278S–94S.

19. Nommsen LA, Lovelady CA, Heinig MJ, et al. Determinants of energy, protein, lipid, and lactose concentration sin human milk during the first 12 mo of lactation: the DARLING study. Am J Clin Nutr 1991;53:457–65.

20. Narang AP, Bains HS, Kansal S, et al. Serial composition of human milk in preterm and term mothers. Indian J Clin Biochem 2006;21:89–94.

21. Anderson GH. The effect of prematurity on milk composition and its physiological basis. Fed Proc 1984;43:2438–42.

22. Zivkovic AM, German JB, Lebrilla CB, et al. Human milk glycobiome and its impact on the infant gastrointestinal microbiota. Proc Natl Acad Sci U S A 2011;108:4653–8.

23. Kulinich A, Liu L. Human milk oligosaccharides: the role in the fine tuning of innate immune responses. Carbohydr Res 2016;432:62–70.

24. Cheng L, Akkerman R, Kong C, et al. More than sugar in the milk: human milk oligosaccharides as essential bioactive molecules in breast milk and current insight in beneficial effects. Crit Rev Food Sci Nutr 2021;61(7):1184–200.

25. Mitoulas LR, Kent JC, Cox DB, et al. Variation in fat, lactose and protein in human milk over 24 h and through the first year of lactation. Br J Nutr 2002;88. 29–37.

26. Demmelmair H, Koletzko B. Lipids in human milk. Best Pract Res Clin Endocrinol Metab 2018;32(1):57–68.

27. Koletzko B. Human milk lipids. Ann Nutr Metab 2016;69(suppl 2):28–40.

28. Ojo-Okunola A, Cacciatore S, Nicol MP, et al. The determinants of the human milk metabolome and its role in infant health. Metabolites 2020;10:77.

29. Mimouni FB, Lubetzky R, Yochpaz S, et al. Preterm human milk macronutrient and energy composition. Clin Perinatol 2017;44(1):165–72. https://doi.org/10.1016/j.clp.2016.11.010.

30. Straarup EM, Lauritzen L, Faerk J, et al. The Stereospecific Triacylglycerol structures and fatty acid profiles of human milk and infant formulas. J Pediatr Gastroenterol Nutr March 2006;42(3):293–9. https://doi.org/10.1097/01.mpg.0000214155.51036.4f.

31. Lyons KE, Ryan CA, Dempsey EM, et al. Breast milk, a source of beneficial microbes and associated benefits for infant health. Nutrients 2020;12(4). https://doi.org/10.3390/nu12041039.

32. Rodríguez JM. The origin of human milk bacteria: is there a bacterial enteromammary pathway during late pregnancy and lactation? Adv Nutr 2014;5(6): 779–84. https://doi.org/10.3945/an.114.007229.

33. Kleinman RE, Walker WA. The enteromammary immune system: an important new concept in breast milk host defense. Dig Dis Sci 1979;24(11):876–82. https://doi.org/10.1007/BF01324906.

34. Biagi E, Quercia S, Aceti A, et al. The bacterial ecosystem of mother's milk and infant's mouth and gut. Front Microbiol 2017;8:1214. https://doi.org/10.3389/fmicb.2017.01214.

35. Goldman AS, Chheda S, Keeney SE, et al. Immunology of human milk and host immunity. In: Polin RA, Fox WH, Abman SH, editors. Fetal and neonatal physiology. Philadelphia: Elsevier; 2011. p. 1690–701. https://doi.org/10.1016/B978-1-4160-3479-7.10158-2.

36. Hayward AR. The human fetus and newborn: development of the immune response. Birth Defects Orig Artic Ser 1983;19(3):289–94.

37. Herrmann K, Carroll K. An exclusively human milk diet reduces necrotizing enterocolitis. Breastfeed Med 2014;9(4):184–90. https://doi.org/10.1089/bfm.2013.0121.

38. Patel AL, Kim JH. Human milk and necrotizing enterocolitis. Semin Pediatr Surg 2018;27(1):34–8. https://doi.org/10.1053/j.sempedsurg.2017.11.007.

39. HMOs and infant intake associated with overweight and obesity and infant growth.pdf | Powered by Box. Available at: https://app.box.com/file/827105430084. Accessed October 8, 2021.

40. Wiciński M, Sawicka E, Gębalski J, et al. Human milk oligosaccharides: health benefits, potential applications in infant formulas, and pharmacology. Nutrients 2020;12(1). https://doi.org/10.3390/nu12010266.

41. Triantis V, Bode L, van Neerven RJJ. Immunological effects of human milk oligosaccharides. Front Pediatr 2018;6:190. https://doi.org/10.3389/fped.2018.00190.

42. Kell DB, Heyden EL, Pretorius E. The biology of lactoferrin, an iron-binding protein that can help defend against viruses and bacteria. Front Immunol 2020;11:1221. https://doi.org/10.3389/fimmu.2020.01221.

43. Oda H, Wakabayashi H, Yamauchi K, et al. Lactoferrin and Bifidobacteria. Biometals 2014;27(5):915–22. https://doi.org/10.1007/s10534-014-9741-8.

44. He Y, Lawlor NT, Newburg DS. Human milk components modulate toll-like receptor-mediated inflammation. Adv Nutr 2016;7(1):102–11. https://doi.org/10.3945/an.115.010090.

45. Tang X, Liu H, Yang S, et al. Epidermal growth factor and intestinal barrier function. Mediators Inflamm 2016;2016:1927348. https://doi.org/10.1155/2016/1927348.

46. Wagner CL, Taylor SN, Johnson D. Host factors in amniotic fluid and breast milk that contribute to gut maturation. Clin Rev Allergy Immunol 2008;34(2):191–204. https://doi.org/10.1007/s12016-007-8032-3.

47. Radulescu A, Zhang H-Y, Chen C-L, et al. Heparin-binding EGF-like growth factor promotes intestinal anastomotic healing. J Surg Res 2011;171(2):540–50. https://doi.org/10.1016/j.jss.2010.06.036.

48. Saito S, Yoshida M, Ichijo M, et al. Transforming growth factor-beta (TGF-beta) in human milk. Clin Exp Immunol 1993;94(1):220–4. https://doi.org/10.1111/j.1365-2249.1993.tb06004.x.

49. Kalliomäki M, Ouwehand A, Arvilommi H, et al. Transforming growth factor-β in breast milk: a potential regulator of atopic disease at an early age. J Allergy Clin Immunol 1999;104(6):1251–7. https://doi.org/10.1016/S0091-6749(99)70021-7.

50. Savino F, Liguori SA, Petrucci E, et al. Evaluation of leptin in breast milk, lactating mothers and their infants. Eur J Clin Nutr 2010;64(9):972–7. https://doi.org/10.1038/ejcn.2010.105.

51. Dundar NO, Anal O, Dundar B, et al. Longitudinal investigation of the relationship between breast milk leptin levels and growth in breast-fed infants. J Pediatr Endocrinol Metab 2005;18(2):181–7. https://doi.org/10.1515/jpem.2005.18.2.181.

52. Savino F, Liguori SA. Update on breast milk hormones: leptin, ghrelin and adiponectin. Clin Nutr 2008;27(1):42–7. https://doi.org/10.1016/j.clnu.2007.06.006.

53. Emami CN, Chokshi N, Wang J, et al. Role of interleukin-10 in the pathogenesis of necrotizing enterocolitis. Am J Surg 2012;203(4):428–35. https://doi.org/10.1016/j.amjsurg.2011.08.016.

54. Melville JM, Moss TJM. The immune consequences of preterm birth. Front Neurosci 2013;7:79. https://doi.org/10.3389/fnins.2013.00079.

55. Abrams SA, Landers S, Noble LM, et al. Donor human milk for the high- risk infant: preparation, safety, and usage options in the United States. Pediatrics 2017;139(1). https://doi.org/10.1542/peds.2016-3440.

56. Moro GE, Arslanoglu S, Bertino E, et al. Human milk in feeding premature infants. J Pediatr Gastroenterol Nutr 2015;61. https://doi.org/10.1097/mpg.0000000000000897.

57. Assad M, Elliott MJ, Abraham JH. Decreased cost and improved feeding tolerance in VLBW infants fed an exclusive human milk diet. J Perinatol 2016;36(3): 216–20. https://doi.org/10.1038/jp.2015.168.

58. Kleinman RE and Greer FR. AAP pediatric nutrition, 8th edition, 2020, Breastfeeding pp 68-69

59. Kleinman RE and Greer FR. AAP pediatric nutrition, 8th edition, 2020, Nutritional Needs of the Preterm Infant pp 142-146

60. Picaud JC, Buffin R. Human milk—treatment and quality of banked human milk. Clin Perinatol 2017;44(1);95–119. https://doi.org/10.1016/j.clp.2016.11.003.

61. Valentine CJ, Dumm M. Pasteurized donor human milk use in the neonatal intensive care unit. Neoreviews 2015;16(3):e152–9. https://doi.org/10.1542/neo.16-3-e152.

62. Haiden N, Ziegler EE. Human milk banking. Ann Nutr Metab 2017;69(2). https://doi.org/10.1159/000452821.

63. Peila C, Moro GE, Bertino E, et al. The effect of holder pasteurization on nutrients and biologically-active components in donor human milk: a review. Nutrients 2016;8(8). https://doi.org/10.3390/nu8080477.

64. Meier P, Patel A, Esquerra-Zwiers A. Donor human milk update: evidence, mechanisms, and priorities for research and practice MOM and DHM: compositional and bioactive differences that impact outcome. J Pediatr 2016. https://doi.org/10.1016/j.jpeds.2016.09.027.

65. Arslanoglu S, Corpeleijn W, Moro G, et al. Donor human milk for preterm infants. J Pediatr Gastroenterol Nutr 2013. https://doi.org/10.1097/MPG.0b013e3182a3af0a.

66. Tully DB, Jones F, Tully MR. Donor milk: what's in it and what's not. J Hum Lact 2001;17(2):152–5. https://doi.org/10.1177/089033440101700212.

67. Lima HK, Wagner-Gillespie M, Perrin MT, et al. Bacteria and bioactivity in Holder pasteurized and shelf-stable human milk products. Curr Dev Nutr 2017;1(8). https://doi.org/10.3945/cdn.117.001438.

68. Lewin A, Delage G, Bernier F, et al. Banked human milk and quantitative risk assessment of Bacillus cereus infection in premature infants: a simulation study. Can J Infect Dis Med Microbiol 2019. https://doi.org/10.1155/2019/6348281.

69. Riskin A. Immunomodulatory constituents of human donor milk. Breastfeed Med 2020;15(9):563–7. https://doi.org/10.1089/bfm.2020.0192.

70. Paulaviciene IJ, Liubsys A, Eidukaite A, et al. The effect of prolonged freezing and holder pasteurization on the macronutrient and bioactive protein compositions of human milk. Breastfeed Med 2020;15(9):583–8. https://doi.org/10.1089/bfm.2020.0219.

71. Dussault N, Cayer MP, Landry P, et al. Girard, Mélissa comparison of the effect of holder pasteurization and high-pressure processing on human milk bacterial load and bioactive factors preservation. J Pediatr Gastroenterol Nutr 2021. https://doi.org/10.1097/MPG.0000000000003065.

72. Meredith-Dennis L, Xu G, Goonatilleke E, et al. Composition and variation of macronutrients, immune proteins, and human milk oligosaccharides in human milk from nonprofit and commercial milk banks. J Hum Lact 2018;34(1):120–9. https://doi.org/10.1177/0890334417710635.

73. Moro GE, Billeaud C, Rachel B, et al. Processing of donor human milk: update and recommendations from the European milk bank association (EMBA). Front Pediatr 2019;7:49. https://doi.org/10.3389/fped.2019.00049.

74. Marx C, Bridge R, Wolf AK, et al. Human milk oligosaccharide composition differs between donor milk and mother's own milk in the NICU. J Hum Lact 2014. https://doi.org/10.1177/0890334413513923.

75. Vázquez DC, García SS, Renau MI, et al. Availability of donor milk for very preterm infants decreased the risk of necrotizing enterocolitis without adversely impacting growth or rates of breastfeeding. Nutrients 2019;11(8). https://doi.org/10.3390/nu11081895.

76. Colaizy TT. Effects of milk banking procedures on nutritional and bioactive components of donor human milk. Semin Perinatol 2021;45(2):151382. https://doi.org/10.1016/j.semperi.2020.151382.

77. Eglash A, Simon L, the Academy of Breastfeeding Medicine. ABM clinical protocol #8: human milk storage information for home use for full-term infants, revised 2017. Breastfeed Med 2017;12(7):390–5. https://doi.org/10.1089/bfm.2017.29047.aje.

78. Quigley M, Embleton ND, Mcguire W. Formula versus donor breast milk for feeding preterm or low birth weight infants. Cochrane Database Syst Rev 2018;2018(6). https://doi.org/10.1002/14651858.CD002971.pub4.

79. Beghetti I, Biagi E, Martini S, et al. Human milk's hidden gift: implications of the milk microbiome for preterm infants' health. Nutrients 2019;11(12):1–13. https://doi.org/10.3390/nu11122944.

80. Hair AB, Hawthorne KM, Chetta KE, et al. Human milk feeding supports adequate growth in infants ≤ 1250 grams birth weight. BMC Res Notes 2013; 6:459. https://doi.org/10.1186/1756-0500-6-459.

81. Huston RK, Markell AM, McCulley EA, et al. Improving growth for infants ≤1250 grams receiving an exclusive human milk diet. Nutr Clin Pract 2018. https://doi.org/10.1002/ncp.10054.

82. Genoni G, Binotti M, Monzani A, et al. Nonrandomized interventional study showed that early aggressive nutrition was effective in reducing postnatal growth restriction in preterm infants. Acta Pediatr 2017;106(10):1589–95. https://doi.org/10.1111/apa.13958.

83. Kantorowska A, Wei JC, Cohen RS, et al. Impact of donor milk availability on breast milk use and necrotizing enterocolitis rates. Pediatrics 2016;137(3). https://doi.org/10.1542/peds.2015-3123.

84. Prolacta introduces the worlds first and only human milk caloric fortifier made from human milk cream for preemies in the NICU - Prolacta bioscience. https://www.prolacta.com/en/prolacta-feed/prolacta-introduces-worlds-first-and-only-human-milk-caloric-fortifier-made-human-milk-cream-preemies-nicu/. Accessed April 18, 2021.

85. Yang I, Corwin EJ, Brennan PA, et al. The infant microbiome: implications for infant health and neurocognitive development. Nurs Res 2016;65(1):76–88.

86. Gopalakrishna K, Hand T. Influence of maternal milk on the neonatal intestinal microbiome. Nutrients 2020;12(823).

87. Moossavi M, et al. Composition and variation of the human milk microbiota are influenced by maternal and early-life factors. Cell Host Microbe 2019;25:324–35.

88. Mohan P, Lal CV, Wagner BD, et al. Airway microbiome and development of bronchopulmonary dysplasia in preterm infants: a systematic review. J Pediatr 2019;204:126–33.

89. Piersigilli F, Van Grambezen B, Hocq C, et al. Nutrients and microbiota in lung diseases of prematurity: the placenta-gut-lung triangle. Nutrients 2020;12.

90. Gray L, O'Hely M, Ranganathan S, et al. The maternal diet, gut bacteria, bacterial metabolites during pregnancy influence offspring asthma. Front Immunol 2017;8(365).
91. Horta BL, Loret de Mola C, Victora CG. Breastfeeding and intelligence: a systematic review and meta-analysis. Acta Paediatr Suppl 2015;104:14–9.
92. Belfort M. Breast milk feeding, brain development, and neurocognitive outcomes: a 7 year longitudinal study in infants born <39 weeks' gestation. J Pediatrc 2016;177:133–9.
93. Keikha M, Bahreynian M, Saleki M, et al. Macro-and micronutrient of human milk composition: are they related to maternal diet? A comprehensive systematic review. Breastfeed Med 2017;12(9).
94. Aumeistere L, Ciprovica I, Zavadska D, et al. Zinc content in breast milk and its association with maternal diet. Nutrients 2018;10(1438).
95. Innis S. Impact of maternal diet on human milk composition and neurological development of infants. Am J Clin Nutr 2014;99(suppl):734S–41S.
96. Holmes A, Schmidlin H, Kurzum E. Breastfeeding considerations for mothers of infants with neonatal abstinence syndrome. Pharmacotherapy 2017;37(7):861–9.
97. Metz T, Stickrath E. Marijuana use in pregnancy and lactation: a review of the evidence. Am J Obstet Gynecol 2015;761–77.
98. Metz T, Borgelt L. Marijuana use in pregnancy and while breastfeeding. Obstet Gynecol 2018;132(5):1198–210.
99. MacVicar S, Humphrey T, Forbes-McKay K. Breastfeeding and the substance-exposed mother and baby. Birth 2018;45:450–8.
100. Lechner B, Vohr B. Neurodevelopment outcomes of preterm infants fed human milk: a systematic review. Clin Perinatol 2017;44:69–83.
101. Manzoni P, Dall'Agnola A, Tomé D, et al. Role of lactoferrin in neonates and infants: an update. Am J Perinatol 2018;35(6):561–5. https://doi.org/10.1055/s-0038-1639359.

Human Milk Fortification: A Practical Analysis of Current Evidence

Erynn M. Bergner, MD[a], Sarah N. Taylor, MD, MSCR[b],
Laura A. Gollins, MBA, RD, LD, CNSC[c], Amy B. Hair, MD[d],*

KEYWORDS

- Preterm infants • Enteral nutrition • Fortification • Human milk

KEY POINTS

- Human milk (HM) is the gold standard for the nutrition of preterm infants. Pasteurized donor human milk (DHM) should be provided for all very low birth weight (VLBW) infants when maternal milk (MM) is not available.
- Optimal timing of HM fortification remains undefined. Fortification strategies should minimize deficits during the transition between parenteral and enteral nutrition.
- Although there seem to be some benefits of using HM-derived fortifiers, evidence to recommend their use over cow milk-derived fortifiers is lacking. Local rates of comorbidities, resources, and MM availability should be considered when implementing fortification practices.
- Individualized fortification is an emerging practice that allows for a more stable provision of nutrient needs. Its implementation, however, is limited by cost, increased resource utilization, and the need for careful attention to laboratory practice and calibration of equipment.
- Higher volume approaches may have benefits for short-term growth. Practitioners should pay careful attention to potential toxicities when implementing this strategy.

INTRODUCTION

Human milk (HM) is the gold standard for preterm infant nutrition.[1] Despite its immune, developmental, and physiologic benefits, HM delivers an inadequate supply of several nutrients, particularly protein, calcium, and phosphorus, to support the growing

[a] Section of Neonatal-Perinatal Medicine, Department of Pediatrics, University of Oklahoma Health Sciences Center, 1200 North Everett Drive, ETNP 7504 Oklahoma City, OK 73104, USA; [b] Section of Neonatology, Department of Pediatrics, Yale School of Medicine, PO Box 208064 New Haven, CT 06520, USA; [c] Neonatal Nutrition Program, Neonatology, Texas Children's Hospital, 6621 Fannin Street, Suite WT6104, Houston, TX 77030, USA; [d] Section of Neonatology, Department of Pediatrics, Baylor College of Medicine, Texas Children's Hospital, 6621 Fannin Street, Suite WT6104, Houston, TX 77030, USA
* Corresponding author.
E-mail address: abhair@texaschildrens.org
Twitter: @ErynnBergner (E.M.B.); @AmyHairMD (A.B.H.)

Clin Perinatol 49 (2022) 447–460
https://doi.org/10.1016/j.clp.2022.02.010
0095-5108/22/© 2022 Elsevier Inc. All rights reserved.

preterm infant. As such, the American Academy of Pediatrics (AAP) and European Society of Pediatric Gastroenterology, Hepatology, and Nutrition (ESPGHAN) recommend that all very low birth weight (VLBW) infants (birth weight <1500 g) receive appropriately fortified HM as the main component of their diet.[2]

In 1977, the AAP issued its first statement on the nutritional needs of low birth weight infants, concluding that optimal growth in this population should mimic the rate of intrauterine growth in the third trimester without imposing stress on the developing metabolic system.[1,3] Deficits in early nutrition place preterm infants at risk for poor growth, and failure to adequately support growth is directly related to long-term neurodevelopmental outcomes.[4,5] Recent evidence also indicates that not only growth but body composition, namely fat-free mass gains, is associated with the development of the preterm brain.[6,7] With the availability of commercial HM fortifiers in the 1980s and 1990s, the use of fortification to provide additional protein, vitamins, and minerals became the standard of care for VLBW infants in an effort to meet intrauterine needs during critical periods of development.[1] In this review, we analyze the current evidence on HM fortification with a focus on current clinically relevant topics and practical analysis of present-day controversies.

DISCUSSION
Considerations

Variability of human milk
HM is a dynamic biofluid with evolving nutrient and bioactive factors.[2,8,9] The variability and concentration of components in maternal milk (MM) and pasteurized donor HM (DHM) is an important consideration when prescribing preterm infants' nutrition as this may alter calculations for nutrient provision, bioavailability, and absorption thus impacting growth during hospitalization.

Maternal milk in comparison to donor human milk for preterm infants
MM has many benefits for preterm infants including protection against necrotizing enterocolitis (NEC), late-onset sepsis, and chronic lung disease in addition to associations with improved neurodevelopmental outcomes.[2,10] Improvements in many of these outcomes demonstrate a dose–response relationship with increasing amount MM correlating with larger effects.[10] When MM is not available, DHM should be used for high-risk infants, including preterm infants less than 1500 g birth weight.[11,12] This recommendation primarily stems from reductions in NEC with DHM in comparison to formula.[13] The use of DHM, however, continues to be associated with growth concerns and has not been demonstrated to improve mortality, long-term growth, or neurodevelopment.[13,14]

It is well-established that preterm milk in early lactation contains higher protein than either term or mature HM.[15,16] Thus, a major concern arises that infants receiving primarily DHM do not receive adequate protein supplementation despite fortification because the protein content in DHM often falls below the reference standard.[17] In addition, the pasteurization process used to prevent viral and bacterial contamination of DHM affects both the macronutrient content and bioactive components of the milk (Table 1). Commercial milk banks often use vat or retort pasteurization while nonprofit milk banks associated with the Human Milk Banking Association of North America (HMBANA) use Holder pasteurization. While all current pasteurization methods are associated with some loss of the milk's bioactive properties, retort sterilization is associated with significant protein, fat, immune-modulating protein, and HM oligosaccharide losses in comparison to Holder or vat pasteurization.[8] Given the multiple factors that can influence HM composition[9,18] in addition to alterations that can occur with

Table 1
Differences in nutrients and bioactive factors in maternal milk versus pasteurized donor HM[8,18,19,70]

Components	Functions	Maternal Milk	Pasteurized Donor Human Milk
Macronutrients, including: Protein Lipid	• Nutritional substrate for growth and development	• Protein content decreases with the duration of lactation. • Lipid content is the most variable of all macronutrients.	• Reduced lipid content secondary to multiple freeze–thaw cycles and container changes. • Reduction or destruction of digestive enzymes (amylases, proteases, lipases). • Higher protein content by holder method compared with vat or retort method. • Highest fat and calculated energy concentration in the vat method and lowest in the retort method.
Growth Factors, including: Epidermal Transforming Vasoactive endothelial	• Maturational, anti-inflammatory, and trophic effect on the gastrointestinal tract	• Content decreases markedly at 1-mo postbirth. • Slower decline seen in earliest gestation/less mature infants.	• Bioactivity varies by growth factor and is reduced by pasteurization.
Bioactive Proteins, including: Immunoglobulins Cytokines Milk Fat Globule Membrane	• Immune modulation • Anti-inflammatory and anti-infective • Gut barrier protection	• Most abundant in colostrum, with higher levels inversely associated with gestational age. • Selective elevation following pathogen exposure in infant environment.	• Lower concentrations than maternal milk with little or no activity in some components • Concentrations of IgA, IgG, and IgM were lowest by retort method and highest by holder method • Lysozyme concentration was the highest by the vat method.
Oligosaccharides	• Prebiotic • Immune modulation • Antimicrobial	• Highest content in colostrum and transitional milk. • Individual variability in number and type.	• Oligosaccharide pattern of donor human milk varies from that of maternal milk but largely preserved in pasteurization and storage • Higher oligosaccharide concentration in Holder method compared with vat or retort method.

storage, handling, and pooling of milk,[19] DHM can have a 2-fold or greater variation in fat, protein, and energy composition and mean values for energy and fat that are frequently below reference standards for HM.[20] Strategies that increase the number of donors in a pool or perform targeted pooling seem to reduce nutrient variation and optimize delivery of bioactive components.[21,22] As pasteurized DHM is typically more mature milk from mothers delivering at term[18] and macronutrient content can be influenced by processing methods,[19] optimization of fortification strategies is particularly important for infants receiving DHM.

Therapeutic Options

Single- and multi-nutrient fortifiers

Multi-nutrient fortifiers supplement the macronutrient (carbohydrate, protein, fat), mineral, and vitamin content of HM. Use of multi-nutrient fortifiers increases in-hospital weight, length, and head circumference velocities without apparent increase in adverse outcomes such as feeding intolerance or NEC.[23] Although limited data are available to assess their influence beyond the neonatal period, numerous studies associate improved in-hospital growth with improved long-term developmental outcomes in former preterm infants.[4,5,24–26] **Table 2** demonstrates the nutrient content attained using common multi-nutrient fortifiers with both preterm and mature term milk.

As individual nutrients can vary greatly within the base milk, single-nutrient fortifiers may play a role in adjusting for deficiencies. A recent series of systematic reviews[27–29] using protein, fat, and carbohydrates as sole single-nutrient fortifiers found no impact of sole single-nutrient fortification on infant outcomes except for low-quality evidence that protein supplementation increases short-term growth. Future studies will likely focus on the use of these single-nutrient fortifiers in conjunction with multi-nutrient fortifiers within the context of individualized fortification strategies.

Standard and individualized fortification

As defined by the European Milk Bank Association (EMBA) working group on HM fortification,[30] standard fortification describes the practice of adding a fixed amount of fortifier to HM based on predetermined assumptions of the base milk's caloric content in order to reach nutritional recommendations. Individualized fortification encompasses both adjustable and targeted fortification. Adjustable fortification modifies initial standard fortification practices by altering the protein fortification based on the infant's blood urea nitrogen (BUN). Targeted fortification uses bedside analysis of the milk the infant is receiving and supplements the individual macronutrients to meet nutritional recommendations. A Cochrane review[31] recently concluded that individualized fortification improves weight, length, and head circumference growth velocity for VLBW infants in comparison to standard fortification practices. Despite initial promising results, evidence of influence on other clinical outcomes remains sparse, although the study of long-term outcomes is underway.[32]

Given wide variations in the macronutrient content of DHM[20] and previously noted growth concerns,[13] individualized fortification strategies could be particularly significant for infants that receive DHM as their primary nutrition source. However, a recent study using this strategy showed that despite receiving similar energy and protein intakes, infants receiving predominantly MM still had significantly better growth than those receiving predominantly DHM, with MM explaining 22.7% of the improved weight gain and 4% of the length gain in multivariate analysis.[33] Thus, individualized fortification cannot fully compensate for the benefits of MM and further optimization is needed.

Targeted fortification also requires increased resource utilization, cost, and careful attention to proper calibration and laboratory technique with infrared spectroscopy

Table 2
Comparison of fortification of preterm versus mature term human milk: total daily nutrients at full volume (160 mL/kg/d)[9,71-79,a]

	Energy (kcal/kg/d)	Protein (g/kg/d)	Fat (g/kg/d)	Sodium (mEq/kg/d)	Calcium (mg/kg/d)	Phosphorous (mg/kg/d)	Iron (mg/kg/d)	Displacement of Human Milk (mL per 100 mL Prepared Feeding)
Recommend Intake (per kg/d)	110–130	3.5–4.5	4.8–6.6	3–5	150–220	75–140	2–3	
Preterm Human Milk (without Fortifier) Week 3/4	123 (98–147)[b]	2.2 (1–3.5)	5.6 (2.6–8.8)	1.1	40	22	0.2	
Week 10/12	106 (62–150)	1.6 (1–2.2)	5.9 (1.3–10.4)	1.1	46	19	0.2	
Mature Term Milk (without fortifier)	107	1.4	5.6	1.2	37	21	0.1	
Enfamil powdered HMF (bovine), (4 packets) Preterm Human Milk[c]	142	3.9	7	1.1	179	101	2.4	2.4
Mature Term Milk	128	3.1	7	1.3	176	99	2.3	
Similac powdered HMF (bovine), (4 packets) Preterm Human Milk[c]	142	3.7	6.1	2.1	221	126	0.7	2.7
Mature Term Milk	128	3	6.1	2.2	218	125	0.6	
Enfamil liquid HMF standard protein (bovine), (4 vials, 20 mL) Preterm Human Milk[c]	142	4.2	7.8	2.6	189	102	2.4	16.7
Mature Term Milk	128	3.5	7.8	2.7	186	102	2.4	
Enfamil liquid HMF high protein (bovine), (4 vials, 20 mL) Preterm Human Milk[c]	142	4.8	7.8	2.6	189	102	2.4	16.7
Mature Term Milk	128	4.2	7.8	2.7	186	102	2.4	
Similac concentrated liquid HMF (bovine), (4 pouches, 20 mL) Preterm Human Milk[c]	141	3.7	6.1	2.2	221	125	0.7	16.7
Mature Term Milk	128	3	6.1	2.2	218	125	0.6	
Similac concentrated liquid hydrolyzed Preterm Human Milk[c]	141	4.5	5.8	2.1	194	109	0.7	16.7
Mature Term Milk	128	3.8	5.8	2.1	190	109	0.6	

(continued on next page)

Table 2
(continued)

		Energy (kcal/kg/d)	Protein (g/kg/d)	Fat (g/kg/d)	Sodium (mEq/kg/d)	Calcium (mg/kg/d)	Phosphorous (mg/kg/d)	Iron (mg/kg/d)	Displacement of Human Milk (mL per 100 mL Prepared Feeding)
protein HMF (bovine), (4 pouches, 20 mL)									
Prolacta +4 donor human milk-derived HMF (20 mL)	Preterm Human Milk[c]	144	3.7	7.5	1	184	102	0.13	20
	Mature Term Milk	128	3	7.5	1	181	102	0.08	
Prolacta +6 donor human milk-derived HMF (30 mL)	Preterm Human Milk[c]	155	4.5	8.5	0.8	194	107	0.11	30
	Mature Term Milk	139	3.8	8.5	1	190	106	0.06	

[a] Values in the table above are calculated from fortified HM prepared according to the manufacturer's directions. For the liquid Similac and Enfamil products, 20 mL of fortifier is added to 100 mL of HM. For the Prolacta +4 product, 20 mL of fortifier is added to 80 mL of HM. For the Prolacta +6 product, 30 mL of fortifier is added to 70 mL of HM.

[b] Values represent mean (+/−2 standard deviations).

[c] Preterm HM calculations with commercial fortifiers are based on Week 3/4 from Gidrewicz et al. 2014.[9] There is significant variability in nutrient composition with preterm MM approaching mature term milk near 12 wk duration of lactation. Nutrient intake is further influenced by milk preparation and feeding delivery methods.

Adapted from Hair, AB. Approach to enteral nutrition in the premature infant. In: UpToDate, Post TW (Ed), UpToDate, Waltham, MA. (Accessed on May 12, 2021) with permission.

devices used in bedside milk analysis. Due to the variability of HM,[9,18] frequent milk analysis is needed to ensure the technique is not unintentionally providing under- or over-nutrition, resulting in a significant increase in time for milk preparation and hospital workforce utilization.[34] In addition, macronutrient results from mid-infrared spectroscopy devices can be influenced by the sample preparation techinique,[35] relative levels of the individual macronutrients in the milk sample,[36] and type of nutrient analyzed.[35,37] Lactose has the least robust correlation in comparison to gold standard laboratory techniques due to the presence of HM oligosaccharides in the sample that can interfere with the measurement. Studies evaluating means to decrease the frequency of milk analysis or laboratory sampling, however, have shown promise.[34,38]

Controversies

Timing of fortification

Three recent systematic reviews[39–41] have evaluated early versus delayed fortification in VLBW infants. Although these reviews had differing selection criteria, none found a significant impact of an early or delayed fortification strategy when evaluating growth, feeding intolerance, morbidities, and mortality. One analysis, however, found a significantly higher duration of hospital stay in the early fortification group.[41] Clinical application of these findings remains difficult due to the wide variation in feeding protocols (**Table 3**) and varying opinions on if early fortification should be defined by volume or postnatal day of fortification.

In the absence of a definite answer, a close look at the transition between primarily parenteral and primarily enteral intakes may provide some guidance in clinical decision making as fortification can compensate for deficits during this critical phase. For instance, Liotto and colleagues[42] demonstrated that VLBW infants with adequate growth velocities (>15 g/kg/d) during the transition phase had higher enteral protein intake during the primarily parenteral phase of feeding advancement and subsequently had higher fat-free mass at term corrected age. This finding is noteworthy as fat-free mass, but not fat mass, gains at term correlate with greater brain size[43] at term and with neurodevelopmental outcomes[6,7] in the at-risk preterm population. Overall energy and protein intakes in the first week of life have additionally been associated with increased fat-free mass at discharge,[44] further speaking toward a role for fortification to fill nutritional gaps in the transition phase.

Table 3
Initiation of human milk fortification in randomized controlled trials since 2010

Author, Year	Volume of Feedings at Time of Fortification (mL/kg/d)	Human Milk or Cow Milk-Derived Fortifier?
Sullivan S et al,[53] 2010	40	Human milk-derived
Moya F et al,[80] 2012	≥ 80	Cow milk-derived
Tillman et al,[81] 2012	At the time of first feed	Cow milk-derived
Kanmaz et al,[82] 2013	90–100	Cow milk-derived
Kim et al,[83] 2015	100	Cow milk-derived
Shah SD et al,[84] 2016	20	Cow milk-derived
O'Connor et al,[55] 2018	100	Cow milk-derived Human milk-derived
Bertino et al,[64] 2019	≥ 80	Cow milk-derived Donkey milk-derived

Several studies have attempted to answer optimal timing of fortification during the transition phase using nutritional modeling approaches and determined fortification at 33% to 67% of volume[45] or 80 mL/kg/d[46] maximized protein and energy intakes. Improvements at this phase could have a significant effect, as growth failure in the transition phase is predictive of growth failure at discharge.[47]

Impact of volume on fortification

Restricted fluid practices have been demonstrated to reduce the rate of morbidities in preterm infants in comparison to liberal fluid practices.[48,49] These studies, however, focus on early life fluid restriction in a predominantly parenteral phase of nutrition. Little is known regarding the influence of enteral fluid volume strategies on common prematurity-related morbidities. A recent meta-analysis[50] found that higher enteral feeding volumes (>180 mL/kg/d fortified HM/preterm formula or >200 mL/kg/d unfortified HM or term formula) may improve weight gain. Evidence was insufficient to draw conclusions on other growth parameters or clinical outcomes. Only one of the 2 studies that involved fortified HM included in this analysis reported overall calories and caloric density of the feeds. In this study, the increased calories received by the higher volume group were attributed to increased volume as overall caloric density of feeds did not differ between the 2 groups.[51] Thus, high-volume strategies provide increased calories via a lower protein-energy ratio than a standard volume-increased fortification approach. As increased protein in the neonatal period is associated with increased lean mass into adulthood in former preterm infants,[48] differences in fortification approaches such as these could have implications for long-term cardiometabolic health. Salas and colleagues[52] provided some reassuring evidence that percent body fat at term did not increase in a clinically meaningful range with a high-volume approach. However, larger sample size investigations and longer-term studies are still needed. Potential toxicities of using high-volume strategies with multi-nutrient fortifiers also remain unknown.

Human milk-derived fortifiers versus cow milk-derived fortifiers

In the past decade, HM-derived fortifiers (HMDF) have emerged as an option to fortify HM. While an exclusive HM diet (MM or DHM fortified with HMDF) has been demonstrated to lower the risk of NEC in comparison to a cow milk-exposed diet (diets containing HM fortified with cow milk-derived fortifier (CMDF) and/or preterm formula),[53] the AAP now recommends all VLBW infants receive HM as 100% of their base diet.[2] This shift away from preterm formula use has now charged clinicians with the decision of which type of fortifier to use within the context of a diet consisting of only MM or DHM. This debate is multifaceted given the increased cost and resource allocation concerns associated with HMDFs. A recent Cochrane review[54] identified only one randomized control trial that compared HMDF to CMDF within an exclusive HM base diet. This study by O'Connor and colleagues[55] did not demonstrate differences in feeding intolerance, NEC, infection, growth, or mortality but was only powered for feeding intolerance. Interestingly, a difference in severe retinopathy of prematurity was identified and warrants further investigation. As the publication of the Cochrane review, Lucas and colleagues[56] performed a subgroup analysis of a prior trial[53] using only infants who received only MM plus either CMDF or HMDF. In this study, exposure to CMDF was associated with a higher risk of NEC and the combined outcome of NEC, surgery, or death in addition to a reduced head circumference. Both of these studies; however, used powdered CMDF. Thus, the newer generation liquid CMDFs that are common in the United States have yet to be compared with HMDFs in a randomized control trial.

Future Directions

Further research on exclusive human milk diets

As the initial studies of exclusive HM diets,[53,57] use of preterm formula has decreased and powdered CMDFs have been largely replaced in the United States with liquid CMDFs containing extensively hydrolyzed protein. Liquid CMDFs were developed due to concerns over bacterial contamination[58,59] and exposure to intact cow-milk protein resulting in pro-inflammatory responses.[60,61] Although evidence does not currently demonstrate a reduction in NEC or sepsis with liquid in comparison to powdered CMDF, a recent systematic review supports improved growth in VLBW infants fortified with hydrolyzed CMDFo.[62] A large-scale randomized control trial is needed to evaluate the efficacy of HMDFs in comparison to newer generation liquid CMDFs and the impact of fortification strategies on long-term cardiometabolic, body composition, and neurodevelopmental outcomes in former preterm infants.

Innovation in human milk-derived fortifier development

Given the high cost and concerns over the displacement of MM involved regarding currently available HMDFs, strategies to improve on means to achieve an exclusive HM diet are key to advancing the field. Schinkel and colleagues[63] recently published promising results on a novel point-of-care HM concentrating device in which multiple measured milk components were concentrated by 20% to 30%. If proven safe for clinical use, strategies such as these may allow for both the delivery of adequate calories and preservation of the beneficial properties of MM for the preterm infant. In addition, these innovations could make fortification strategies more feasible in low-resource settings.

Alternate protein sources

Due to the cost of HMDFs and pro-inflammatory concerns of preterm formulas and CMDF made from mature bovine protein, investigations into alternate protein sources are important avenues of exploration in the field of HM fortification. Donkey milk-derived fortifiers have been developed due to biological similarity to HM. Initial studies indicate that infants who receive it have improved feeding intolerance,[64] reduced gastroesophageal reflux frequency,[65] and achieved similar growth[66] and neurodevelopmental outcomes[67] at 18 months in comparison to CMDF. Similarly, bovine colostrum has also emerged as a novel alternative to supplement MM in early life as it is a rich source of protein and bioactive factors. Initial results demonstrate feasibility and tolerance of administration in preterm infants[68] and an influence on the gut microbiome.[69] Further research and comparisons to current practices are needed to determine the role the strategies could play in neonatal nutrition.

CLINICS CARE POINTS

- Human milk (HM) is the gold standard for the nutrition of preterm infants.
- Pasteurized donor human milk (DHM) should be provided for all VLBW infants when maternal milk (MM) is not available.
- Optimal timing of HM fortification remains undefined. Fortification strategies should minimize deficits during the transition between parenteral and enteral nutrition.
- Although there seem to be some benefits of using HMDFs, evidence to recommend their use over CMDFs is lacking. Local rates of comorbidities, resources, and MM availability should be considered when implementing fortification practices.
- Individualized fortification is an emerging practice that allows for a more stable provision of nutrient needs. Its implementation, however, is limited by cost, increased resource

utilization, and the need for careful attention to laboratory practice and calibration of equipment.

- Higher volume approaches may have benefits for short-term growth. Practitioners should pay careful attention to potential toxicities when implementing this strategy.

DISCLOSURE

The authors have nothing to disclose.

REFERENCES

1. Greer FR. Feeding the premature infant in the 20th century. J Nutr 2001;131(2): 426s–30s.
2. American Academy of Pediatrics Section on Breastfeeding. Breastfeeding and the use of human milk. Pediatrics 2012;129(3):e827–41.
3. American Academy of Pediatrics, Committee on Nutrition. Nutritional needs of low-birth-weight infants. Pediatrics 1977;60(4):519–30.
4. Ehrenkranz RA, Dusick AM, Vohr BR, et al. Growth in the neonatal intensive care unit influences neurodevelopmental and growth outcomes of extremely low birth weight infants. Pediatrics 2006;117(4):1253–61.
5. Franz AR, Pohlandt F, Bode H, et al. Intrauterine, early neonatal, and postdischarge growth and neurodevelopmental outcome at 5.4 years in extremely preterm infants after intensive neonatal nutritional support. Pediatrics 2009;123(1): e101–9.
6. Ramel SE, Gray HL, Christiansen E, et al. Greater early gains in fat-free mass, but not fat mass, are associated with improved neurodevelopment at 1 year corrected age for prematurity in very low birth weight preterm infants. J Pediatr 2016;173:108–15.
7. Pfister KM, Zhang L, Miller NC, et al. Early body composition changes are associated with neurodevelopmental and metabolic outcomes at 4 years of age in very preterm infants. Pediatr Res 2018;84(5):713–8.
8. Meredith-Dennis L, Xu G, Goonatilleke E, et al. Composition and variation of macronutrients, immune proteins, and human milk oligosaccharides in human milk from nonprofit and commercial milk banks. J Hum Lact 2018;34(1):120–9.
9. Gidrewicz DA, Fenton TR. A systematic review and meta-analysis of the nutrient content of preterm and term breast milk. BMC Pediatr 2014;14:216.
10. Schanler RJ. Outcomes of human milk-fed premature infants. Semin Perinatol 2011;35(1):29–33.
11. American academy of pediatrics committe on nutrition, Section on breastfeeding, Committee on fetus and newborn. Donor human milk for the high-risk infant: preparation, safety, and usage options in the United States. Pediatrics 2017;139(1): e20163440.
12. Arslanoglu S, Corpeleijn W, Moro G, et al. Donor human milk for preterm infants: current evidence and research directions. J Pediatr Gastroenterol Nutr 2013; 57(4):535–42.
13. Quigley M, Embleton ND, McGuire W. Formula versus donor breast milk for feeding preterm or low birth weight infants. Cochrane Database Syst Rev 2019; 7(7):Cd002971.

14. O'Connor DL, Gibbins S, Kiss A, et al. Effect of supplemental donor human milk compared with preterm formula on neurodevelopment of very low-birth-weight infants at 18 months: a randomized clinical trial. Jama 2016;316(18):1897–905.

15. Lemons JA, Moye L, Hall D, et al. Differences in the composition of preterm and term human milk during early lactation. Pediatr Res 1982;16(2):113–7.

16. Atkinson SA, Anderson GH, Bryan MH. Human milk: comparison of the nitrogen composition in milk from mothers of premature and full-term infants. Am J Clin Nutr 1980;33(4):811–5.

17. Radmacher PG, Adamkin DH. Fortification of human milk for preterm infants. Semin Fetal neonatal Med 2017;22(1):30–5.

18. Meier P, Patel A, Esquerra-Zwiers A. Donor human milk update: evidence, mechanisms, and priorities for research and practice. J Pediatr 2017;180:15–21.

19. Colaizy TT. Effects of milk banking procedures on nutritional and bioactive components of donor human milk. Semin Perinatol 2021;45(2):151382.

20. Perrin MT, Belfort MB, Hagadorn JI, et al. The nutritional composition and energy content of donor human milk: a systematic review. Adv Nutr (Bethesda, Md) 2020; 11(4):960–70.

21. Friend LL, Perrin MT. Fat and protein variability in donor human milk and associations with milk banking processes. Breastfeed Med 2020;15(6):370–6.

22. Young BE, Murphy K, Borman LL, et al. Milk bank pooling practices impact concentrations and variability of bioactive components of donor human milk. Front Nutr 2020;7:579115.

23. Brown JV, Embleton ND, Harding JE, et al. Multi-nutrient fortification of human milk for preterm infants. Cochrane Database Syst Rev 2016;5:Cd000343.

24. Shah PS, Wong KY, Merko S, et al. Postnatal growth failure in preterm infants: ascertainment and relation to long-term outcome. J Perinatal Med 2006;34(6): 484–9.

25. Belfort MB, Rifas-Shiman SL, Sullivan T, et al. Infant growth before and after term: effects on neurodevelopment in preterm infants. Pediatrics 2011;128(4): e899–906.

26. Zozaya C, Díaz C, Saenz de Pipaón M. How should we define postnatal growth restriction in preterm infants? Neonatology 2018;114(2):177–80.

27. Amissah EA, Brown J, Harding JE. Fat supplementation of human milk for promoting growth in preterm infants. Cochrane Database Syst Rev 2020;8:Cd000341.

28. Amissah EA, Brown J, Harding JE. Carbohydrate supplementation of human milk to promote growth in preterm infants. Cochrane Database Syst Rev 2020;9(9): Cd000280.

29. Amissah EA, Brown J, Harding JE. Protein supplementation of human milk for promoting growth in preterm infants. Cochrane Database Syst Rev 2020;9(9): Cd000433.

30. Arslanoglu S, Boquien CY, King C, et al. Fortification of human milk for preterm infants: update and recommendations of the european milk bank association (EMBA) working group on human milk fortification. Front Pediatr 2019;7:76.

31. Fabrizio V, Trzaski JM, Brownell EA, et al. Individualized versus standard diet fortification for growth and development in preterm infants receiving human milk. Cochrane Database Syst Rev 2020;11(11):Cd013465.

32. Belfort MB, Woodward LJ, Cherkerzian S, et al. Targeting human milk fortification to improve very preterm infant growth and brain development: study protocol for Nourish, a single-center randomized, controlled clinical trial. BMC Pediatr 2021; 21(1):167.

33. de Halleux V, Pieltain C, Senterre T, et al. Growth benefits of own mother's milk in preterm infants fed daily individualized fortified human milk. Nutrients 2019; 11(4):772.

34. Rochow N, Fusch G, Zapanta B, et al. Target fortification of breast milk: how often should milk analysis be done? Nutrients 2015;7(4):2297–310.

35. Fusch G, Kwan C, Kotrri G, et al. Bed Side" human milk analysis in the neonatal intensive care unit: a systematic review. Clin Perinatol 2017;44(1):209–67.

36. Kwan C, Fusch G, Bahonjic A, et al. Infrared analyzers for breast milk analysis: fat levels can influence the accuracy of protein measurements. Clin Chem Lab Med 2017;55(12):1931–5.

37. Parat S, Groh-Wargo S, Merlino S, et al. Validation of mid-infrared spectroscopy for macronutrient analysis of human milk. J Perinatol 2017;37(7):822–6.

38. Minarski M, Maas C, Engel C, et al. Calculating protein content of expressed breast milk to optimize protein supplementation in very low birth weight infants with minimal effort-a secondary analysis. Nutrients 2020;12(5):1231.

39. Alyahya W, Simpson J, Garcia AL, et al. Early versus delayed fortification of human milk in preterm infants: a systematic review. Neonatology 2020;117(1): 24–32.

40. Thanigainathan S, Abiramalatha T. Early fortification of human milk versus late fortification to promote growth in preterm infants. Cochrane Database Syst Rev 2020;7(7):Cd013392.

41. Basu S, Upadhyay J, Singh P, et al. Early versus late fortification of breast milk in preterm infants: a systematic review and meta-analysis. Eur J Pediatr 2020; 179(7):1057–68.

42. Liotto N, Amato O, Piemontese P, et al. Protein intakes during weaning from parenteral nutrition drive growth gain and body composition in very low birth weight preterm infants. Nutrients 2020;12(5):1298.

43. Bell KA, Matthews LG, Cherkerzian S, et al. Associations of growth and body composition with brain size in preterm infants. J Pediatr 2019;214:20–6, e22.

44. Ramel SE, Haapala J, Super J, et al. Nutrition, illness and body composition in very low birth weight preterm infants: implications for nutritional management and neurocognitive outcomes. Nutrients 2020;12(1):145.

45. Falciglia GH, Murthy K, Holl JL, et al. Energy and protein intake during the transition from parenteral to enteral nutrition in infants of very low birth weight. J Pediatr 2018;202:38–43, e31.

46. Brennan AM, Kiely ME, Fenton S, et al. Standardized parenteral nutrition for the transition phase in preterm infants: a bag that fits. Nutrients 2018;10(2):170.

47. Miller M, Vaidya R, Rastogi D, et al. From parenteral to enteral nutrition: a nutrition-based approach for evaluating postnatal growth failure in preterm infants. JPEN J Parenter enteral Nutr 2014;38(4):489–97.

48. Bell EF, Acarregui MJ. Restricted versus liberal water intake for preventing morbidity and mortality in preterm infants. Cochrane Database Syst Rev 2014; 2014(12):Cd000503.

49. Abbas S, Keir AK. In preterm infants, does fluid restriction, as opposed to liberal fluid prescription, reduce the risk of important morbidities and mortality? J paediatrics Child Health 2019;55(7):860–6.

50. Abiramalatha T, Thomas N, Thanigainathan S. High versus standard volume enteral feeds to promote growth in preterm or low birth weight infants. Cochrane Database Syst Rev 2021;3(3):Cd012413.

51. Travers CP, Wang T, Salas AA, et al. Higher- or usual-volume feedings in infants born very preterm: a randomized clinical trial. J Pediatr 2020;224:66–71, e61.

52. Salas AA, Travers CP, Jerome ML, et al. Percent body fat content measured by plethysmography in infants randomized to high- or usual-volume feeding after very preterm birth. J Pediatr 2021;230:251–4, e253.
53. Sullivan S, Schanler RJ, Kim JH, et al. An exclusively human milk-based diet is associated with a lower rate of necrotizing enterocolitis than a diet of human milk and bovine milk-based products. J Pediatr 2010;156(4):562–567 e561.
54. Premkumar MH, Pammi M, Suresh G. Human milk-derived fortifier versus bovine milk-derived fortifier for prevention of mortality and morbidity in preterm neonates. Cochrane Database Syst Rev 2019;2019(11).
55. O'Connor DL, Kiss A, Tomlinson C, et al. Nutrient enrichment of human milk with human and bovine milk-based fortifiers for infants born weighing <1250 g: a randomized clinical trial. Am J Clin Nutr 2018;108(1):108–16.
56. Lucas A, Boscardin J, Abrams SA. Preterm infants fed cow's milk-derived fortifier had adverse outcomes despite a base diet of only mother's own milk. Breastfeed Med 2020;15(5):297–303.
57. Cristofalo EA, Schanler RJ, Blanco CL, et al. Randomized trial of exclusive human milk versus preterm formula diets in extremely premature infants. J Pediatr 2013; 163:1592–5.
58. Centers for Disease Control and Prevention. Enterobacter sakazakii infections associated with the use of powdered infant formula–Tennessee, 2001. MMWR Morbidity mortality weekly Rep 2002;51(14):297–300.
59. Jason J. Prevention of invasive Cronobacter infections in young infants fed powdered infant formulas. Pediatrics 2012;130(5):e1076–84.
60. Chatterton DE, Nguyen DN, Bering SB, et al. Anti-inflammatory mechanisms of bioactive milk proteins in the intestine of newborns. Int J Biochem Cell Biol 2013;45(8):1730–47.
61. Bæk O, Brunse A, Nguyen DN, et al. Diet modulates the high sensitivity to systemic infection in newborn preterm pigs. Front Immunol 2020;11:1019.
62. Bridges KM, Newkirk M, Byham-Gray L, et al. Comparative effectiveness of liquid human milk fortifiers: a systematic review and meta-analysis. Nutr Clin Pract 2021;36(6):1144–62.
63. Schinkel ER, Nelson ER, Young BE, et al. Concentrating human milk: an innovative point-of-care device designed to increase human milk feeding options for preterm infants. J Perinatol 2021;41(3):582–9.
64. Bertino E, Cavallarin L, Cresi F, et al. A novel donkey milk-derived human milk fortifier in feeding preterm infants: a randomized controlled trial. J Pediatr Gastroenterol Nutr 2019;68(1):116–23.
65. Cresi F, Maggiora E, Pirra A, et al. Effects on gastroesophageal reflux of donkey milk-derived human milk fortifier versus standard fortifier in preterm newborns: additional data from the fortilat study. Nutrients 2020;12(7):2142.
66. Peila C, Spada E, Bertino E, et al. The "Fortilat" randomized clinical trial follow-up: auxological outcome at 18 months of age. Nutrients 2020;12(12):3730.
67. Peila C, Spada E, Deantoni S, et al. The "Fortilat" randomized clinical trial follow-up: neurodevelopmental outcome at 18 months of Age. Nutrients 2020;12(12): 3807.
68. Juhl SM, Ye X, Zhou P, et al. Bovine colostrum for preterm infants in the first days of life: a randomized controlled pilot trial. J Pediatr Gastroenterol Nutr 2018;66(3): 471–8.
69. Jiang PP, Muk T, Krych L, et al. Gut colonization in preterm infants supplemented with bovine colostrum in the first week of life: an explorative pilot study. JPEN J Parenter enteral Nutr 2021;46(3):592–9.

70. Parker M. Human Milk feeding and fortification of human milk for premature infants. In: UptoDate, Post TW (ed), UpToDate, Waltham, MA. (Accessed on July 7th, 2021.)

71. American Academy of Pediatrics. Current recommendations of advisable nutrient intakes for fully enterally fed VLBW infants. In: Kleinman RE, Greer FR, editors. Pediatric nutrition. 8th edition.; 2019.

72. Koletzo B, Poindexter BB, Uauy R. Nutrition in the preterm infant: scientific basis and practical guidelines. Cinncinati, OH: Digital Educational Publishing Inc; 2005.

73. Mead Johnson Nutrition. Enfamil® human milk fortifier powder. Available at: https://www.hcp.meadjohnson.com/products/premature-low-birth-weight-formulas/enfamil-human-milk-fortifier-powder/. Accessed June 15, 2021.

74. Abbott. Similac® Human milk fortifier powder. Available at: https://abbottnutrition.com/similac-human-milk-fortifier-powder. Accessed November 22, 2020.

75. Mead Johnson Nutrition. Enfamil® liquid human milk fortifier standard protein. Available at: https://www.hcp.meadjohnson.com/products/premature-low-birth-weight-formulas/enfamilreg-human-milk-fortifier-liquid-standard-protein/. Accessed June 15, 2021.

76. Mead Johnson Nutrition. Enfamil® liquid human milk fortifier high protein. Available at: https://www.hcp.meadjohnson.com/products/premature-low-birth-weight-formulas/enfamilreg-human-milk-fortifier-liquid-high-protein/. Accessed June 15, 2021.

77. Abbott. Similac® Human milk fortifier concentrated liquid. Available at: https://abbottnutrition.com/similac-human-milk-fortifier-concentrated-liquid. Accessed June 15, 2021.

78. Abbott. Similac® Human milk fortifier hydrolyzed protein concentrated liquid. Available at: https://abbottnutrition.com/similac-human-milk-fortifier-hydrolyzed-protein-concentrated-liquid. Accessed June 15, 2021.

79. Prolacta® Bioscience. Preterm nutrition products. Available at: https://www.prolacta.com/en/products/preterm-nutrition-products/#fortifier. Accessed June 15, 2021.

80. Moya F, Sisk PM, Walsh KR, et al. A new liquid human milk fortifier and linear growth in preterm infants. Pediatrics 2012;130(4):e928–35.

81. Tillman S, Brandon DH, Silva SG. Evaluation of human milk fortification from the time of the first feeding: effects on infants of less than 31 weeks gestational age. J Perinatol : official J Calif Perinatal Assoc 2012;32(7):525–31.

82. Kanmaz HG, Mutlu B, Canpolat FE, et al. Human milk fortification with differing amounts of fortifier and its association with growth and metabolic responses in preterm infants. J Hum Lact 2013;29(3):400–5.

83. Kim JH, Chan G, Schanler R, et al. Growth and tolerance of preterm infants fed a new extensively hydrolyzed liquid human milk fortifier. J Pediatr Gastroenterol Nutr 2015;61(6):665–71.

84. Shah SD, Dereddy N, Jones TL, et al. Early versus delayed human milk fortification in very low birth weight infants-a randomized controlled trial. J Pediatr 2016; 174:126–31, e121.

Long-Term Impact of Early Nutritional Management

Catherine O. Buck, MD*, Angela M. Montgomery, MD, MSEd

KEYWORDS

- Preterm • Growth • Neurodevelopment • Energy • Protein • Human milk

KEY POINTS

- Growth patterns which follow growth measures over time are the strongest indicators of neurodevelopmental outcomes in preterm infants.
- More information is needed regarding use of body composition measures that indicate the right balance of brain growth with fat tissue development.
- Early protein energy intake and use of human milk are critical components of the preterm infant diet that may improve neurodevelopmental outcomes.

INTRODUCTION

Extremely preterm infants are born at a time of critical brain development. After 24 weeks' gestation, total and regional brain volumes increase 1.5- to nearly 4-fold through term age, respectively.[1,2] Concurrently, there is important maturation of the cortical gray matter, rapid development of white matter cell types, and growth of cortical connections.[3,4] In preterm infants, brain maturation is impaired in comparison with infants born at term, demonstrating the vulnerability of these cell types at this critical stage of development.[5]

Although advances in neonatal care have led to a decrease in the incidence of severe cerebral palsy, the incidence of suboptimal neurodevelopment in extremely preterm infants has remained overall unchanged.[6–8] Recent studies have shown that rates of other motor, language, and behavioral impairments among infants born preterm have increased over time.[9] Preterm infants are vulnerable to brain injury secondary to alteration of the expected cerebral neurodevelopmental trajectory.[10] Optimizing early nutrition for preterm infants may promote neurodevelopment through enhanced brain growth.[11]

Research continues to work toward identifying the optimal diet and the optimal growth pattern to reduce growth faltering, optimize neurodevelopmental outcomes,

Department of Pediatrics, Yale School of Medicine, PO Box 208064, 333 Cedar Street, New Haven, CT 06520, USA
* Corresponding author.
E-mail address: Catherine.Buck@yale.edu
Twitter: @catybuck (C.O.B.); @amontgom09 (A.M.M.)

Clin Perinatol 49 (2022) 461–474
https://doi.org/10.1016/j.clp.2022.02.014
0095-5108/22/© 2022 Elsevier Inc. All rights reserved.

and prevent metabolic sequalae of prematurity and growth that occurs too fast. This article reviews the available evidence regarding the link between early nutrition and growth targets in extremely preterm infants with long-term clinical outcomes. Such nutritional targets may be beneficial in clinical practice to optimize the neurodevelopmental outcomes of the preterm infant.

EARLY GROWTH TARGETS AND NEURODEVELOPMENT

The goal of growth monitoring of the preterm infant is to model healthy, normal fetal and newborn growth while balancing the quantity and quality of the nutrients provided. In clinical practice, most growth parameters are measured weekly. Preterm infant growth curves and tables, many of which were determined based on intrauterine growth or gestational age–specific birthweights of varying populations, are widely used in the clinical setting to assess growth patterns.[12–15] It is recommended that use of these reference curves includes an evaluation of the proportionality of growth, and incorporation of z scores (standard deviation scores) into the clinical growth assessment.

Delivery of early nutrition should target preterm infant growth patterns that are associated with optimal long-term outcomes. Most research regarding preterm infant growth and neurodevelopmental outcomes shows that growth trajectories, rather than a measurement at a certain time, are associated with decreased risk of suboptimal neurodevelopmental outcome (**Table 1**).[16–22] Change in weight z score from birth to 36 weeks corrected age and/or hospital discharge has been associated with Bayley Scales of Infant Development (BSID) scores at age 18 to 24 months[16,17] and mental processing at age 5 years.[22] Weight gain velocity, calculated as either grams/kilogram/day or grams/day, is also an important predictor of neurodevelopmental outcome.[21,23] In extremely low birth weight infants, Ehrenkranz and colleagues[20] showed that those in the highest quartile of weight gain through hospital discharge had higher BSID scores at 18 to 22 months, increased odds of having a normal neurologic examination, and a decreased risk of cerebral palsy.

Preterm infant head growth is also an important predictor of neurodevelopmental outcome. Change in head circumference and head circumference z score are positively associated with psychomotor scores at 18 to 24 months corrected age,[21,24] and motor and cognitive scores on the BSID at age 16 to 36 months.[25] Two-year outcomes from the INERBIO-21st study have also found that faltering of fetal head growth near 25 weeks' gestational age was associated with increased risk of suboptimal neurodevelopmental outcome at 2 years of age.[26] Linear growth, which represents lean body mass, is linked to head growth and neurodevelopmental outcomes in preterm infants. Ramel and colleagues[27] found that length at hospital discharge predicted language outcomes at age 24 months. Length gain velocity has been associated with psychomotor scores on the BSID at 18 months corrected age,[21] and suboptimal gains in length z scores through hospital discharge have been associated with an increased risk of abnormal neurodevelopmental examination at 2 years of age.[28]

Although body mass index (BMI) and other indicators of fat mass and adiposity are important indicators of later health, it is unclear in the preterm infant how these measures may predict later outcomes. In some studies, BMI change through discharge has been associated with measures of brain size,[29] and predicted BSID scores at age 18 months in very preterm infants.[21] BMI curves have been created for use in the preterm infant population.[30] In one study, infants with linear growth restriction and high BMI had worse language scores, and higher risk of neurodevelopmental impairment at age 22 to 26 months.[31] Additionally, lean mass (by air displacement plethysmography) at term age has been associated with brain volumes and brain

Table 1
Preterm infant growth patterns neurodevelopmental outcomes

Growth Pattern/Target	Neurodevelopmental Outcome	Reference
Weight z score near term age	Ø BSID at 18–24 mo	Zozaya et al,[16] 2018 Shah et al,[17] 2006
Weight gain velocity	+ BSID at 24 mo + BSID, normal neurologic examination at 18–22 mo - Risk of cerebral palsy at 18–22 mo + Processing speed at 4 y	Belfort et al,[21] 2011 Ehrenkranz et al,[20] 2006 Pfister et al,[19] 2018
Change in weight z score	+ BSID at 18–24 mo	Zozaya et al,[16] 2018 Shah et al,[17] 2006
Length at term age	+ Speech on BSID at 24 mo	Ramel et al,[27] 2012
Length gain velocity	+ Processing speed at 4 y + Psychomotor index on BSID at 18 mo	Pfister et al,[19] 2018 Belfort et al,[21] 2011
Change in length z score	- Abnormal neurologic examination at 24 mo	Simon et al,[28] 2018
Change in head circumference	+ Composite motor and cognitive scores at 16–36 mo + Neuromotor and psychomotor assessment at 24 mo + Normal neurologic examination at 5 y - Risk of impaired mobility at age 5 y	Raghuram et al,[25] 2017 Sicard et al,[24] 2017 Franz et al,[22] 2009
Change in body mass index	+ BSID at 18 mo + Brain size at term age (BMI z scores)	Belfort et al,[21] 2011 Bell et al,[29] 2019
Change in fat mass	Ø BSID at 12 mo Ø Processing speed at 4 y	Ramel et al,[33] 2016 Pfister et al,[19] 2018
Change in fat-free mass	+ BSID at 12 mo + Processing speed at 4 y	Ramel et al,[33] 2016 Pfister et al,[19] 2018

Ø = no significant association; + = positive association; - = inverse association.
Abbreviations: BMI, body mass index; BSID, Bayley Scales of Infant Development.

size at hospital discharge.[29,32] Fat-free mass gain from birth to term age, but not fat mass gain, has been associated with BSID-II scores at age 12 months[33] and processing speed at age 4 years.[19] As validated research measures of body composition move into clinical practice, investigation of how bedside tools can evaluate the appropriate amount and type of fat tissue development in very preterm infants, and the link to nutritional management and longitudinal outcomes is also needed.

Although weight and length gain trajectories over time are the strongest indicators of neurodevelopmental outcome in preterm infants, it remains unknown which is the best growth pattern for predicting long-term outcomes.[34] Much of the evidence for growth patterns, such as weight gain velocity and length gains over time, pull from observational cohort data. As growth trajectories are followed clinically, it must be recognized that there may be inaccuracies in the development of the standardized curves that are used in the clinical setting. Additionally, clinical tools for assessing malnutrition and patterns of growth faltering have been developed, but require further validation and longitudinal follow-up.[35]

PRETERM INFANT NUTRITION AND NEURODEVELOPMENT

The National Institutes for Health and the Academy of Nutrition and Dietetics "Pre-B project" recently reviewed the existing literature regarding preterm infant nutrition and created evidenced-based nutrition guidelines for the very preterm population.[36] General recommendations of the guideline include optimization of early protein intake to 3.5 to 4 g/kg/d, use of fortified mother's milk when available, and advising close attention to infant growth when pasteurized donor human milk is provided. Daily nutritional management of the preterm infant should balance known short- and long-term benefits of specific components of the parenteral and enteral diet prescribed by the clinical team (**Table 2**).

Protein Energy

In a Cochrane review of 21 studies, higher amino acid intake in the first 24 hours of life (>2 g/kg/d) was associated with a reduction in infant growth faltering (defined as weight <10th percentile at discharge) in very preterm infants.[37] The authors were unable to evaluate the benefit of higher protein intake on neurodevelopment. Many studies evaluating differences in early protein intake in very preterm infants have not found associations with neurodevelopmental outcomes.[38–41] In an observational study, Stephens and colleagues[42] found that each 1 g/kg/d increase in protein intake over the first postnatal week was associated with an eight-point increase in mental development index on the BSID at 18 months. In a randomized trial, Balakrishnan and colleagues[43] found no difference in BSID scores at 18 to 24 months when groups were randomized to receive starting parenteral nutrition protein at either 0.5 or 3 g/kg/d, and advanced to goal thereafter. In a similar study, Blanco and colleagues[40] found that infants randomized to receive higher starting parenteral nutrition had worse growth outcomes through 2 years of age. Overall neurodevelopmental outcomes at age 2 were similar between groups in that study.

There is heterogeneity in the existing literature with regards to the amount of protein studied and the variability of other macronutrients altered, making it difficult to understand the independent effect of protein alone on the growth and neurodevelopmental outcomes. Results from the PRoVIDe trial, which aims to evaluate the effect of an early intravenous protein supplement specifically on neurodevelopment at age 2 years in preterm infants, are pending.[44] An analysis of the initial results found that with each 1 g/kg/d increase in protein intake over the first 14 days, there was a positive association with change in head circumference z score through hospital discharge.[45]

Energy and Lipid Intake

Increased energy intake via early parenteral nutrition in very preterm infants has been associated with improved head growth in the first month.[46] Higher protein energy in the first postnatal week may also be predictive of some developmental outcomes in very preterm infants. In an observational study, Shim and colleagues[47] found that preterm infants who received early, aggressive nutrition (higher protein targets and enteral feeding initiated by 24 hours of life) had higher weight at term corrected age, lower rates of growth faltering through age 18 months, and were more likely to have normal language scores at 18 months. In another cohort, cumulative lipid and energy intake in the first 2 postnatal weeks was associated with the developmental quotient at age 12 months.[48]

Fatty acids and other lipids are essential to growth, adipose development, and brain development in the preterm infant. Long-chain polyunsaturated fatty acids, such as DHA and AA, are particularly important in supporting brain maturation. However,

Table 2
Early nutrient targets and neurodevelopmental outcomes

Nutritional Target	Neurodevelopmental Outcome	Reference
Enteral/parenteral protein in 1st week	+ Mental developmental index at 18 mo Ø BSID at 18–24 mo	Stephens et al,[42] 2009 Balakrishnan et al,[91] 2018 Buddhavarapu et al,[38] 2016 Blanco et al,[40] 2012 Burattini et al,[92] 2013
Enteral/parenteral protein in 1st month	Ø BSID outcome at 24 mo	Power et al,[93] 2019 Cester et al,[94] 2014
Energy intake	+ Normal language development (Denver screen) at 18 mo + Developmental quotient at 12 mo	Shim et al,[47] 2014 dit Trolli et al,[48] 2012
Lipid type: DHA and AA	+ Problem solving, recognition memory at 6 mo + Attention capacity at 20 mo	Henriksen et al,[53] 2008
Human milk dose	Ø BSID at 12 mo + BSID at 18–22 mo, 30 mo + Sequential processing, motor performance at 5 y + IQ, mathematics performance, working memory at 7 y Ø Neurodevelomental outcome after social risk adjustment + Verbal IQ at 7–8 y + Reading scores at 11 y + Full-scale IQ in males in adolescence	Vohr et al,[59] 2006; Vohr et al,[58] 2007 Belfort et al,[61] 2016 Furman et al,[95] 2004 Pinelli et al,[96] 2003 O'Connor & Unger,[74] 2013 Tanaka et al,[97] 2009 Horwood et al,[98] 2001 Johnson et al,[99] 2011 Isaacs et al,[100] 2010
Human milk at discharge	- Suboptimal neurodevelopmental assessment at 2 and 5 y - Risk of severe cognitive deficiency at 5 y	Beaino et al,[101] 2011 Roze et al,[102] 2012
Donor human milk	Ø BSID (Cochrane review) Ø BSID at 18–22 mo	Quigley et al,[64] 2018 Brown et al,[103] 2016

Ø = no significant association; + = positive association; - = inverse association.

studies of enteral supplementation of long-chain polyunsaturated fatty acids have not consistently shown neurodevelopmental benefit in very preterm infants.[49–52] One randomized trial of DHA and AA supplementation of enteral feeds during the newborn hospitalization found a correlation between DHA/AA supplementation and cognitive development at age 6 months,[53] but not at age 20 months.[54]

Enteral Nutrition and Human Milk

Mother's own milk is the preferred feeding source for preterm infants because it is associated with numerous short- and long-term health benefits and improved neurodevelopmental outcomes.[55] Mother's milk contains numerous bioactive factors that confer health benefits compared with formula feeds including improvements in gastrointestinal function, digestion, host defenses, and neurodevelopment. The specific nutrients in breast milk thought to play an important role in impacting brain development of preterm infants include oligosaccharides, polyunsaturated fatty acids, and lactoferrin.[56] Several studies of preterm infants have shown that consumption of mother's milk during neonatal intensive care unit (NICU) hospitalization, compared with preterm formula, is associated with improved neurodevelopment in a dose–response relationship.[57–60]

Vohr and colleagues[59] demonstrated that hospitalized preterm infants receiving mother's milk were more likely to have a Bayley Mental Development Index greater than or equal to 85, higher mean Bayley Psychomotor Development Index and Bayley Behavior Rating Scale percentile scores at 18 months compared with the no human milk group. The authors also noted a dose–response relationship and for every 10 mL/kg/d increase in human milk intake, the Bayley Mental Development Index increased by 0.53 points, the Bayley Psychomotor Development Index increased by 0.63 points, the Behavior Rating Scale percentile score increased by 0.82 points, and the likelihood of rehospitalization decreased by 6%.[59] These beneficial effects of mother's milk intake on neurodevelopment persisted at 30 months of age.[58] In another longitudinal prospective study, Belfort and colleagues[61] found that predominant mother's milk feeding in the first 28 days for very preterm infants was associated with greater deep nuclear gray matter volume at term equivalent age and with better performance at age 7 years of age on IQ, academic achievement, working memory, and motor function tests.

Despite the numerous short- and long-term benefits of mother's own milk, alternative forms of enteral nutrition including donor breast milk or preterm formula are often necessary for preterm infants. Human pasteurized donor milk should be given when mother's milk is not available, is insufficient, or is contraindicated, because pasteurized donor milk is associated with improved feeding tolerance and decreased risk of necrotizing enterocolitis when compared with preterm formula.[62] Although pasteurized donor breast milk may retain some of the health benefits of mother's own milk for preterm infants, it does not seem to confer the same short-term growth or long-term neurodevelopmental gains.[63] In preterm infants, feeding with preterm formula compared with donor breast milk results in higher rates of weight gain, linear growth, and head growth.[64] Feeding with preterm formula may ensure more consistent delivery of necessary nutrients and better support growth compared with donor breast milk over the NICU hospitalization. The balance of risks and benefits of feeding formula versus donor breast milk for preterm infants requires further investigation.

Despite the many benefits of mother's milk and pasteurized donor milk, the nutritional requirements of preterm infants in the NICU cannot be met with human milk alone. Preterm infants require more protein, energy, fatty acids, minerals, and micronutrients than term newborns for appropriate growth and development and human milk fortification is necessary to meet these requirements.[55,65–67] Commercially available fortifiers vary by form (powder vs liquid), protein content and structure, macronutrient composition, lipid content, and source (bovine vs human).[68,69] The optimal timing to initiate fortification and duration to continue fortification have not been established.[70] Many NICUs initiate fortification when feeding volumes are between 80 and 100 mL/kg/d and continue fortification for at least the duration of the infant's NICU hospitalization. The amount of fortification provided should be based on individual preterm infant growth patterns and on overall protein and energy intake, especially for those receiving pasteurized donor milk.[71,72]

POSTDISCHARGE NUTRITIONAL GOALS IN PRETERM INFANTS

Poor growth is a common outcome of the NICU hospitalization, and many preterm infants are in a state of suboptimal nutrition at the time of discharge. Growth faltering at and beyond the time of discharge may be caused by oral feeding difficulty and/or increased metabolic demands requiring increased caloric intake to establish a return to standardized growth curves. With increasing evidence that postdischarge nutrition plays a role in improving long-term growth and neurodevelopmental outcomes, numerous studies have examined different types of postdischarge nutrition for the preterm infant.[73–76]

Continuing feeding with mother's milk postdischarge should remain the goal because of the many health and developmental benefits. However, only half of very low birth weight infants are being fed mother's milk at the time of hospital discharge and many mothers are unable to provide sufficient milk to meet the needs of their preterm infant.[77] The postdischarge diet must meet the protein, energy, and mineral needs for linear growth and correct for deficiencies of micronutrients. Breastmilk alone may not meet the nutritional needs for many preterm infants after discharge. Continuing fortification of mother's milk and/or supplementation with nutrient-enriched postdischarge formula are ways to support the unique nutritional needs of preterm infants. Although studies on the impact of this practice on short- and long-term growth and long-term neurodevelopment are inconclusive, a recent review did demonstrate that increased protein after discharge resulted in increased growth and lean mass accretion at 1 year, most notably in boys.[75]

For preterm infants receiving mother's milk postdischarge, the question remains about how or if to provide fortification and/or supplementation. The decision regarding fortification or supplementation for infants receiving mother's milk should be individualized to a particular infants' clinical history and growth. Serial monitoring of growth parameters, including weight, length, and head circumference on validated growth curves, is critical.[78] Fortification and/or supplementation with nutrient-enriched postdischarge formula should be considered until infants demonstrate adequate catch-up growth.[79]

For infants receiving formula feedings postdischarge, the benefit of using postdischarge nutrient-enriched formula remains uncertain. Recent reviews of infants receiving postdischarge formula compared with standard term formula did not find consistent evidence of improved growth parameters or neurodevelopment up to 12 to 18 months postterm.[76] Given emerging evidence that postdischarge nutrition plays a role in long-term growth and development, it is reasonable to consider nutrient-enriched formula until preterm infants have achieved adequate catch-up growth.

POTENTIAL TRADE-OFFS: RISK OF CARDIOMETABOLIC DISEASE IN PRETERM INFANTS

Although the goal of preterm infant nutritional management and monitoring is aimed to optimize brain growth and neurodevelopmental outcome, there may be other trade-offs, such as too much catch-up growth and/or adverse cardiometabolic outcomes. After hospital discharge, there is some evidence that more rapid BMI and fat mass gains in infancy are associated with worse IQ[80] and lower working memory in childhood,[81] respectively. There is also evidence that early growth trajectories may be related to later cardiometabolic outcomes in very preterm infants.[18,80,82–85] In one cohort, weight gain in the first 14 postnatal days was associated with insulin resistance and cardiovascular disease risk at age 13 to 16 years.[82] Additionally, weight for length gains through 36 weeks corrected gestational age have been associated with body fat percentage and waist circumference at age 21 years.[83] Follow-up data from very preterm infants in the Neonatal Research Network shows that weight gain velocity through age 18 months predicted risk of obesity[85] and high blood pressure at age 6 to 7 years.[86]

In the pediatric population, growth indicators, such as BMI, change over time, and phenotypes of fat development (eg, visceral fat) are associated with obesity and cardiometabolic risk.[87–89] At term corrected age, preterm infants have overall higher body fat percentage and increased intra-abdominal fat compared with infants born at term.[90] However, it is unclear how these differences relate to preterm infant growth and/or neurodevelopment after hospital discharge.[33,80] Before validated measures of body composition in the preterm infant are adapted for clinical use, studies must examine which methods and which patterns are predictive of longitudinal preterm infant growth, cardiometabolic, and neurodevelopmental outcomes.

SUMMARY

Particular attention to the early nutritional management and growth monitoring of the extremely preterm infant is a critical element in neonatal care that targets optimal neurodevelopment. Optimization of early protein energy, use of human milk, and growth targets from birth to after hospital discharge that follow measures over time are the strongest indicators of neurodevelopmental outcome in very preterm infants. Use of standardized growth curves, avoiding growth faltering, and assessment of the proportionality of growth over time are essential elements in the tracking of growth over time. Although the specific effects of early protein targets of neurodevelopmental outcomes are unknown, optimization of early protein energy and early enteral feeds may be beneficial in promoting brain growth and preterm infant neurodevelopment. Mother's own milk during NICU hospitalization is associated with improved neurodevelopmental outcomes, and the goal of postdischarge nutrition in the very preterm infant should be to continue mother's own milk feeding. Future research is needed regarding the optimal supplementation, fortification, and growth targets after hospital discharge to promote a balance of neurodevelopment and metabolic outcomes in preterm infants.

CLINICS CARE POINTS

- Trajectories of preterm infant growth, including weight, length, and head circumference, are stronger predictors of preterm neurodevelopmental outcomes than measures at hospital discharge or term corrected age.

- Optimization of early parenteral and enteral protein energy in the nutritional management of the very preterm infant is important to reduce risk of suboptimal neurodevelopmental outcome.

- Consumption of mother's milk during NICU hospitalization, compared with preterm formula, is associated with improved neurodevelopment in a dose–response relationship.

- Nutrition in the postdischarge period may have beneficial longer term effects on overall growth trajectory and neurodevelopment.

- Although maintaining mother's milk postdischarge should remain the goal because of its known health benefits, the role of fortification, supplementation, or feeding with nutrient-enriched postdischarge formula on growth and development remains uncertain.

DISCLOSURE

The authors have nothing to disclose.

REFERENCES

1. Clouchoux C, Guizard N, Evans AC, et al. Normative fetal brain growth by quantitative in vivo magnetic resonance imaging. Am J Obstet Gynecol 2012;206(2): 173.e1-8.
2. Cormack BE, Harding JE, Miller SP, et al. The influence of early nutrition on brain growth and neurodevelopment in extremely preterm babies: a narrative review. Nutrients 2019;11(9):2029.
3. Volpe JJ. Brain injury in premature infants: a complex amalgam of destructive and developmental disturbances. Lancet Neurol 2009;8(1):110–24.
4. Dubois J, Benders M, Cachia A, et al. Mapping the early cortical folding process in the preterm newborn brain. Cereb Cortex 2008;18(6):1444–54.
5. Lubsen J, Vohr B, Myers E, et al. Microstructural and functional connectivity in the developing preterm brain. Semin Perinatol 2011;35(1):34–43.
6. Pascal A, Govaert P, Oostra A, et al. Neurodevelopmental outcome in very preterm and very-low-birthweight infants born over the past decade: a meta-analytic review. Dev Med Child Neurol 2018;60(4):342–55.
7. Adams-Chapman I, Heyne RJ, DeMauro SB, et al. Neurodevelopmental impairment among extremely preterm infants in the neonatal research network. Pediatrics 2018;141(5).
8. Allotey J, Zamora J, Cheong-See F, et al. Cognitive, motor, behavioural and academic performances of children born preterm: a meta-analysis and systematic review involving 64 061 children. BJOG 2018;125(1):16–25.
9. McGowan EC, Vohr BR. Neurodevelopmental follow-up of preterm infants: what is new? Pediatr Clin North Am 2019;66(2):509–23.
10. Back SA, Miller SP. Brain injury in premature neonates: a primary cerebral dysmaturation disorder? Ann Neurol 2014;75(4):469–86.
11. Hsiao CC, Tsai ML, Chen CC, et al. Early optimal nutrition improves neurodevelopmental outcomes for very preterm infants. Nutr Rev 2014;72(8):532–40.
12. Fenton TR, Kim JH. A systematic review and meta-analysis to revise the Fenton growth chart for preterm infants. Bmc Pediatr 2013;13.
13. Villar J, Giuliani F, Bhutta ZA, et al. Postnatal growth standards for preterm infants: the preterm postnatal follow-up study of the INTERGROWTH-21(st) project. Lancet Glob Health 2015;3(11):e681–91.
14. Olsen IE, Groveman SA, Lawson ML, et al. New intrauterine growth curves based on United States data. Pediatrics 2010;125(2):e214–24.
15. Ehrenkranz RA, Younes N, Lemons JA, et al. Longitudinal growth of hospitalized very low birth weight infants. Pediatrics 1999;104(2 Pt 1):280–9.
16. Zozaya C, Diaz C, Saenz de Pipaon M. How should we define postnatal growth restriction in preterm infants? Neonatology 2018;114(2):177–80.
17. Shah PS, Wong KY, Merko S, et al. Postnatal growth failure in preterm infants: ascertainment and relation to long-term outcome. J Perinat Med 2006;34(6): 484–9.
18. Pfister KM, Ramel SE. Linear growth and neurodevelopmental outcomes. Clin Perinatol 2014;41(2):309–21.
19. Pfister KM, Zhang L, Miller NC, et al. Early body composition changes are associated with neurodevelopmental and metabolic outcomes at 4 years of age in very preterm infants. Pediatr Res 2018;84(5):713–8.
20. Ehrenkranz RA, Dusick AM, Vohr BR, et al. Growth in the neonatal intensive care unit influences neurodevelopmental and growth outcomes of extremely low birth weight infants. Pediatrics 2006;117(4):1253–61.

21. Belfort MB, Rifas-Shiman SL, Sullivan T, et al. Infant growth before and after term: effects on neurodevelopment in preterm infants. Pediatrics 2011;128(4): e899–906.

22. Franz AR, Pohlandt F, Bode H, et al. Intrauterine, early neonatal, and postdischarge growth and neurodevelopmental outcome at 5.4 years in extremely preterm infants after intensive neonatal nutritional support. Pediatrics 2009;123(1): e101–9.

23. Fenton TR, Anderson D, Groh-Wargo S, et al. An attempt to standardize the calculation of growth velocity of preterm infants-evaluation of practical bedside methods. J Pediatr 2018;196:77–83.

24. Sicard M, Nusinovici S, Hanf M, et al. Fetal and postnatal head circumference growth: synergetic factors for neurodevelopmental outcome at 2 years of age for preterm infants. Neonatology 2017;112(2):122–9.

25. Raghuram K, Yang J, Church PT, et al. Head growth trajectory and neurodevelopmental outcomes in preterm neonates. Pediatrics 2017;140(1):e20170216.

26. Villar J, Gunier RB, Tshivuila-Matala COO, et al. Fetal cranial growth trajectories are associated with growth and neurodevelopment at 2 years of age: INTERBIO-21st Fetal Study. Nat Med 2021;27(4):647–52.

27. Ramel SE, Demerath EW, Gray HL, et al. The relationship of poor linear growth velocity with neonatal illness and two-year neurodevelopment in preterm infants. Neonatology 2012;102(1):19–24.

28. Simon L, Theveniaut C, Flamant C, et al. In preterm infants, length growth below expected growth during hospital stay predicts poor neurodevelopment at 2 years. Neonatology 2018;114(2):135–41.

29. Bell KA, Matthews LG, Cherkerzian S, et al. Associations of growth and body composition with brain size in preterm infants. J Pediatr 2019;214:20–6.e22.

30. Olsen IE, Lawson ML, Ferguson AN, et al. BMI curves for preterm infants. Pediatrics 2015;135(3):e572–81.

31. Meyers JM, Tan S, Bell EF, et al. Neurodevelopmental outcomes among extremely premature infants with linear growth restriction. J Perinatol 2019; 39(2):193–202.

32. Paviotti G, De Cunto A, Zennaro F, et al. Higher growth, fat and fat-free masses correlate with larger cerebellar volumes in preterm infants at term. Acta Paediatr 2017;106(6):918–25.

33. Ramel SE, Gray HL, Christiansen E, et al. Greater early gains in fat-free mass, but not fat mass, are associated with improved neurodevelopment at 1 year corrected age for prematurity in very low birth weight preterm infants. J Pediatr 2016;173:108–15.

34. Rochow N, Landau-Crangle E, So HY, et al. Z-score differences based on cross-sectional growth charts do not reflect the growth rate of very low birth weight infants. PLoS One 2019;14(5):e0216048.

35. Goldberg DL, Becker PJ, Brigham K, et al. Identifying malnutrition in preterm and neonatal populations: recommended indicators. J Acad Nutr Diet 2018; 118(9):1571–82.

36. Fenton TR, Griffin IJ, Groh-Wargo S, et al. Very low birthweight preterm infants: a 2020 evidence analysis center evidence-based nutrition practice guideline. J Acad Nutr Diet 2021;122(1):182–206.

37. Osborn DA, Schindler T, Jones LJ, et al. Higher versus lower amino acid intake in parenteral nutrition for newborn infants. Cochrane Database Syst Rev 2018;3: CD005949.

38. Buddhavarapu S, Manickaraj S, Lodha A, et al. Does high protein intake during first week of life improve growth and neurodevelopmental outcome at 18 months corrected age in extremely preterm infants? Indian J Pediatr 2016;83(9):915–21.
39. Cester EA, Bloomfield FH, Taylor J, et al. Do recommended protein intakes improve neurodevelopment in extremely preterm babies? Arch Dis Child Fetal Neonatal Ed 2015;100(3):F243–7.
40. Blanco CL, Gong AK, Schoolfield J, et al. Impact of early and high amino acid supplementation on ELBW infants at 2 years. J Pediatr Gastroenterol Nutr 2012; 54(5):601–7.
41. Bellagamba MP, Carmenati E, D'Ascenzo R, et al. One extra gram of protein to preterm infants from birth to 1800 g: a single-blinded randomized clinical trial. J Pediatr Gastroenterol Nutr 2016;62(6):879–84.
42. Stephens BE, Walden RV, Gargus RA, et al. First-week protein and energy intakes are associated with 18-month developmental outcomes in extremely low birth weight infants. Pediatrics 2009;123(5):1337–43.
43. Balakrishnan M, Jennings A, Przystac L, et al. Growth and neurodevelopmental outcomes of early, high-dose parenteral amino acid intake in very low birth weight infants: a randomized controlled trial. JPEN J Parenter Enteral Nutr 2018;42(3):597–606.
44. Bloomfield FH, Crowther CA, Harding JE, et al. The ProVIDe study: the impact of protein intravenous nutrition on development in extremely low birthweight babies. BMC Pediatr 2015;15:100.
45. Cormack BE, Jiang Y, Harding JE, et al. Relationships between neonatal nutrition and growth to 36 weeks' corrected age in ELBW babies-secondary cohort analysis from the provide trial. Nutrients 2020;12(3):760.
46. Morgan C, McGowan P, Herwitker S, et al. Postnatal head growth in preterm infants: a randomized controlled parenteral nutrition study. Pediatrics 2014; 133(1):e120–8.
47. Shim SY, Ahn HM, Cho SJ, et al. Early aggressive nutrition enhances language development in very low-birthweight infants. Pediatr Int 2014;56(6):845–50.
48. dit Trolli SE, Kermorvant-Duchemin E, Huon C, et al. Early lipid supply and neurological development at one year in very low birth weight (VLBW) preterm infants. Early Hum Dev 2012;88(Suppl 1):S25–9.
49. Makrides M, Gibson RA, McPhee AJ, et al. Neurodevelopmental outcomes of preterm infants fed high-dose docosahexaenoic acid: a randomized controlled trial. JAMA 2009;301(2):175–82.
50. Collins CT, Gibson RA, Anderson PJ, et al. Neurodevelopmental outcomes at 7 years' corrected age in preterm infants who were fed high-dose docosahexaenoic acid to term equivalent: a follow-up of a randomised controlled trial. BMJ Open 2015;5(3):e007314.
51. Moon K, Rao SC, Schulzke SM, et al. Long-chain polyunsaturated fatty acid supplementation in preterm infants. Cochrane Database Syst Rev 2016;12: CD000375.
52. Carlson SE, Werkman SH, Tolley EA. Effect of long-chain n-3 fatty acid supplementation on visual acuity and growth of preterm infants with and without bronchopulmonary dysplasia. Am J Clin Nutr 1996;63(5):687–97.
53. Henriksen C, Haugholt K, Lindgren M, et al. Improved cognitive development among preterm infants attributable to early supplementation of human milk with docosahexaenoic acid and arachidonic acid. Pediatrics 2008;121(6): 1137–45.

54. Westerberg AC, Schei R, Henriksen C, et al. Attention among very low birth weight infants following early supplementation with docosahexaenoic and arachidonic acid. Acta Paediatr 2011;100(1):47–52.

55. Bhatia J. Human milk and the premature infant. Ann Nutr Metab 2013;62(Suppl 3):8–14.

56. Pei JJ, Tang J. [A review on the relationship between breast milk nutrients and brain development in preterm infants]. Zhongguo Dang Dai Er Ke Za Zhi 2019; 21(6):607–12.

57. Lechner BE, Vohr BR. Neurodevelopmental outcomes of preterm infants fed human milk: a systematic review. Clin Perinatol 2017;44(1):69–83.

58. Vohr BR, Poindexter BB, Dusick AM, et al. Persistent beneficial effects of breast milk ingested in the neonatal intensive care unit on outcomes of extremely low birth weight infants at 30 months of age. Pediatrics 2007;120(4):e953–9.

59. Vohr BR, Poindexter BB, Dusick AM, et al. Beneficial effects of breast milk in the neonatal intensive care unit on the developmental outcome of extremely low birth weight infants at 18 months of age. Pediatrics 2006;118(1):e115–23.

60. Belfort MB. Human milk and preterm infant brain development. Breastfeed Med 2018;13(S1):S23–5.

61. Belfort MB, Anderson PJ, Nowak VA, et al. Breast milk feeding, brain development, and neurocognitive outcomes: a 7-year longitudinal study in infants born at less than 30 weeks' gestation. J Pediatr 2016;177:133–9.e131.

62. Committee On N, Section On B, Committee On F, Committee On N, Section On B, Committee On F, Newborn. Donor human milk for the high-risk infant: preparation, safety, and usage options in the United States. Pediatrics 2017;139(1): e20163440.

63. Hård AL, Nilsson AK, Lund AM, et al. Review shows that donor milk does not promote the growth and development of preterm infants as well as maternal milk. Acta Paediatr 2019;108(6):998–1007.

64. Quigley M, Embleton ND, McGuire W. Formula versus donor breast milk for feeding preterm or low birth weight infants. Cochrane Database Syst Rev 2018;6(6):Cd002971.

65. Bhatia J. Human milk for preterm infants and fortification. Nestle Nutr Inst Workshop Ser 2016;86:109–19.

66. Mangili G, Garzoli E. Feeding of preterm infants and fortification of breast milk. Pediatr Med Chir 2017;39(2):158.

67. Radmacher PG, Adamkin DH. Fortification of human milk for preterm infants. Semin Fetal Neonatal Med 2017;22(1):30–5.

68. Gao C, Miller J, Collins CT, et al. Comparison of different protein concentrations of human milk fortifier for promoting growth and neurological development in preterm infants. Cochrane Database Syst Rev 2020;11(11):Cd007090.

69. Premkumar MH, Pammi M, Suresh G. Human milk-derived fortifier versus bovine milk-derived fortifier for prevention of mortality and morbidity in preterm neonates. Cochrane Database Syst Rev 2019;2019(11):CD013145.

70. Alyahya W, Simpson J, Garcia AL, et al. Early versus delayed fortification of human milk in preterm infants: a systematic review. Neonatology 2020;117(1): 24–32.

71. Brownell EA, Matson AP, Smith KC, et al. Dose-response relationship between donor human milk, mother's own milk, preterm formula, and neonatal growth outcomes. J Pediatr Gastroenterol Nutr 2018;67(1):90–6.

72. Lin YH, Hsu YC, Lin MC, et al. The association of macronutrients in human milk with the growth of preterm infants. PLoS One 2020;15(3):e0230800.

73. Nzegwu NI, Ehrenkranz RA. Post-discharge nutrition and the VLBW infant: to supplement or not supplement? A review of the current evidence. Clin Perinatol 2014;41(2):463–74.

74. O'Connor DL, Unger S. Post-discharge nutrition of the breastfed preterm infant. Semin Fetal Neonatal Med 2013;18(3):124–8.

75. Teller IC, Embleton ND, Griffin IJ, et al. Post-discharge formula feeding in preterm infants: a systematic review mapping evidence about the role of macronutrient enrichment. Clin Nutr 2016;35(4):791–801.

76. Young L, Embleton ND, McGuire W. Nutrient-enriched formula versus standard formula for preterm infants following hospital discharge. Cochrane Database Syst Rev 2016;12:CD004696.

77. Parker MG, Greenberg LT, Edwards EM, et al. National trends in the provision of human milk at hospital discharge among very low-birth-weight infants. JAMA Pediatr 2019;173(10):961–8.

78. Lapillonne A, O'Connor DL, Wang D, et al. Nutritional recommendations for the late-preterm infant and the preterm infant after hospital discharge. J Pediatr 2013;162(3 Suppl):S90–100.

79. Fernandes AI, Gollins LA, Hagan JL, et al. Very preterm infants who receive transitional formulas as a complement to human milk can achieve catch-up growth. J Perinatol 2019;39(11):1492–7.

80. Belfort MB, Gillman MW, Buka SL, et al. Preterm infant linear growth and adiposity gain: trade-offs for later weight status and intelligence quotient. J Pediatr 2013;163(6):1564–9.e1562.

81. Scheurer JM, Zhang L, Plummer EA, et al. Body composition changes from infancy to 4 years and associations with early childhood cognition in preterm and full-term children. Neonatology 2018;114(2):169–76.

82. Singhal A, Fewtrell M, Cole TJ, et al. Low nutrient intake and early growth for later insulin resistance in adolescents born preterm. Lancet 2003;361(9363):1089–97.

83. Kerkhof GF, Willemsen RH, Leunissen RW, et al. Health profile of young adults born preterm: negative effects of rapid weight gain in early life. J Clin Endocrinol Metab 2012;97(12):4498–506.

84. Vohr BR, Allan W, Katz KH, et al. Early predictors of hypertension in prematurely born adolescents. Acta Paediatr 2010;99(12):1812–8.

85. Vohr BR, Heyne R, Bann CM, et al. Extreme preterm infant rates of overweight and obesity at school age in the SUPPORT neuroimaging and neurodevelopmental outcomes cohort. J Pediatr 2018;200:132–9.e133.

86. Vohr BR, Heyne R, Bann C, et al. High blood pressure at early school age among extreme preterms. Pediatrics 2018;142(2):e20180269.

87. Lowe WL Jr, Scholtens DM, Kuang A, et al. Hyperglycemia and Adverse Pregnancy Outcome Follow-up Study (HAPO FUS): maternal gestational diabetes mellitus and childhood glucose metabolism. Diabetes Care 2019;42(3):372–80.

88. Gademan MG, Vermeulen M, Oostvogels AJ, et al. Maternal prepregnancy BMI and lipid profile during early pregnancy are independently associated with offspring's body composition at age 5-6 years: the ABCD study. PLoS One 2014;9(4):e94594.

89. Ouyang F, Parker MG, Luo ZC, et al. Maternal BMI, gestational diabetes, and weight gain in relation to childhood obesity: the mediation effect of placental weight. Obesity (Silver Spring) 2016;24(4):938–46.

90. Johnson MJ, Wootton SA, Leaf AA, et al. Preterm birth and body composition at term equivalent age: a systematic review and meta-analysis. Pediatrics 2012; 130(3):E640–9.

91. Balakrishnan M, Jennings A, Przystac L, et al. Growth and Neurodevelopmental Outcomes of Early, High-Dose Parenteral Amino Acid Intake in Very Low Birth Weight Infants: A Randomized Controlled Trial. JPEN J Parenter Enteral Nutr. 2018;42(3):597–606.

92. Burattini I, Bellagamba MP, Spagnoli C, et al. Targeting 2.5 versus 4 g/kg/day of amino acids for extremely low birth weight infants: a randomized clinical trial. J Pediatr. 2013;163(5):1278–82, e1271.

93. Power VA, Spittle AJ, Lee KJ, et al. Nutrition, Growth, Brain Volume, and Neurodevelopment in Very Preterm Children. J Pediatr 2019;215:50–5.e3.

94. Cester EA, Bloomfield FH, Taylor J, et al. Do recommended protein intakes improve neurodevelopment in extremely preterm babies? Arch Dis Child Fetal Neonatal Ed 2015;100(3):F243–7.

95. Furman L, Minich N. Efficiency of breastfeeding as compared to bottle-feeding in very low birth weight (VLBW, <1.5 kg) infants. J Perinatol 2004;24(11):706–13.

96. Pinelli J, Saigal S, Atkinson SA. Effect of breastmilk consumption on neurodevelopmental outcomes at 6 and 12 months of age in VLBW infants. Adv Neonatal Care 2003;3(2):76–87.

97. Tanaka K, Kon N, Ohkawa N, et al. Does breastfeeding in the neonatal period influence the cognitive function of very-low-birth-weight infants at 5 years of age? Brain Dev 2009;31(4):288–93.

98. Horwood LJ, Darlow BA, Mogridge N. Breast milk feeding and cognitive ability at 7-8 years. Arch Dis Child Fetal Neonatal Ed 2001;84(1):F23–7.

99. Johnson S, Wolke D, Hennessy E, et al. Educational outcomes in extremely preterm children: neuropsychological correlates and predictors of attainment. Dev Neuropsychol 2011;36(1):74–95.

100. Isaacs EB, Fischl BR, Quinn BT, et al. Impact of breast milk on intelligence quotient, brain size, and white matter development. Pediatr Res 2010;67(4):357–62.

101. Beaino G, Khoshnood B, Kaminski M, et al. Predictors of the risk of cognitive deficiency in very preterm infants: the EPIPAGE prospective cohort. Acta Paediatr 2011;100(3):370–8.

102. Roze JC, Darmaun D, Boquien CY, et al. The apparent breastfeeding paradox in very preterm infants: relationship between breast feeding, early weight gain and neurodevelopment based on results from two cohorts, EPIPAGE and LIFT. BMJ Open 2012;2(2):e000834.

103. Brown JV, Embleton ND, Harding JE, et al. Multi-nutrient fortification of human milk for preterm infants. Cochrane Database Syst Rev 2016;(5):CD000343.

Infant Nutrition in Low-and-Middle-Income Countries

Aamir Javaid, BS[a], Sana Syed, MD, MSCR, MSDS[b],*

KEYWORDS

- Nutrition • Breastfeeding • Infant • Environmental enteropathy
- low-and-middle-income countries

KEY POINTS

- Approximately 144 million (21%) children less than 5 years of age worldwide have faltering linear growth, known as stunting, indicating chronic undernutrition.
- Around 45% of deaths among children less than 5 years of age are linked to undernutrition, mostly in low-and-middle-income countries (LMICs). Simultaneously, rates of childhood obesity are increasing in these countries.
- Optimizing nutrition within the 1,000 days from conception to a child's second birthday, with an emphasis on appropriate breastfeeding practices, increases the likelihood of giving a child the best start to life.
- While traditional metrics of malnutrition have focused on identifying distinct clinical subcategories such as stunting and wasting, a recent shift has been toward understanding the interplay between overlapping clinical phenotypes and the numerous related factors, among them water quality and sanitation, chronic diarrheal illnesses, and the generational consequences of malnutrition.
- Future research directed toward better biomarkers of chronic malnutrition before acute clinical symptoms develop will help direct targeted efforts toward at-risk populations, both through personalized nutritional interventions and structural community-level change.

INTRODUCTION

Malnutrition refers to an imbalance in a person's energy or nutrient intake and can range from undernutrition, overnutrition, and micronutrient-related imbalances. The burden of infant malnutrition, and particularly undernutrition, is greatest in low-and-middle-income countries (LMICs). Since the 1970s, undernutrition has been measured

[a] Department of Medicine, University of Virginia School of Medicine, Charlottesville, VA USA Address: 409 Lane Road, Room 2035B, Charlottesville, VA 22908, USA; [b] Division of Pediatric Gastroenterology and Hepatology, Department of Pediatrics, University of Virginia, 409 Lane Road, Room 2035B, Charlottesville, VA 22908, USA
* Corresponding author.
E-mail address: ss8xj@virginia.edu

Clin Perinatol 49 (2022) 475–484
https://doi.org/10.1016/j.clp.2022.02.011
0095-5108/22/© 2022 Elsevier Inc. All rights reserved.

Abbreviations	
LMICs	Low-and-middle-income Countries
RUTF	Ready-to-Use Therapeutic Food
WHO	World Health Organization
UNICEF	United Nations' Children's Fund
WASH	Water, Sanitation, and Hygiene

by 3 broad phenotypes: stunting (low-height-for-age), wasting (low-weight-for-height or low mid-upper arm circumference), and underweight (low weight-for-age). Children with stunting or wasting have traditionally been treated differently, both with regard to immediate therapeutic approaches and policy-level guidance and financing. Children with wasting are at high risk of short-term mortality which can be acutely corrected with nutritional therapy, whereas stunting reflects long-term nutritional deficiencies more amenable to community-level interventions rather than short-term nutritional corrections.[1]

While these categories have been useful for identifying at-risk populations for under-nutrition, some experts have begun to argue that they draw artificial boundaries which may not capture the full spectrum of undernutrition and related conditions. Children may be born with wasting, stunting, or some combination of the 2 and pass from one state to another throughout their lives.[2,3] Furthermore, current metrics of wasting and stunting may not be adequate for identifying and targeting efforts toward the larger number of children who are at risk for or in the process of becoming undernour-ished. More emphasis is being placed on the complex interplay and numerous factors that influence infant weight or growth faltering, including maternal factors throughout adolescence and pregnancy, epigenetics, and comorbid pathologies such as repeated infections with underlying environmental enteropathy.

In this article, we discuss the epidemiology of infant malnutrition, consensus guide-lines for the management of acute malnutrition, guideline-recommended infant feeding practices, and future areas of research and policy implementation to achieve the Sustainable Development Goal to end all forms of malnutrition by 2030.[4]

EPIDEMIOLOGY OF MALNUTRITION

In 2020, approximately 149 million (22%) children less than 5 years of age worldwide had faltering linear growth, known as stunting, and around 45 million (15%) children had wasting.[5] Overall, the prevalence of stunting has declined over the last 30 years (39.3% in 1990%–22% in 2020), due, in part, to improvements in education, socioeco-nomic status, sanitation, family planning, and access to maternal health services.[6] The number of countries whereby the prevalence of stunting is ≥ 30% has decreased from 67 in 2000 to 33 in 2020, mostly concentrated in sub-Saharan Africa and South Asia. Meanwhile, severe wasting is most prevalent in South Asia, with 25 million children affected (75% of all children with severe wasting).

Infant malnutrition is disproportionately prevalent in LMICs. While less than half of all children less than 5 years of age live in LMICs, nearly two-thirds of all children with stunting and three-quarters of all children with wasting live there.[5] Undernutrition ac-counts for approximately 45% of deaths among children less than 5 years of age.[7]

Approximately 39 million (5.7%) children are overweight, which has been steadily increasing over the last 2 decades. While the relative percentage of overweight chil-dren in LMICs has not changed over the last 2 decades, South-East Asia and Northern

Africa were the only global subregions with a significant increase in the percentage of overweight children since 2000.[5]

DIAGNOSIS AND MANAGEMENT OF ACUTE MALNUTRITION

While acute malnutrition can manifest in many ways and be comorbid with other conditions, it is traditionally defined based on criteria for wasting. Moderate acute malnutrition is defined as a weight-for-height z-score between −2 and −3 or mid-upper arm circumference between 115 and 125 mm while severe acute malnutrition is weight-for-height z-score less than −3 or mid-upper arm circumference less than 115 mm.[8] Moderate acute malnutrition affects approximately 32.7 million children (4.8% of all children less than 5 years of age) worldwide and 14.3 million children suffer from severe acute malnutrition. Moderate and severe acute malnutrition are most prevalent in resource-limited regions of the globe, especially sub-Saharan Africa and South Asia (including Afghanistan, Bangladesh, India, Nepal, and Pakistan).[5]

Severe acute malnutrition can be further categorized into clinical subtypes based on the presence (kwashiorkor) or absence (marasmus) of edema, although mixed clinical phenotypes also occur (referred to as marasmic kwashiorkor). Nonedematous severe wasting, or marasmus, is characterized by:

- Head appearing large relative to the body
- Staring eyes
- Irritable affect
- Emaciated, weak appearance
- Bradycardia, hypotension, hypothermia
- Dry, thin skin
- Shrunken arms, thighs, and buttocks; redundant skin folds caused by loss of subcutaneous fat
- Thin, sparse hair, easily plucked. Intermediate periods of inadequate dietary intake can result in alternating bands of lost hair color and normal pigmentation, known as flag signs.

Edematous severe wasting, or kwashiorkor, is characterized by symmetric bilateral pitting edema that begins in the most dependent regions (presacral, genital, preorbital) and proceeds cranially, with or without anasarca. Muscle atrophy is usually seen, with or without increased body fat. Other features include:

- Apathetic, listless affect
- Rounded prominence of the cheeks ("moon face")
- Pursed mouth
- Thin, dry, peeling skin with confluent areas of hyperkeratosis and hyperpigmentation
- Dry, dull, hypopigmented hair that falls out or is easily plucked
- Distended abdomen, hepatomegaly, dilated intestinal loops
- Bradycardia, hypotension, hypothermia
- Loose inner inguinal skin folds, despite generalized edema

Most international consensus guidelines recommend community-based management of acute malnutrition except in select cases whereby inpatient care is indicated, such as children with no appetite, failure of outpatient therapy, and challenging social situations such as untreated HIV or tuberculosis. Furthermore, most infants less than 6 months are also initially managed inpatient so appropriate breastfeeding counseling can be offered.[8,9]

Community-based management of acute malnutrition entails a decentralized system whereby resources such as high caloric and micronutrient-rich ready-to-use therapeutic food (RUTF) are kept available with counseling provided to caregivers to optimize prevention and prevent relapse. Multiple RUTF formulations exist; the most common is a mixture of peanuts, sugar, oil, and powdered milk with vitamin and mineral supplementation.[10] Feeding protocol is typically at a dose of 175 kcal/kg/d and given in small frequent doses driven by the child's appetite. The only other foods a child should be offered are breast milk and water. Lastly, a brief empiric course of oral antibiotics (usually amoxicillin or cefdinir) is recommended by the World Health Organization (WHO), as children frequently have underlying bacterial infections.[8,11] Children should return for follow-up every 1 to 2 weeks and are considered treated once the weight-for-height z-score becomes ≥ -2 or mid-upper arm circumference ≥ 125 mm with no edema for at least 1 to 2 weeks.[8]

COMMON MICRONUTRIENT DEFICIENCIES IN LOW-AND-MIDDLE-INCOME COUNTRIES

Although all nutrients are necessary for neurodevelopment, the key nutrients essential for early brain growth include vitamins A, D, B6, B12, protein, zinc, iron, choline, folate, iodine, and long-chain polyunsaturated fatty acids. Moreover, supplementation of zinc, iron, and vitamin D are usually necessary during breastfeeding within the first 6 months.[12] See **Table 1** for common micronutrient deficiencies and their symptoms.

Table 1
Signs and symptoms of common micronutrient deficiencies

Micronutrient	Signs/Symptoms of Deficiency
Vitamin A	Dry skin, night blindness, corneal degradation, conjunctival keratinization
Vitamin B1 (thiamine)	Beriberi, Wernicke–Korsakoff syndrome
Vitamin B2 (riboflavin)	Angular stomatitis, cheilitis, corneal vascularization
Vitamin B3 (niacin)	Pellagra (diarrhea, dermatitis, dementia)
Vitamin B5 (pantothenate)	Dermatitis, enteritis, alopecia, adrenal insufficiency
Vitamin B6 (pyridoxine)	Convulsions, irritability, peripheral neuropathy, sideroblastic anemia (always supplement with isoniazid for tuberculosis)
Vitamin B9 (folate)	Glossitis, megaloblastic anemia without neurologic changes
Vitamin B12 (cobalamin)	Megaloblastic anemia with neurologic changes (optic neuropathy, subacute combined degeneration), glossitis,
Vitamin C	Scurvy, swollen gums, anemia, bruising, immunosuppression, poor wound healing
Vitamin D[a]	Rickets, hypocalcemia, tetany
Vitamin E	Hemolytic anemia, posterior column degeneration
Vitamin K	Increased PT, PTT, normal bleeding time
Biotin	Dermatitis, enteritis
Selenium	Cardiomyopathy, impaired macrophage phagocytosis
Zinc[a]	Dysgeusia, impaired wound healing, alopecia, hypogonadism
Iron[a]	Microcytic anemia, fatigue, weakness
Iodine	Hypothyroidism, goiter, fatigue, constipation

[a] indicates commonly associated with exclusively breastfed infants.

THE FIRST 1,000 DAYS

Multiple consensus guidelines recommend optimizing nutrition within the first 1000 days from conception to 2 years of age to ensure children have the best trajectory for a healthy life. The crux of the guidelines is appropriate breastfeeding. It is estimated that more than 820,000 lives of children less than 5 years of age could be saved every year if all children were optimally breastfed in the first 2 years of life.[5] The WHO and United Nations' Children's Fund (UNICEF) recommend 1-6-24 breastfeeding: introduction within the first hour of life, exclusive breastfeeding to 6 months, and continued breastfeeding for up to 24 or more months of age.[5]

Only 44% of infants less than 6 months are exclusively breastfed. Breastfeeding has innumerable benefits for the infant and mother. Early initiation of breastfeeding within the first hour of birth has been shown to reduce newborn mortality, and continued breastfeeding protects the newborn from acquired diarrheal or other illnesses. Breastfed infants are less likely to be overweight or obese than adolescents. Breastfeeding improves IQ, school attendance, and is associated with higher income in adult life.[13,14] Improving child development and reducing health costs through breastfeeding results in economic gains for individual families as well as benefits for national per capita gross domestic product. Breast milk can also be a critical source of energy and nutrient needs during illness and reduces mortality among malnourished children. For mothers, breastfeeding has been associated with a reduced risk of ovarian and breast cancers and helps space pregnancies by preventing ovulation through the lactation amenorrhea method.

The guidelines support complementary feeding starting at 6 months of age. Around this time, the infant's energy and nutritional requirements begin to exceed that provided by breast milk alone, and foods should start to be introduced. Breast milk can provide half or more of a child's energy needs between the ages of 6 and 12 months and one-third of energy needs between 12 and 24 months. The guidelines recommend continuing frequent, on-demand breastfeeding until at least 2 years and, at 6 months, starting with small amounts of food and gradually increasing food consistency and variety. They recommend 2 to 3 meals per day for infants 6 to 8 months old, 3 to 4 meals per day for infants 9 to 23 months of age, with additional 1 to 2 snacks as required. Responsive feeding involves feeding slowly, patiently, encourage children to eat without forcing, and talking to children and maintaining eye contact while feeding. They also encourage the use of fortified foods and vitamin–mineral supplements as needed. During illness, it is recommended to increase fluid intake with increased breastfeeding and offering soft, favorite foods.[5] Unfortunately, few children receive nutritionally adequate and safe complementary foods; in many countries, less than 25% of infants 6 to 23 months of age meet the criteria of dietary diversity and feeding frequency that are appropriate for their age.[5]

In special or difficult circumstances, it is encouraged for mothers and babies to remain together whenever possible and to use the most appropriate feeding options available. Breastfeeding is preferred in almost all circumstances, including low-birth weight and premature infants, malnourished infants, and adolescent mothers. They also recommend continued breastfeeding for infants born to HIV-infected mothers on antiretroviral therapy, exclusively in the first 6 months and then until at least 12 months of age.[5]

BEYOND THE FIRST 1,000 DAYS: CHRONIC DIARRHEAL ILLNESSES AND ENDEMIC MALNUTRITION

Approximately 33% of reproductive age women have anemia and 15% to 20% of all babies are born with low birthweight,[15] suggesting that the causes of endemic malnutrition cannot be solved only through efforts focused on the first 1000 days of life. Emerging research has identified chronic diarrheal illnesses and underlying inflammation as highly prevalent in regions of endemic malnutrition and stunting, as seen in many LMICs.

There were approximately 1.7 billion episodes of early childhood diarrhea in 2016 resulting in around 800,000 deaths.[16–18] While there has been a substantial reduction in diarrheal-related mortality in recent years due to the recognition of the acute symptoms and appropriate treatment with oral rehydration therapy, the long-term consequences of repeated subclinical enteral infections are only beginning to be appreciated.

Environmental enteropathy refers to disorders of chronic intestinal inflammation common among children in low-resource settings exposed to repeated enteral infections. It is associated with malabsorption, increased intestinal permeability, and mucosal and systemic inflammation which can lead to poor vaccine response,[19,20] faltering child growth[21,22] and cognitive development,[23,24] and eventually manifest in a variety of conditions only beginning to be recognized, including obesity, diabetes, and metabolic syndrome later in life.[25–27]

Because environmental enteropathy lacks obvious acute symptoms, there is no consensus definition for diagnosis and the global disease burden is unclear.[17] Smaller studies have demonstrated the prevalence in low resource settings; for example, in a cohort of 200 adults in Zambia, all jejunal biopsies demonstrated some degree of abnormal villous height and crypt depth.[28] Another study of 57 preschool children in India with chronic diarrhea showed 75% of them had abnormal jejunal histology with 66% demonstrating villous atrophy.[29]

The hallmark of environmental enteropathy is small bowel villous blunting on intestinal biopsy; however, such testing is not feasible in most clinical settings and an active area of research is to identify minimally invasive blood, stool, or urine biomarkers. Most current biomarkers are nonspecific, such as markers of intestinal absorptive dysfunction (eg, lactulose, mannitol), barrier dysfunction (eg, alpha-1-antitrypsin), intestinal inflammation (eg, calprotectin), systemic inflammation (eg, TNF-alpha, IL-6), and microbe translocation (eg, LPS), among others.[19,30,31] New molecular tools detecting transcriptomic[32] and metabolomic[33] changes in the gut microbiome are being explored for more sensitive detection of environmental enteropathy and prediction of growth faltering. In a recent study of 42 children with environmental enteropathy in rural Pakistan and 52 undernourished North American controls from birth to 24 months, the Pakistani cohort had duodenal transcriptomic suppression of antioxidant and lipid metabolism genes, induction of antimicrobial response genes, hypermethylation of epithelial metabolism and barrier function genes, and hypomethylation of immune response and cell proliferation. The methylome changes, in particular, are significant because they suggest that the effects of malnutrition may not just be acquired during life but perhaps can even be passed down through successive generations before a baby is even born.[34]

Prevention of environmental enteropathy can be achieved through striving for safe water, sanitation, and hygiene (WASH) practices. The acute consequences of inadequate WASH practices were estimated to cause 13% of deaths among children less than 5 years of age, although the true impact of related endemic malnutrition may be even greater.[18] Low-cost strategies to improve access to safe drinking water include building and improving water supply systems such as wells and applying strategies to purify drinking water such as through water filters. Sanitation efforts to separate human excreta from human contact involve systemic optimization of toilets and waste containment systems, waste transportation through sewers, and final disposal.

Hygiene interventions, some of which have been underscored in the COVID-19 pandemic, include hand washing, proper cooking and storage of food, and specific interventions for the prevention of particular diseases (shoe wearing for soil helminths, face masks for respiratory illnesses, sleeping nets for mosquito-borne illnesses, or animal management for zoonotic diseases).[35]

FUTURE DIRECTIONS

Current definitions of child malnutrition will only detect it once it has progressed to a clear and significant clinical phenotype, while the underlying causes likely had been in effect for months or years beforehand. There is need for increased understanding of the distal factors driving endemic malnutrition and better methods to measure and manage them. Such approaches might involve more specific minimally invasive biomarkers for early manifestations of malnutrition such as environmental enteropathy, greater coordination between interventions targeting malnutrition in children, adolescent women and mothers, and WASH interventions. Future research also aimed at elucidating the interactions between wasting, stunting, and other clinical manifestations of malnutrition may help with the reduction of the associated risks of morbidity and mortality. A more holistic approach to infant malnutrition will aid with the reduction of the short-term consequences as well as help to foster long-term global prosperity so that 1 day we can eliminate malnutrition in all its forms worldwide.[2]

CLINICS CARE POINTS

- Malnutrition refers to an imbalance in a person's energy or nutrient intake and can range between undernutrition, overnutrition, and micronutrient-related imbalances.

- Undernutrition has traditionally been defined by phenotypes of stunting (low-height-for-age) and wasting (low-weight-for-height or low mid-upper arm circumference)

- Acute malnutrition, or wasting, can be further characterized as moderate (weight-for-height z-score between −2 and −3 or mid-upper arm circumference between 115 and 125 mm) and severe (weight-for-height z-score < −3 or mid-upper arm circumference < 115 mm)

- Wasting has been further subdivided into edematous (kwashiorkor) and nonedematous (marasmus) phenotypes

- Management of acute malnutrition is typically handled in the outpatient setting using a community-based management approach through ready-to-use-food administered at 175 kcal/kg/d given in small frequent doses driven by the child's appetite, counseling of caregivers, and weekly to biweekly follow-up until symptoms have resolved for at least 1 to 2 weeks

- Indications for inpatient management include children with no appetite, failure of outpatient therapy, and challenging social situations such as untreated HIV or tuberculosis. Most infants less than 6 months are also initially managed inpatient so appropriate breastfeeding counseling can be offered

- A brief empiric course of oral antibiotics (usually amoxicillin or cefdinir) is typically recommended in acute malnutrition, as children frequently have underlying bacterial infections

- International consensus guidelines focus on nutrition in the first 1000 days from conception to 2 years of age

- Recommended breastfeeding guidelines are 1-6-24: start within 1st hour of birth, exclusive breastfeeding to 6 months, continued breastfeeding for first 24 months

- Complimentary feeding can be initiated after 6 months with continued frequent, on-demand breastfeeding in addition to introducing small amounts of food and gradually increasing food consistency and variety

- Some experts have begun to recognize malnutrition as a spectrum of disorders with potentially overlapping phenotypes that children pass between throughout their lives. The causes may potentially begin even before conception.

- Chronic diarrheal illnesses and subclinical inflammation can cause disorders of the small bowel known as environmental enteropathy and in the long term can lead to stunting and acute malnutrition.

- Water, sanitation, and hygiene (WASH) practices are the best way to prevent environmental enteropathy.

- Future research should be directed toward better understanding the interplay between stunting, wasting, and other manifestations of malnutrition as well as the development of better biomarkers for the measurement and management of the distal causes of malnutrition, including chronic diarrheal illnesses, genomic and transcriptomic patterns, and environmental safety, among others.

DISCLOSURE

The authors have nothing to disclose.

REFERENCES

1. Bergeron G, Castleman T. Program responses to acute and chronic malnutrition: divergences and convergences. Adv Nutr 2012;3(2):242–9.
2. Wells JC, Briend A, Boyd EM, et al. Beyond wasted and stunted—a major shift to fight child undernutrition. The Lancet Child Adolesc Health 2019;3(11):831–4.
3. Schoenbuchner SM, Dolan C, Mwangome M, et al. The relationship between wasting and stunting: a retrospective cohort analysis of longitudinal data in Gambian children from 1976 to 2016. Am J Clin Nutr 2019;110(2):498–507.
4. Sharma D. Achieving sustainable development nutrition targets: the challenge for South Asia. J Glob Health 2020;10(1):010303.
5. Organization WH. UNICEF/WHO/The World Bank Group joint child malnutrition estimates: levels and trends in child malnutrition: key findings of the 2020 edition. 2020.
6. Vaivada T, Akseer N, Akseer S, et al. Stunting in childhood: an overview of global burden, trends, determinants, and drivers of decline. Am J Clin Nutr 2020; 112(Suppl 2):777s–91s.
7. Liu L, Johnson HL, Cousens S, et al. Global, regional, and national causes of child mortality: an updated systematic analysis for 2010 with time trends since 2000. Lancet 2012;379(9832):2151–61.
8. World Health O. Technical note: supplementary foods for the management of moderate acute malnutrition in infants and children 6–59 months of age. Geneva: World Health Organization; 2012.
9. Trehan I, Manary MJ. Management of severe acute malnutrition in low-income and middle-income countries. Arch Dis Child 2015;100(3):283–7.
10. Manary MJ. Local production and provision of ready-to-use therapeutic food (RUTF) spread for the treatment of severe childhood malnutrition. Food Nutr Bull 2006;27(3 Suppl):S83–9.
11. Trehan I, Goldbach HS, LaGrone LN, et al. Antibiotics as part of the management of severe acute malnutrition. N Engl J Med 2013;368(5):425–35.

12. Schwarzenberg SJ, Georgieff MK. Advocacy for improving nutrition in the first 1000 Days to support childhood development and adult health. Pediatrics 2018;141(2).
13. Victora CG, Bahl R, Barros AJ, et al. Breastfeeding in the 21st century: epidemiology, mechanisms, and lifelong effect. Lancet 2016;387(10017):475–90.
14. Rollins NC, Bhandari N, Hajeebhoy N, et al. Why invest, and what it will take to improve breastfeeding practices? Lancet 2016;387(10017):491–504.
15. Resolution WHA65.6. Comprehensive implementation plan on maternal, infant and young child nutrition. Sixty-fifth World Health Assembly Geneva, 21–26 May 2012 Resolutions and decisions, annexes. 2012:12-13.
16. Walker CLF, Rudan I, Liu L, et al. Global burden of childhood pneumonia and diarrhoea. Lancet (London, England) 2013;381(9875):1405–16.
17. GBD 2015 Mortality and Causes of Death Collaborators. Global, regional, and national life expectancy, all-cause mortality, and cause-specific mortality for 249 causes of death, 1980-2015: a systematic analysis for the Global Burden of Disease Study 2015. Lancet 2016;388(10053):1459–544.
18. Water S, Hygiene and Health WHO Team. Water, sanitation, hygiene and health: a primer for health professionals. World Health Organization; 2019.
19. Naylor C, Lu M, Haque R, et al. Environmental enteropathy, oral vaccine failure and growth faltering in infants in Bangladesh. EBioMedicine 2015;2(11):1759–66.
20. Gilmartin AA, Petri WA Jr. Exploring the role of environmental enteropathy in malnutrition, infant development and oral vaccine response. Philos Trans R Soc Lond B Biol Sci 2015;370(1671).
21. Rogawski ET, Bartelt LA, Platts-Mills JA, et al. Determinants and impact of Giardia infection in the first 2 Years of life in the MAL-ED birth cohort. J Pediatr Infect Dis Soc 2017;6(2):153–60.
22. Amour C, Gratz J, Mduma E, et al. Epidemiology and impact of Campylobacter infection in children in 8 low-resource settings: results from the MAL-ED study. Clin Infect Dis 2016;63(9):1171–9.
23. Eppig C, Fincher CL, Thornhill R. Parasite prevalence and the worldwide distribution of cognitive ability. Proc Biol Sci 2010;277(1701):3801–8.
24. Pinkerton R, Oriá RB, Lima AA, et al. Early childhood diarrhea Predicts cognitive Delays in later childhood Independently of malnutrition. Am J Trop Med Hyg 2016;95(5):1004–10.
25. Rogawski ET, Guerrant RL. The burden of enteropathy and "subclinical" infections. Pediatr Clin North Am 2017;64(4):815–36.
26. Guerrant RL, DeBoer MD, Moore SR, et al. The impoverished gut–a triple burden of diarrhoea, stunting and chronic disease. Nat Rev Gastroenterol Hepatol 2013; 10(4):220–9.
27. DeBoer MD, Chen D, Burt DR, et al. Early childhood diarrhea and cardiometabolic risk factors in adulthood: the Institute of nutrition of Central America and Panama nutritional supplementation longitudinal study. Ann Epidemiol 2013; 23(6):314–20.
28. Kelly P, Menzies I, Crane R, et al. Responses of small intestinal architecture and function over time to environmental factors in a tropical population. Am J Trop Med Hyg 2004;70(4):412–9.
29. Mishra OP, Dhawan T, Singla PN, et al. Endoscopic and histopathological evaluation of preschool children with chronic diarrhoea. J Trop Pediatr 2001;47(2): 77–80.
30. Korpe PS, Petri WA Jr. Environmental enteropathy: critical implications of a poorly understood condition. Trends Mol Med 2012;18(6):328–36.

31. Guerrant RL, Leite AM, Pinkerton R, et al. Biomarkers of environmental enteropathy, inflammation, stunting, and Impaired growth in children in Northeast Brazil. PLoS One 2016;11(9):e0158772.

32. Yu J, Ordiz MI, Stauber J, et al. Environmental enteric dysfunction includes a broad spectrum of inflammatory responses and epithelial Repair Processes. Cell Mol Gastroenterol Hepatol 2016;2(2):158–74.e151.

33. Mayneris-Perxachs J, Lima AA, Guerrant RL, et al. Urinary N-methylnicotinamide and β-aminoisobutyric acid predict catch-up growth in undernourished Brazilian children. Sci Rep 2016;6:19780.

34. Haberman Y, Iqbal NT, Ghandikota S, et al. Mucosal genomics implicate lymphocyte activation and lipid metabolism in refractory environmental enteric dysfunction. Gastroenterology 2021;160(6):2055–71.e50.

35. Ngure FM, Reid BM, Humphrey JH, et al. Water, sanitation, and hygiene (WASH), environmental enteropathy, nutrition, and early child development: making the links. Ann New York Acad Sci 2014;1308(1):118–28.

Nutritional Supplements to Improve Outcomes in Preterm Neonates

Mohan Pammi, MD, PhD, MRCPCH[a],*, Ravi M. Patel, MD, MSc[b]

KEYWORDS

- Immunity • Preterm • Necrotizing enterocolitis • Neonate • Nutrition

KEY POINTS

- Strategies to optimize the developing gut microbiome in the preterm infant to decrease the risk of necrotizing enterocolitis (NEC) and improve nutritional outcomes include the use of probiotics, prebiotics, synbiotics, and paraprobiotics.
- Low–to–moderate-certainty evidence suggests that probiotics decrease NEC, mortality, and late-onset sepsis. Absence of a Food and Drug Administration-approved product and quality control are barriers against recommending the routine use of probiotics.
- Among nutrients that enhance immunity or prevent deficiencies, high-certainty evidence is lacking to support the benefits of routine supplementation of most nutrients on short-term or long-term morbidity or mortality in preterm infants.
- Based on data from large, randomized trials, vitamin A may reduce the risk of bronchopulmonary dysplasia (BPD) whereas docosahexaenoic acid supplementation may increase the risk of BPD.
- Based on data from meta-analyses of small trials, zinc supplementation may reduce mortality and arginine supplementation may reduce necrotizing enterocolitis. These findings warrant confirmation in larger studies.

INTRODUCTION

Let food be thy medicine, and medicine thy food

—Hippocrates

Preterm infants are at increased risk of mortality and morbidity.[1–3] Nutrition-related morbidities include poor growth, immune deficiency, nutritional deficiencies, and adverse long-term neurodevelopment, especially in extremely preterm and small-

[a] Section of Neonatology, Department of Pediatrics Baylor College of Medicine & Texas Children's Hospital Houston, TX 77030, USA; [b] Division of Neonatal-Perinatal Medicine, Department of Pediatrics, Emory University School of Medicine and Children's Healthcare of Atlanta, 2015 Uppergate Drive NE, Atlanta, GA 30322, USA
* Corresponding author. 6621, Fannin Street, Houston, TX 77030.
E-mail address: mohanv@bcm.edu

Clin Perinatol 49 (2022) 485–502
https://doi.org/10.1016/j.clp.2022.02.012
0095-5108/22/© 2022 Elsevier Inc. All rights reserved.

for-gestational-age infants.[4–6] Nutritional supplements, therefore, have been used to enhance growth and development, and decrease infection (immune nutrients).[7] In this review, we discuss the evidence supporting the use of nutrients that enhance preterm infants' immune status, optimize the microbiome, improve growth and development, and influence the risk of necrotizing enterocolitis (NEC), sepsis, and other outcomes (**Fig. 1**). NEC is a major cause of mortality (15%–30%) and significant long-term morbidity in preterm infants who survive the first few days after birth.[8,9] NEC is seen in 6% of very low birth weight (VLBW; birth weight <1500 g) infants and it accounts for 1 in 10 neonatal intensive care unit deaths.[9–12] The pathogenesis of NEC is not clear but microbial dysbiosis, formula feeding, and excessive inflammation have been implicated.[12] Furthermore, a clear definition of this disease remains elusive and it likely represents several different diseases with the final outcome of intestinal injury or necrosis.[13] A major endogenous source of infection in late-onset sepsis in the gastrointestinal tract,[14,15] and hence enteral nutrition and immune nutrients may influence the incidence of late-onset sepsis.

Nutrients that Optimize the Intestinal Microbiome

The Intestinal Microbiome in Preterm Infants

Before birth, the fetus is bathed in the amniotic fluid that may not be sterile[16] although uncertainty[17] exists about a fetal microbiome. Rather, the fetal–maternal unit is constantly exposed to microbes and microbial metabolites that may originate from the vagina and mother's gastrointestinal tract including the mouth.[18] The microbial milieu in the meconium of babies may determine the development of sepsis and NEC.[19] La Rosa and colleagues observed an orchestrated, patterned progression of gut microbiota toward an abundance of *Clostridia* with increasing gestational age.[20] Antibiotics, feeding, and mode of delivery caused abrupt shifts in microbiota but did not change this predestined progression. Microbial dysbiosis in the gastrointestinal tract and an exaggerated inflammatory response have been implicated in the development of NEC.[21–23] Excessive toll-like receptor-4 (TLR4) signaling in response to lipopolysaccharides[24,25] and an exaggerated inflammatory response[22,23] in preterm infants have been reported. The microbial dysbiosis theory of NEC is supported by studies demonstrating that NEC cannot be produced in germ free animals.[24,26] In addition, it is supported by an association between early antibiotic use and NEC.[27,28] Other studies comparing gut microbiota in infants with NEC and controls have discussed a Proteobacteria bloom positively associated[29] and anaerobes (especially *Negativicutes*) negatively associated with NEC.[30] In our meta-analyses of microbiome studies in preterm infants evaluating infants with NEC versus controls who did not develop NEC, we

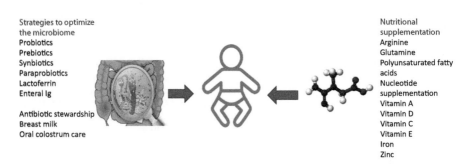

Strategies to optimize the microbiome
Probiotics
Prebiotics
Synbiotics
Paraprobiotics
Lactoferrin
Enteral Ig

Antibiotic stewardship
Breast milk
Oral colostrum care

Nutritional supplementation
Arginine
Glutamine
Polyunsaturated fatty acids
Nucleotide supplementation
Vitamin A
Vitamin D
Vitamin C
Vitamin E
Iron
Zinc

Fig. 1. An overview of nutritional supplements to improve clinical outcomes in preterm infants.

found gradual shifts in the relative abundances of multiple phyla at about 27 weeks corrected gestational age, in which decreased abundances of *Firmicutes* and *Bacteroidetes* and increased abundances of *Proteobacteria* precede the diagnosis of NEC.[31] If microbial dysbiosis is implicated in the development of NEC, then optimization of the microbiome may be a promising strategy in preventing it.

Probiotics. The World Health Organization defines probiotics as "live microorganisms, which when administered in adequate amounts confer a health benefit on the host."[32] A probiotic should be without pathogenic or toxic activity to the host and must have a beneficial effect on the host. Moreover, a probiotic formulation must have genetic stability, remain viable when reaching the colon and colonize the host.[2,10] Probiotics prevent colonization with pathogenic microorganisms by competition with pathogen adhesion, production of antimicrobial substances, improvement in the intestinal mucosal barrier integrity, and immunomodulation (biological plausibility).[11]

In the most recent Cochrane review, by Sharif and colleagues, 56 trials in which 10,812 infants participated were included. Trials varied by the formulation of the probiotics administered, and the most commonly used preparations contained *Bifidobacterium* spp., *Lactobacillus* spp., *Saccharomyces* spp., and *Streptococcus* spp. alone or in combinations. Meta-analysis suggested that probiotics reduce the risk of NEC [RR 0.54, 95% CI 0.45–0.65; 54 trials, 10,604 infants; number needed to treat for an additional beneficial outcome (NNTB) 33, 95% CI 25–50, low certainty of evidence (CoE)]. Sensitivity analysis of trials at low risk of bias suggest a decreased NEC risk (RR 0.70, 95% CI 0.55–0.89; 16 trials, 4597 infants; NNTB 50, 95% CI 33–100, low CoE). Meta-analyses suggested that probiotics reduce mortality (RR 0.76, 95% CI 0.65–0.89; 51 trials, 10,170 infants; NNTB 50, 95% CI 50–100, moderate certainty of evidence), and late-onset invasive infection (RR 0.89, 95% CI 0.82–0.97; 47 trials, 9762 infants; NNTB 50, 95% CI 33–100, moderate certainty of evidence). However, the authors caution clinicians on the low quality of evidence, variations in the formulations used, and the lack of quality control of the formulation.

In a network meta-analysis (NMA), van den Akker and colleagues evaluated 51 trials with 11,231 infants for the strain-specific effects of probiotics.[33] They evaluated 25 different strains, of which 3 demonstrated significant reduction in mortality, 7 reduced NEC, and 2 reduced late-onset sepsis. However, the assessment of treatment effects of individual strains was limited by imprecision in effect estimates, owing to small sample sizes of the included trials. This NMA served as the basis of a conditional recommendation from the European Society for Pediatric Gastroenterology Hepatology and Nutrition Working Group for Probiotics and Prebiotics, based on the low CoE, for two strains to prevent NEC: *Lactobacillus rhamnosus* GG ATCC53103 or *Bifidobacterium infantis* Bb-02, *Bifidobacterium lactis* Bb-12, and *Streptococcus thermophilus* TH-4.[34] Chi and colleagues evaluated the effects of probiotics and synbiotics in an NMA of preterm infants.[35] This NMA included 45 randomized trials with 12,320 participants that evaluated 14 different interventions or placebo. The NMA demonstrated that *Lactobacillus* plus prebiotic, *Bifidobacterium* plus prebiotic, and *Bifidobacterium* plus *Lactobacillus* were each associated with a lower risk of mortality and NEC, compared with the placebo. In addition, *Lactobacillus* plus prebiotic, compared with the placebo, was associated with a lower risk of sepsis.

The clinical report from the American Academy of Pediatrics Committee on Fetus and Newborn concludes poor reporting of adverse effects and the nonavailability of pharmaceutical-grade probiotics as major barriers in recommending the routine use of probiotics.[36] The Canadian Pediatric Society states that there is no evidence for probiotic use in infants weighing less than 1000 g and in infants weighing more than

1000 g administering live microorganisms should be approached with caution.[37] Along with promotion of breastfeeding, probiotics can be considered for the prevention of NEC in preterm infants weighing more than 1 kg who are at risk for NEC.[37,38]

Prebiotics—human milk and non-human synthetic oligosaccharides. Prebiotics are defined as substrates selectively utilized by host microorganisms conferring a health benefit to the host.[39] A prebiotic is a substrate that the host ingests that is not digested in the upper intestinal tract and has the potential to selectively stimulate the growth of beneficial bacteria by fermentation. The fermentation bioproducts have a beneficial effect on the host by reducing the colonic pH, increasing the abundance of short-chain fatty acids (SCFAs), and modulating the immune system.[11]

Human milk oligosaccharides (HMOs) are multifunctional glycans naturally present in human milk. HMOs have great structural diversity and about 15 structures of HMO have been identified.[40] Human milk contains three major types of HMO: neutral, neutral N-containing, and acid; the content of HMOs in human milk varies between women and during stages in lactation.[41] All HMOs are derived from an extension of lactose biosynthesis in the Golgi apparatus of the cell.[42] HMOs are resistant to gastric acid and pancreatic enzymes and are metabolized by microbes in the gut. However, less than 1% of the HMOs are absorbed into the circulation. HMOs by themselves have anti-infective effects by preventing pathogen adhesion, acting as decoy for pathogens and altering the microbiome in the intestine. HMOs are fermented by microbes, producing acetic acid, which reduces the pH in the intestine. HMOs can indirectly increase SCFA production (butyrate and propionate), which are a source of energy for enterocytes and maintain the intestinal barrier function.[40] Nonhuman milk oligosaccharides, which have been manufactured to function in a similar manner to oligosaccharides in breast milk,[43] include neutral short-chain galacto-oligosaccharides (GOS), long-chain fructo-oligosaccharides (FOS), and pectin-derived acidic oligosaccharides. Nonhuman oligosaccharides may have direct effects on the immune system.[43]

Chi and colleagues performed a systematic review of the effects of prebiotics on preterm outcomes including 18 random controlled trials (RCTs) ($n = 1322$).[44] Prebiotics decreased the incidence of sepsis (RR 0.64, 95% CI: 0.51, 0.78), mortality (RR, 0.58, 95% CI: 0.36, 0.94), length of hospital stay [mean difference (MD): –5.18, 95% CI: –8.94, –1.11], and time to full enteral feeding (MD: –0.99, 95% CI: –1.15, 0.83). No significant differences were found in NEC (RR = 0.79, 95% CI: 0.44, 1.44) or feeding intolerance (RR = 0.87, 95% CI: 0.52, 1.45). No adverse effects were reported.

Synbiotics. Synbiotics, a term first introduced by Gibson and Roberfroid in 1995,[45] are "mixtures of probiotics and prebiotics that beneficially affect the host by improving the survival and implantation of live microbial dietary supplements in the gastrointestinal tract, by selectively stimulating the growth and/or by activating the metabolism of one or a limited number of health-promoting bacteria, thus improving host welfare." Synbiotics are believed to act synergistically to increase overall gut health by offering more benefits than the use of either a probiotic or prebiotic agent alone.

In adults, ingestion of synbiotics improved insulin metabolism in patients with type 2 diabetes and symptoms in patients with irritable bowel syndrome and inflammatory bowel disease.[15–17] In children, synbiotics decreased weight in obese patients, improved symptoms of atopic dermatitis, and decreased sepsis and NEC rates in patients with congenital heart disease.[10,18,19]

Four placebo-controlled studies have been reported on the use of synbiotics in preterm infants.[46–49] One study that used a combination of the probiotic B lactis and the prebiotic inulin described a lower incidence of NEC and reduced mortality in both the probiotic and synbiotic study arms, but with no beneficial effects observed in infants administered the prebiotic alone.[46] The synbiotics did not have any additive effect compared with the use of probiotics alone in this trial. Another trial reported that infants administered a synbiotic preparation containing *L. acidophilus*, *Bifidobacterium longum*, *Bifidobacterium bifidum*, *S. thermophiles*, and FOS had a lower incidence and reduced severity of NEC.[47] An RC study of preterm infants weighing more than 1000 g administered a synbiotic preparation containing 8 probiotic strains (mixture of various strains of *Lactobacillus* and *Bifidobacterium*), in combination with FOS, did not show beneficial effects on the severity of NEC, sepsis, or mortality.[48] Another RCT in preterm VLBW infants born at less than or equal to 32 weeks investigated the effects of *Lactobacillus* and *Bifidobacterium* together with oligosaccharides and lactoferrin and found no effects on NEC or sepsis.[49] The NMA by Chi and colleagues provided additional information on prebiotics in combination with probiotics, with findings suggesting that the synbiotic combinations may have greater treatment effectiveness than probiotic supplementation alone.[35] The impact of human milk feeding which contains prebiotics (e.g., oligosaccharides) in combination with probiotics or synbiotics was not evaluated in this review.

Paraprobiotics. One of the challenges of using live microorganisms in extremely preterm infants who may have poor gut barrier and prone to translocation is probiotic-related sepsis. An alternative is using derivatives of probiotics that are not viable and where quality control with nonviable material is stricter.[50] Paraprobiotics (ghost probiotics) are defined as "non-viable microbial cells (intact or broken) or crude cell extracts (i.e., with complex chemical composition), which, when administered (orally or topically) in adequate amounts, confer a benefit on the human or animal consumer."[51] Several methods have been used to inactivate probiotic organism including heat, chemicals (e.g., formalin), gamma or ultraviolet rays, and sonication. Each method may alter the probiotic differently including its effect on the host, and heat inactivated probiotics has been the most studied.[51,52]

Clinical studies comparing nonviable with viable probiotic strains showed similar effects but studies were small, lacked a control group, and used nonstandardized strains.[53] A systematic review of trials of inactivated microbes of probiotic strains, for prevention ($n = 14$) or treatment ($n = 26$) of various diseases, in adults and children compared modified microbes with either placebo (44%) or the same probiotic strain (39%) or standard treatment (17%). Modified microbes were similar to the probiotic group in effectiveness and adverse effects.[52] Meta-analysis of data from 5 RCTs showed significant benefits of modified *L acidophilus* [standard mean difference (SMD): -0.81, 95% CI: -1.44, -0.17] as an adjuvant in treatment of acute diarrhea.[52] To the best of our knowledge, no clinical trials of paraprobiotics have been performed in preterm Infants.

Enteral Lactoferrin supplementation. Lactoferrin is a multifunctional glycoprotein, found in high concentrations in human colostrum, with lower concentrations found in human breast milk, tears, saliva, seminal fluid, vaginal secretions, and joint fluid, and in neutrophil granules.[54] Lactoferrin is protective in animal models of systemic and intestinal infection.[55–57] In an animal model of colitis, lactoferrin reduces intestinal injury and inflammation.[58] The systemic effects of enteral lactoferrin are thought to be indirect and probably are initiated by contact with intestinal epithelial cells and gut-associated lymphoid tissue (GALT). Lactoferrin modulates cytokine and chemokine production by GALT cells, which then enter the systemic circulation and influence circulating leukocytes.[59,60] Lactoferrin receptors on enterocytes modulate cell differentiation and proliferation,[61] making lactoferrin a promising agent for the prevention or treatment of NEC and sepsis in preterm neonates. Lactoferrin may act synergistically with probiotics enhancing their growth and inhibiting the colonization or growth of bacteria that compete with probiotics in the intestinal niche.[62,63]

In a systematic review and meta-analysis of enteral lactoferrin supplementation performed using Cochrane methodology, we identified 13 reports of 12 RCTs that enrolled 5425 preterm infants and evaluated lactoferrin supplementation of enteral feeds compared with placebo.[64] Meta-analysis suggests that enteral lactoferrin decreases culture-positive late-onset sepsis (RR 0.82, 95% CI 0.74–0.91; NNTB 25, 95% CI 17–50; 12 studies, 5425 participants, low CoE) including fungal sepsis (RR 0.23, 95% CI, 0.10, 0.54; NNTB 100, 95% CI 50–100; 6 studies, 3266 participants; low CoE).[64] Lactoferrin supplementation decreased length of hospital stay (mean difference [MD] −2.38 days, 95% CI, −4.67, −0.09: 3 studies, 1079 participants, low CoE). A sensitivity analysis including studies of good methodological quality suggests a decrease in late-onset sepsis with enteral lactoferrin supplementation (RR 0.87 95% CI, 0.78, 0.97: 9 studies, 4702 participants, low CoE). We did not find any differences in NEC stage II or III (typical RR 0.90, 95% CI, 0.69, 1.17; 7 studies, 4874 participants; low CoE) or all-cause mortality (typical RR 0.97, 95% CI 0.79, 1.20; 11 studies, 5510 participants; very low CoE). Ochoa and colleagues found no differences in neurodevelopmental outcomes at 24 months of age by the validated Mullen and Bayley III developmental test (292 participants, low CoE).[65] No adverse effects due to enteral lactoferrin was reported after use in 5425 preterm infants. The optimal timing of prophylaxis (how early after birth), dosage (150–300 mg/kg/d) or the duration of prophylaxis (8 weeks or more) that provides optimal benefit without adverse effects for preterm neonates remains unclear.

Enteral immunoglobulin supplementation for prevention of necrotizing enterocolitis. In early studies in the late 1980s, benefit of enteral immunoglobulin (Ig) preventing NEC was reported. Anti-infective and anti-inflammatory effects of IgA and IgG were proposed mechanisms of action of enteral Ig. Eibl and colleagues reported no NEC in the first 28 days of life in 88 infants (800–2000 g) who received 600 mg/d of human-derived oral IgA-IgG but 6 cases were reported in 91 control infants not receiving treatment ($P = .01$).[66] Rubaltelli and colleagues studied 132 newborns with birth weight less than 1500 g or gestational age less than 34 weeks and reported no cases of NEC in 65 patients in the treatment group (500 mg monomeric IgG orally during the first 2 weeks of life) but 4 cases of NEC in 67 patients in the control group.[67] However, in a multicenter, double-blind, placebo-controlled trial (768 infants to receive human IgG 1200 mg/kg daily and 761 to receive placebo, for up to 28 days), Ig did not reduce the incidence of NEC (43/768 in the intervention group vs 41/768 in the control group).[68]

In an updated Cochrane review, Foster and colleagues in 2016[69] summarized current evidence on enteral Ig from 3 eligible trials (including 2095 neonates). Enteral administration of IgG or an IgG/IgA combination did not result in a significant reduction in the incidence of definite NEC (RR 0.84, 95% CI 0.57–1.25, 3 studies, 1840 infants), suspected NEC (RR 0.84, 95% CI 0.49–1.46; 1 study, 1529 infants), need for surgery (RR 0.21, 95% CI 0.02–1.75; 2 studies, 311 infants) or death from NEC (RR 1.10, 95% CI 0.47–2.59, 3 studies, 1840 infants).

Nutrients that Enhance Immunity or Prevent Deficiencies

Preterm infants miss accretion of nutrients during the final trimester of pregnancy and are often at risk for nutritional deficiencies. Additionally, studies of breastmilk have allowed identification of nutrients that have important immunomodulatory or nutritional beneficial effects. In this section, we review studies of nutrient supplementation to enhance immunity or prevent nutritional deficiencies that have been studied in preterm infants to improve clinical outcomes.

Arginine

Several mechanistic studies have highlighted the importance of the intestinal microcirculation in NEC.[70–72] Arginine is a precursor to nitric oxide, which is important in endothelial vascular regulation and is the most potent vasodilator in the newborn intestine.[73] Arginine has been shown in a proclinical piglet model to protect the intestinal epithelial barrier through nitric oxide-dependent mechanisms.[74] Decreased serum arginine at 7 and 14 days of life has been reported among infants who go on to develop NEC compared with those without NEC.[75] In addition, in a piglet model of NEC, a continuous infusion of L-arginine was shown to reduce intestinal injury, with a decrease in necrosis despite the presence of intestinal inflammation.[76] A Cochrane systematic review and meta-analysis summarized 3 randomized trials (n = 285 neonates) and reported that arginine supplementation reduced the risk of any stage of NEC (RR 0.38; 95% CI 0.23–0.64) and potentially stage 3 NEC (RR 0.13; 95% CI 0.02–1.03), as well as NEC-related death (RR 0.18; 95% CI 0.03–1.00).[77] In this review, there were no significant side effects reported and no significant differences in long-term outcomes, based on data from a single trial that reported long-term follow-up data. Although arginine is a promising treatment to prevent NEC, trials to date have been limited by small sample sizes with imprecision in estimates of effect (low CoE).

Glutamine

Glutamine is an amino acid that is abundant in both blood and human milk.[78] As with arginine, low plasma levels of glutamine at 7 and 14 days after birth have been associated with an increased risk of NEC.[75] In a study of 84 adults needing intensive care, glutamine supplementation in parenteral nutrition improved survival at 6 months (57% vs 29%; P = .049) and in a study of 45 adults receiving bone marrow transplantation, glutamine supplementation in parenteral nutrition reduced clinical infection (P = .04).[79] These studies suggest the potential benefit of glutamine supplementation in critical ill patients. Of note, glutamine is not provided by standard parenteral amino acid solutions. These data were the basis for a pilot study showing that glutamine supplementation increased plasma glutamine concentrations,[80] which was followed by a large, double-masked, multicenter randomized trial conducted by the NICHD Neonatal Research Network (NRN).[81] In this trial, 1433 infants with a birth weight of 401 to 1000 g were randomized to a control amino acid solution (TrophAmine) or a solution with 20% glutamine. Glutamine had no effect on the primary outcome of death or late-onset sepsis (relative risk of 1.07; 95% CI 0.97–1.17), nor did it have any benefit in reducing feeding tolerance, NEC or improving growth. Infants who received glutamine had a longer duration of parenteral nutrition supplementation (32.1 vs 29.8 days; P = .05). A Cochrane systematic review and meta-analysis summarized 12 randomized trials (n = 2877 subjects) that evaluated glutamine supplementation in preterm infants.[82] The review reported no significant evidence that glutamine supplementation reduced the risk of adverse outcomes in preterm infants, with no significant effect on mortality (RR 0.97; 95% CI 0.08–1.17), neurodevelopmental impairment at 18 to 24 months (RR 1.07; 95% CI 0.59–1.92) or invasive infection (RR 0.94; 95% CI 0.86–1.04). These findings do not support the use of glutamine to improve neonatal outcomes.

Polyunsaturated fatty acids

Fatty acids have variable lengths of carbon chains, with different degrees of saturation and location of double bonds. Polyunsaturated fatty acids (PUFAs), particularly long chain omega-3 and omega-6 fatty acids, are named based on the location of these bonds. Long chain PUFAs (LCPUFAs), such as arachidonic acid (AA) and docosahexaenoic acid (DHA), have been shown to accumulate in the brain during intrauterine development.[83] Previous studies have reported differences in DHA and AA in formula versus breast milk,[84] which may be one potential factor that could explain the potential cognitive benefit associated with breastfeeding.[85] In addition, higher DHA levels have been associated with better visual acuity.[86] A Cochrane systematic review and meta-analysis summarized 17 randomized trials ($n = 2260$ subjects) that evaluated LCPUFA supplementation to preterm infants.[87] The review reported no evidence that LCPUFA improved neurodevelopmental outcomes measured using the Bayley Scales of Infant Development Mental Development Index or Psychomotor Developmental Index. In addition, there was no effect on measures of visual acuity. Similar findings were reported for LCPUFA supplementation for term infants.[88] More recently, a large randomized trial evaluated the effect of DHA supplementation on the risk of bronchopulmonary dysplasia (BPD),[89] based on pre-clinical studies showing the effects of DHA on suppression of inflammation,[90] improved lung growth when DHA was supplemented to the mother and increases in surfactant production.[91] This trial showed a higher risk of BPD among infants randomized to enteral DHA supplementation, compared with a control, soy-based emulsion (RR 1.13; 95% CI 1.02–1.25). One limitation was the lack of AA supplementation, in addition to DHA, with some studies and statements suggesting that the ratio of AA:DHA is important.[92,93] These data suggest the need for caution in supplementation of DHA alone to preterm infants and the need for additional studies to determine how the AA:DHA balance might influence important neonatal outcomes.

Nucleotide supplementation

Human milk has a number of nucleotides that have potential gastrointestinal and immunologic effects.[94] The potential immunomodulatory effects of dietary nucleotides are supported by a randomized trial of 370 full-term infants, in which those infants supplemented with nucleotides, chosen based on the pattern of those nucleosides available in human milk, had a greater immune response to vaccination, compared with those infants not supplemented.[95] In term infants, nucleotide supplementation has been shown to increase the rate of weight gain and transiently increase short-term head growth.[96] Nucleotides have been added to some infant formulas since the mid-1980s.[97] However, evidence to demonstrate that nucleotide supplementation reduces morbidity or mortality in preterm infants is lacking. Of note, nucleotides may influence the amounts of some PUFAs[98] but have no effect on 2,3-DPG concentrations.[99]

Iron

Iron is an essential micronutrient for hematopoiesis and brain development, with deficiencies resulting in anemia and linked to neurobehavioral problems.[100,101] Current recommendations in the United States support the intake of at least 2 mg/kg/d of enteral iron through 12 months of age for preterm infants,[102] with similar recommendations of 2 to 3 mg/kg/d by the European Society for Pediatric Gastroenterology, Hepatology, and Nutrition Committee on Nutrition.[103] However, data are scarce from clinical trials to guide recommendations for enteral iron supplementation.[104] In a randomized trial of 2 mg/kg/d of enteral iron supplementation with a multivitamin preparation, compared with a multivitamin alone, there was no effect on the hematocrit at 36 weeks' postmenstrual age, the number of transfusions, BPD, sepsis, medical NEC or surgical NEC in VLBW infants.[105] Another randomized trial of 204 infants with birth weight less than 1301 g compared the effect of early enteral iron supplementation as soon as infants were feeding greater than 100 mL/kg/d of enteral feeding to initiation at 61 days of life.[106] This trial showed no difference in ferritin concentrations at 61 days of life, but a greater proportion of infants with late supplementation, compared to early supplementation, had iron deficiency (40% vs 15%; $P = .0009$) and a greater transfusion volume after 14 days of age (mean of 32 mL/kg vs 16 mL/kg; $P = .002$). A Cochrane systematic review and meta-analysis summarized 26 randomized trials ($n = 2726$ subjects) that evaluated enteral iron supplementation to no supplementation or different regimens of supplementation in preterm infants.[107] The review reported slightly higher hemoglobin levels and iron stores, but no improvement in growth or neurodevelopmental outcomes among infants receiving enteral iron supplementation, compared with no supplementation. A more recent systematic review reported similar findings.[108]

There are some observational studies that report potential concerns with higher doses of enteral iron supplementation. One study of 80 VLBW infants reported an association between higher doses of enteral iron supplementation and a greater abundance of bacteria with functional potential for ferroptosis and epithelial invasion.[109] Another observational study of 598 VLBW infants reported that higher doses of cumulative enteral iron exposure were associated with a higher risk of BPD, although residual confounding was possible.[110] Both of these studies, although at risk for confounding biases, highlight the need for additional studies to determine the optimal dose of iron and the safety of higher doses of enteral iron supplementation.

Zinc

Zinc is a trace element important for the functional activity of a number of proteins in a wide number of metabolic pathways, including those involved in immunity and growth.[111,112] As most of the zinc for a fetus accrues in the third trimester, preterm infants have low zinc stores and may become deficient. A Cochrane systematic review and meta-analysis summarized 5 randomized trials (n = 482 subjects) that evaluated zinc supplementation in preterm infants.[113] Enteral zinc supplementation was associated with decreased all-cause mortality (RR 0.55; 95% CI 0.31–0.97) and improved weight gain, but there was no significant difference in BPD, retinopathy of prematurity (ROP), sepsis, or NEC. A separate study not included in this review of 1154 full-term, small-for-gestational-age infants in India showed micronutrient supplementation that included enteral zinc reduced mortality (rate ratio 0.32; 95% CI 0.12–0.89),[114] providing some additional clinical data on the potential benefits of micronutrient supplementation in high-risk populations. However, the effect in this trial could not be specifically attributed to zinc given other micronutrients were also supplemented. There is currently an ongoing single-center trial of 126 infants evaluating the effect of enteral zinc supplementation on BPD at a single US center (ClinicalTrials.gov Identifier: NCT03532555). These studies suggest the potential benefit of zinc supplementation on mortality although, given the imprecision in estimates and the small size of the trials, additional studies are needed to increase the confidence in the effect estimates of zinc supplementation on mortality in preterm infants.

Vitamin A

Extremely LBW infants have low amounts of plasma and tissue vitamin A,[115] which is associated with the risk of BPD. In a small RCT of 40 very low birth weight infants, intramuscular vitamin A was shown to reduce the risks of BPD,[116] with the intramuscular route resulting in higher plasma vitamin A concentrations compared with the enteral route.[117] These findings were confirmed in a large, multicenter randomized trial of 807 infants conducted by the NRN, in which intramuscular vitamin A injections reduced the risk of BPD (RR 0.89; 95% CI 0.80–0.99).[118] A Cochrane systematic review and meta-analysis summarized 10 randomized trials ($n = 1460$ subjects) and found that vitamin A decreased the risk of BPD but had no effect on long-term outcome based on the follow-up of 1 trial.[119] More recently, a trial of 188 infants evaluated a water-soluble enteral vitamin A formulation and reported no effect on the severity of BPD, evaluated using a shift of the pulse oximeter saturation versus inspired oxygen curve.[120] A secondary analysis of the NRN vitamin A trial suggested that the effect of vitamin A was greater among infants with a lower baseline risk of BPD.[121] One explanation is the attributable fraction of BPD due to vitamin A deficiency might be greater for more mature infants whereas those infants who are more immature with a higher baseline risk of BPD could have a number of other potential etiologies for BPD that would not be modified by vitamin A supplementation. Most US centers do not use vitamin A to prevent BPD[122] despite vitamin A being one of the few medications available that safely prevent BPD.[123]

Vitamin C
Vitamin C is important in tissue repair and immune function and is contained in some infant multivitamin preparations. However, there are limited data on the effect of vitamin C supplementation in preterm infants. One double-blind randomized trial of 56 subjects found no difference in clinical outcomes such as NEC, hemolysis, weight gain or transfusion among infants randomized to vitamin C (50 mg/d), compared with placebo.[124] Another randomized trial of 119 infants who weighed less than 1500 g at birth or at less than 32 weeks' gestation showed no difference in various measures of the severity of lung disease or ROP.[125] Of note, 19% of infants who received higher doses of vitamin C received oxygen at 36 weeks' postmenstrual age, compared with 41% of infants who received lower doses of vitamin C, although this was not statistically significant. Currently, evidence to recommend routine vitamin C supplementation is lacking.

Vitamin D
Vitamin D deficiency can occur in early life and lead to rickets; supplementation of 400 IU/d is now universally recommended to breastfeeding newborns in the United States.[126] Vitamin D deficiency is also common among preterm infants.[127] Among extremely preterm infants, higher doses of up to 1000 IU/d may be needed to maintain serum 25-hydroxy vitamin D (25(OH)D) concentrations above 25 ng/mL, as shown in a randomized trial of 100 infants.[128] However, in this trial, higher doses of vitamin D were not associated with any improvement in neonatal outcomes, including no significant effect on respiratory disease, NEC, intraventricular hemorrhage (IVH), ROP, or infection. Of note, death was increased in infants supplemented with 200 IU/d, but not 800 IU/day, and this may have been a chance finding given the number of secondary outcomes tested. A systematic review of 12 trials found no differences between 800 and 1000 IU/d and 400 IU/d on 25(OH)D concentrations, but higher doses did increase length and head growth and IgA and IgG levels.[129] The European Society of Pediatric Gastroenterology, Hepatology and Nutrition Committee on Nutrition recommends a vitamin D intake of 800 to 1000 IU/d. Although vitamin D deficiency may be associated with respiratory morbidity,[130] there is no clear evidence that supplementation improves respiratory outcomes, such as BPD.

Vitamin E

Deficiency of vitamin E, an antioxidant, has been associated with hemolytic anemia in preterm infants,[131] with a number of early studies evaluating its use in prevention of ROP[132,133] or intracranial hemorrhage.[134,135] However, one concern was the finding of an increased risk of sepsis among infants receiving vitamin E treatment for more than 1 week.[133] These risks and benefits are summarized in a Cochrane systematic review and meta-analysis of 26 randomized trials, with a wide variation in sample sizes and outcomes reported among trials.[136] The meta-analysis showed that vitamin E supplementation had no evidence of effect on mortality before discharge (RR 0.97; 95% CI 0.83–1.14) but increased the risk of sepsis (RR 1.53; 95% CI 1.13–2.08) while reducing the risks of any intracranial hemorrhage (RR 0.85; 95% CI 0.73–0.99) and potentially reducing the risks of severe ROP in a subset of infants who were examined (RR 0.58; 95% CI 0.34–1.00). Of note, there was no effect on severe IVH (RR 0.91; 95% CI 0.60–1.38). Vitamin E supplementation is not widely used, potentially because of the risk of sepsis, along with unclear benefit in reducing severe IVH. A trial of a single dose of vitamin E soon after birth showed some improvement in alpha-tocopherol levels, but inconsistent enough that 30% of supplemented infants had levels below target,[137] and larger such trials have yet to be conducted.

FUNDING

M. Pammi is funded by NIH grants, R03HD098482 and R21HD091718 not related to this review and funders had no role in this manuscript. Ravi Patel discloses funding from the NIH (UG1 HD027851 and K23 HL128942) and serves on the data safety monitoring board of an ongoing trial by Infant Bacterial Therapeutics and Premier Research.

CLINICS CARE POINTS

- Evidence from small trials suggest zinc supplementation may reduce mortality and arginine supplementation may reduce necrotizing enterocolitis but these findings need to be confirmed in well-designed trials with adequate sample sizes.

- Currently, high certainty evidence is lacking for the use of Immunonutrients for use in preterm neonates to decrease the morbidity of NEC or Late-onset sepsis. Low to moderate quality evidence suggests that probiotics decrease NEC, mortality and late-onset sepsis but availability of pharmaceutical grade product is a barrier to routine use. Vitamin A supplementation decreases chronic lung disease or death modestly in VLBW infants but does not improve neurodevelopmental outcomes.

REFERENCES

1. Glass HC, et al. Outcomes for extremely premature infants. Anesth Analg 2015; 120:1337–51.
2. Rysavy MA, et al. Assessment of an Updated neonatal research network extremely preterm birth outcome model in the Vermont oxford network. JAMA Pediatr 2020;174:e196294.
3. Chawla S, et al. Association of neurodevelopmental outcomes and neonatal morbidities of extremely premature infants with differential exposure to antenatal steroids. JAMA Pediatr 2016;170:1164–72.

4. Han J, et al. Associations of early nutrition with growth and body composition in very preterm infants: a prospective cohort study. Eur J Clin Nutr 2022;76(1): 103–10.

5. Ramel SE, Haapala J, Super J, et al. Nutrition, illness and body composition in very low birth weight preterm infants: implications for nutritional management and neurocognitive outcomes. Nutrients 2020;12(1):145.

6. Roggero P, Liotto N, Menis C, et al. New insights in preterm nutrition. Nutrients 2020;12(6):1857.

7. Zhou P, Li Y, Ma LY, et al. The role of immunonutrients in the prevention of necrotizing enterocolitis in preterm very low birth weight infants. Nutrients 2015;7: 7256–70.

8. Neu J, Walker WA. Necrotizing enterocolitis. New Engl J Med 2011;364:255–64.

9. Fanaroff AA, et al. Trends in neonatal morbidity and mortality for very low birthweight infants. Am J Obstet Gynecol 2007;196:147 e141–148.

10. Han SM, et al. Trends in incidence and outcomes of necrotizing enterocolitis over the last 12 years: a multicenter cohort analysis. J Pediatr Surg 2020;55: 998–1001.

11. Jacob J, Kamitsuka M, Clark RH, et al. Etiologies of nicu deaths. Pediatrics 2015;135:e59–65.

12. Lin PW, Stoll BJ. Necrotising enterocolitis. Lancet 2006;368:1271–83.

13. Gordon PV, Swanson JR, MacQueen BC, et al. A critical question for nec researchers: can we create a consensus definition of nec that facilitates research progress? Semin perinatol 2017;41:7–14.

14. Carl MA, et al. Sepsis from the gut: the enteric habitat of bacteria that cause late-onset neonatal bloodstream infections. Clin Infect Dis 2014;58:1211–8.

15. Tarr PI, Warner BB. Gut bacteria and late-onset neonatal bloodstream infections in preterm infants. Semin Fetal Neonatal Med 2016;21:388–93.

16. DiGiulio DB. Diversity of microbes in amniotic fluid. Semin Fetal Neonatal Med 2012;17:2–11.

17. Kennedy KM, et al. Fetal meconium does not have a detectable microbiota before birth. Nat Microbiol 2021;6:865–73.

18. Aagaard K, et al. The placenta harbors a unique microbiome. Sci Translational Med 2014;6:237ra265.

19. Heida FH, et al. A necrotizing enterocolitis-associated gut microbiota is present in the meconium: results of a prospective study. Clin Infect Dis 2016;62:863–70.

20. La Rosa PS, et al. Patterned progression of bacterial populations in the premature infant gut. Proc Natl Acad Sci U S A 2014;111:12522–7.

21. Claud EC, Walker WA. Bacterial colonization, probiotics, and necrotizing enterocolitis. J Clin Gastroenterol 2008;42(Suppl 2):S46–52.

22. Nanthakumar NN, Fusunyan RD, Sanderson I, et al. Inflammation in the developing human intestine: a possible pathophysiologic contribution to necrotizing enterocolitis. Proc Natl Acad Sci U S A 2000;97:6043–8.

23. Nanthakumar N, et al. The mechanism of excessive intestinal inflammation in necrotizing enterocolitis: an immature innate immune response. PLoS One 2011;6:e17776.

24. Afrazi A, et al. New insights into the pathogenesis and treatment of necrotizing enterocolitis: toll-like receptors and beyond. Pediatr Res 2011;69:183–8.

25. Morowitz MJ, Poroyko V, Caplan M, et al. Redefining the role of intestinal microbes in the pathogenesis of necrotizing enterocolitis. Pediatrics 2010;125: 777–85.

26. Musemeche CA, Kosloske AM, Bartow SA, et al. Comparative effects of ischemia, bacteria, and substrate on the pathogenesis of intestinal necrosis. J Pediatr Surg 1986;21:536–8.
27. Cotten CM, et al. Prolonged duration of initial empirical antibiotic treatment is associated with increased rates of necrotizing enterocolitis and death for extremely low birth weight infants. Pediatrics 2009;123:58–66.
28. Alexander VN, Northrup V, Bizzarro MJ. Antibiotic exposure in the newborn intensive care unit and the risk of necrotizing enterocolitis. J Pediatr 2011;159: 392–7.
29. Torrazza RM, Neu J. The altered gut microbiome and nocrotizing enterocolitis. Clin Perinatol 2013;40:93–108.
30. Warner BB, et al. Gut bacteria dysbiosis and necrotising enterocolitis in very low birthweight infants: a prospective case-control study. Lancet 2016;387(10031): 1928–36.
31. Pammi M, et al. Intestinal Dysbiosis in preterm infants preceding necrotizing enterocolitis: a systematic review and meta-analysis. Microbiome 2017;5:31.
32. (WHO)., F. a. A. O. F. W. H. O.. Guidelines for the evaluation of probiotics in food: report of a joint fao/whoworking group on drafting guidelines for the evaluation of probiotics in food 2002. 2002. Available at: https://www.who.int/foodsafety/fs_management/en/probiotic_guidelines.pdf.
33. van den Akker CHP, et al. Probiotics for preterm infants: a strain-specific systematic review and network meta-analysis. J Pediatr Gastroenterol Nutr 2018; 67:103–22.
34. van den Akker CHP, et al. Probiotics and preterm infants: a position paper by the European Society for Paediatric Gastroenterology Hepatology and Nutrition Committee on Nutrition and the European Society for Paediatric Gastroenterology Hepatology and Nutrition working group for probiotics and prebiotics. J Pediatr Gastroenterol Nutr 2020;70:664–80.
35. Chi C, et al. Effects of probiotics in preterm infants: a network meta-analysis. Pediatrics 2021;147.
36. Poindexter B. Use of probiotics in preterm infants. Pediatrics 2021;147.
37. Marchand V. Using probiotics in the paediatric population. Paediatr Child Health 2012;17:575–6.
38. Marchand V, Canadian Paediatric Society, N. a. G. C.. Using probiotics in the paediatric population. Position statement of the Canadian paediatric society. 2019. Available at: https://www.cps.ca/en/documents/position/probiotics-in-the-paediatric-population.
39. Gibson GR, et al. Expert consensus document: the international scientific association for probiotics and prebiotics (isapp) consensus statement on the definition and scope of prebiotics. Nat Rev Gastroenterol Hepatol 2017;14:491–502.
40. Wiciński M, Sawicka E, Gębalski J, et al. Human milk oligosaccharides: health benefits, potential applications in infant formulas, and pharmacology. Nutrients 2020;12.
41. Bode L. Human milk oligosaccharides: every baby needs a sugar mama. Glycobiology 2012;22:1147–62.
42. Bode L. The functional biology of human milk oligosaccharides. Early Hum Dev 2015;91:619–22.
43. Eiwegger T, et al. Prebiotic oligosaccharides: in vitro evidence for gastrointestinal epithelial transfer and immunomodulatory properties. Pediatr Allergy Immunol 2010;21:1179–88.

44. Chi C, Buys N, Li C, et al. Effects of prebiotics on sepsis, necrotizing enterocolitis, mortality, feeding intolerance, time to full enteral feeding, length of hospital stay, and stool frequency in preterm infants: a meta-analysis. Eur J Clin Nutr 2019;73:657–70.

45. Gibson GR, Roberfroid MB. Dietary modulation of the human colonic microbiota: introducing the concept of prebiotics. J Nutr 1995;125:1401–12.

46. Dilli D, et al. The propre-save study: effects of probiotics and prebiotics alone or combined on necrotizing enterocolitis in very low birth weight infants. J Pediatr 2015;166:545–51, e541.

47. Sreenivasa B, Kumar PS, Suresh Babu MT, et al. Role of synbiotics in the prevention of necrotizing enterocolitis in preterm neonates: a randomized controlled trial. Int J Contemp Pediatr 2015;2:127–30.

48. Nandhini LP, et al. Synbiotics for decreasing incidence of necrotizing enterocolitis among preterm neonates - a randomized controlled trial. J Matern Fetal Neonatal Med 2016;29:821–5.

49. Serce Pehlevan O, Benzer D, Gursoy T, et al. Synbiotics use for preventing sepsis and necrotizing enterocolitis in very low birth weight neonates: a randomized controlled trial. Clin Exp Pediatr 2020;63:226–31.

50. Deshpande G, Athalye-Jape G, Patole S. Para-probiotics for preterm neonates-the next frontier. Nutrients 2018;10.

51. Taverniti V, Guglielmetti S. The immunomodulatory properties of probiotic microorganisms beyond their viability (ghost probiotics: proposal of paraprobiotic concept). Genes Nutr 2011;6:261–74.

52. Zorzela L, Ardestani SK, McFarland LV, et al. Is there a role for modified probiotics as beneficial microbes: a systematic review of the literature. Benef Microbes 2017;8:739–54.

53. Lahtinen SJ. Probiotic viability - does it matter? Microb Ecol Health Dis 2012;23.

54. Legrand D. Overview of lactoferrin as a natural immune modulator. J Pediatr 2016;173(Suppl):S10–5.

55. Venkatesh MP, Pham D, Kong L, et al. Prophylaxis with lactoferrin, a novel antimicrobial agent, in a neonatal rat model of coinfection. Adv Ther 2007;24: 941–54.

56. Zagulski T, Lipinski P, Zagulska A, et al. Lactoferrin can protect mice against a lethal dose of escherichia coli in experimental infection in vivo. Br J Exp Pathol 1989;70:697–704.

57. Edde L, et al. Lactoferrin protects neonatal rats from gut-related systemic infection. Am J Physiol 2001;281:G1140–50.

58. Togawa J, et al. Lactoferrin reduces colitis in rats via modulation of the immune system and correction of cytokine imbalance. Am J Physiol Gastrointest Liver Physiol 2002;283:G187–95.

59. Bellamy W, Takase M, Wakabayashi H, et al. Antibacterial spectrum of lactoferricin b, a potent bactericidal peptide derived from the n-terminal region of bovine lactoferrin. J Appl Bacteriol 1992;73:472–9.

60. Tomita M, Takase M, Wakabayashi H, et al. Antimicrobial peptides of lactoferrin. Adv Exp Med Biol 1994;357:209–18.

61. Buccigrossi V, et al. Lactoferrin induces concentration-dependent functional modulation of intestinal proliferation and differentiation. Pediatr Res 2007;61: 410–4.

62. Strunk T, et al. Probiotics and antimicrobial protein and peptide levels in preterm infants. Acta Paediatr 2017;106(11):1747–53.

63. Chen PW, Liu ZS, Kuo TC, et al. Prebiotic effects of bovine lactoferrin on specific probiotic bacteria. Biometals 2017;30:237–48.
64. Pammi M, Suresh G. Enteral lactoferrin supplementation for prevention of sepsis and necrotizing enterocolitis in preterm infants. Cochrane database Syst Rev 2020;3:Cd007137.
65. Ochoa TJ, et al. Randomized controlled trial of bovine lactoferrin for prevention of sepsis and neurodevelopment impairment in infants weighing less than 2000 grams. J Pediatr 2020;219:118–25.e5.
66. Eibl MM, Wolf HM, Fürnkranz H, et al. Prevention of necrotizing enterocolitis in low-birth-weight infants by iga-igg feeding. New Engl J Med 1088;319·1–7.
67. Rubaltelli FF, Benini F, Sala M. Prevention of necrotizing enterocolitis in neonates at risk by oral administration of monomeric Igg. Dev Pharmacol Ther 1991;17: 138–43.
68. Lawrence G, et al. Enteral human igg for prevention of necrotising enterocolitis: a placebo-controlled, randomised trial. Lancet (London, England) 2001;357: 2090–4.
69. Foster JP, Seth R, Cole MJ. Oral immunoglobulin for preventing necrotizing enterocolitis in preterm and low birth weight neonates. Cochrane database Syst Rev 2016;4:Cd001816.
70. Downard CD, et al. Altered intestinal microcirculation is the critical event in the development of necrotizing enterocolitis. J Pediatr Surg 2011;46:1023–8.
71. Yazji I, et al. Endothelial tlr4 activation impairs intestinal microcirculatory perfusion in necrotizing enterocolitis via enos-no-nitrite signaling. Proc Natl Acad Sci U S A 2013;110:9451–6.
72. Watkins DJ, Besner GE. The role of the intestinal microcirculation in necrotizing enterocolitis. Semin Pediatr Surg 2013;22:83–7.
73. Nair J, Lakshminrusimha S. Role of no and other vascular mediators in the etiopathogenesis of necrotizing enterocolitis. Front Biosci (Schol Ed) 2019;11:9–28.
74. Chapman JC, Liu Y, Zhu L, et al. Arginine and citrulline protect intestinal cell monolayer tight junctions from hypoxia-induced injury in piglets. Pediatr Res 2012;72:576–82.
75. Becker RM, et al. Reduced serum amino acid concentrations in infants with necrotizing enterocolitis. J Pediatr 2000;137:785–93.
76. Di Lorenzo M, Bass J, Krantis A. Use of l-arginine in the treatment of experimental necrotizing enterocolitis. J Pediatr Surg 1995;30:235–40, discussion 240-231.
77. Shah PS, Shah VS, Kelly LE. Arginine supplementation for prevention of necrotising enterocolitis in preterm infants. Cochrane database Syst Rev 2017;4. CD004339.
78. Bulus N, Cersosimo E, Ghishan F, et al. Physiologic importance of glutamine. Metabolism 1989;38:1–5.
79. ziegler t r, et al. Clinical and metabolic efficacy of glutamine-supplemented parenteral nutrition after bone marrow transplantation. a randomized, double-blind, controlled study. Ann Intern Med 1992;116:821–8.
80. Poindexter BB, et al. Effect of parenteral glutamine supplementation on plasma amino acid concentrations in extremely low-birth-weight infants. Am J Clin Nutr 2003;77:737–43.
81. Poindexter BB, et al. Parenteral glutamine supplementation does not reduce the risk of mortality or late-onset sepsis in extremely low birth weight infants. Pediatrics 2004;113:1209–15.

82. Moe-Byrne T, Brown JV, McGuire W. Glutamine supplementation to prevent morbidity and mortality in preterm infants. Cochrane database Syst Rev 2016; 4:CD001457.
83. Clandinin MT, et al. Intrauterine fatty acid accretion rates in human brain: implications for fatty acid requirements. Early Hum Dev 1980;4:121–9.
84. Clark KJ, Makrides M, Neumann MA, et al. Determination of the optimal ratio of linoleic acid to alpha-linolenic acid in infant formulas. J Pediatr 1992;120: S151–8.
85. Lucas A, Morley R, Cole TJ, et al. Breast milk and subsequent intelligence quotient in children born preterm. Lancet 1992;339:261–4.
86. Makrides M, Simmer K, Goggin M, et al. Erythrocyte docosahexaenoic acid correlates with the visual response of healthy, term infants. Pediatr Res 1993;33: 425–7.
87. Moon K, Rao SC, Schulzke SM, et al. Longchain polyunsaturated fatty acid supplementation in preterm infants. Cochrane database Syst Rev 2016;12: CD000375.
88. Jasani B, Simmer K, Patole SK, et al. Long chain polyunsaturated fatty acid supplementation in infants born at term. Cochrane database Syst Rev 2017;3: CD000376.
89. Collins CT, et al. Docosahexaenoic acid and bronchopulmonary dysplasia in preterm infants. N Engl J Med 2017;376:1245–55.
90. Serhan CN, Chiang N, Van Dyke TE. Resolving inflammation: dual anti-inflammatory and pro-resolution lipid mediators. Nat Rev Immunol 2008;8: 349–61.
91. Blanco PG, et al. Oral docosahexaenoic acid given to pregnant mice increases the amount of surfactant in lung and amniotic fluid in preterm fetuses. Am J Obstet Gynecol 2004;190:1369–74.
92. Akinsulire O, et al. Early enteral administration of a complex lipid emulsion supplement prevents postnatal deficits in docosahexaenoic and arachidonic acids and increases tissue accretion of lipophilic nutrients in preterm piglets. JPEN J Parenter enteral Nutr 2020;44:69–79.
93. Koletzko B, et al. Should formula for infants provide arachidonic acid along with dha? a position paper of the european academy of paediatrics and the child health foundation. Am J Clin Nutr 2020;111:10–6.
94. Yu VY. Scientific rationale and benefits of nucleotide supplementation of infant formula. Paediatr Child Health 2002;38:543–9.
95. Pickering LK, et al. Modulation of the immune system by human milk and infant formula containing nucleotides. Pediatrics 1998;101:242–9.
96. Wang L, Mu S, Xu X, et al. Effects of dietary nucleotide supplementation on growth in infants: a meta-analysis of randomized controlled trials. Eur J Nutr 2019;58:1213–21.
97. Carver JD, Stromquist CI. Dietary nucleotides and preterm infant nutrition. J Perinatol 2006;26:443–4.
98. Wang L, Liu J, Lv H, et al. Effects of nucleotides supplementation of infant formulas on plasma and erythrocyte fatty acid composition: a meta-analysis. PLoS One 2015;10:e0127758.
99. Scopesi F, et al. Lack of effect of dietary nucleotide supplementation on erythrocyte 2,3-diphosphoglycerate concentration. a study on preterm neonates. J Matern Fetal Neonatal Med 2006;19:343–6.
100. Georgieff MK. Iron assessment to protect the developing brain. Am J Clin Nutr 2017;106:1588S–93S.

101. Rao R, Georgieff MK. Iron therapy for preterm infants. Clin Perinatol 2009;36: 27–42.

102. Baker RD, Greer FR, Committee on Nutrition American Academy of P. Diagnosis and prevention of iron deficiency and iron-deficiency anemia in infants and young children (0-3 years of age). Pediatrics 2010;126:1040–50.

103. Agostoni C, et al. Enteral nutrient supply for preterm infants: commentary from the european society of paediatric gastroenterology, hepatology and nutrition committee on nutrition. J Pediatr Gastroenterol Nutr 2010;50:85–91.

104. Buchanan GR, Paucity of clinical trials in iron deficiency: lessons learned from study of vlbw infants. Pediatrics 2013;131:e582–4.

105. Taylor TA, Kennedy KA. Randomized trial of iron supplementation versus routine iron intake in vlbw infants. Pediatrics 2013;131:e433–8.

106. Franz AR, Mihatsch WA, Sander S, et al. Prospective randomized trial of early versus late enteral iron supplementation in infants with a birth weight of less than 1301 grams. Pediatrics 2000;106:700–6.

107. Mills RJ, Davies MW. Enteral iron supplementation in preterm and low birth weight infants. Cochrane Database Syst Rev 2012;3:CD005095.

108. McCarthy EK, Dempsey EM, Kiely ME. Iron supplementation in preterm and low-birth-weight infants: a systematic review of intervention studies. Nutr Rev 2019; 77:865–77.

109. Ho T, Sarkar A, Szalacha L, et al. Intestinal microbiome in preterm infants influenced by enteral iron dosing. J Pediatr Gastroenterol Nutr 2021;72:e132–8.

110. Patel RM, et al. Enteral iron supplementation, red blood cell transfusion, and risk of bronchopulmonary dysplasia in very-low-birth-weight infants. Transfusion 2019;59:1675–82.

111. Terrin G, et al. Zinc in early life: a key element in the fetus and preterm neonate. Nutrients 2015;7:10427–46.

112. Vallee BL, Auld DS. Zinc coordination, function, and structure of zinc enzymes and other proteins. Biochemistry 1990;29:5647–59.

113. Staub E, Evers K, Askie LM. Enteral zinc supplementation for prevention of morbidity and mortality in preterm neonates. Cochrane database Syst Rev 2021;3:CD012797.

114. Sazawal S, et al. Zinc supplementation in infants born small for gestational age reduces mortality: a prospective, randomized, controlled trial. Pediatrics 2001; 108:1280–6.

115. Shenai JP, Chytil F, Stahlman MT. Liver vitamin a reserves of very low birth weight neonates. Pediatr Res 1985;19:892–3.

116. Shenai JP, Kennedy KA, Chytil F, et al. Clinical trial of vitamin a supplementation in infants susceptible to bronchopulmonary dysplasia. J Pediatr 1987;111: 269–77.

117. Rush MG, Shenai JP, Parker RA, et al. Intramuscular versus enteral vitamin a supplementation in very low birth weight neonates. J Pediatr 1994;125:458–62.

118. Tyson JE, et al. Vitamin a supplementation for extremely-low-birth-weight infants. national institute of child health and human development neonatal research network. N Engl J Med 1999;340:1962–8.

119. Darlow BA, Graham PJ, Rojas-Reyes MX. Vitamin A supplementation to prevent mortality and short- and long-term morbidity in very low birth weight infants. Cochrane Database Syst Rev 2016;8:CD000501.

120. Rakshasbhuvankar AA, et al. Enteral vitamin a for reducing severity of bronchopulmonary dysplasia: a randomized trial. Pediatrics 2021;147.

121. Rysavy MA, et al. Should vitamin a injections to prevent bronchopulmonary dysplasia or death be reserved for high-risk infants? reanalysis of the national institute of child health and human development neonatal research network randomized trial. J Pediatr 2021;236:78–85.e5.

122. Tolia VN, Murthy K, McKinley PS, et al. The effect of the national shortage of vitamin a on death or chronic lung disease in extremely low-birth-weight infants. JAMA Pediatr 2014;168:1039–44.

123. Jensen EA, Foglia EE, Schmidt B. Evidence-based pharmacologic therapies for prevention of bronchopulmonary dysplasia: application of the grading of recommendations assessment, development, and evaluation methodology. Clin Perinatol 2015;42:755–79.

124. Doyle J, et al. Does Vitamin C cause hemolysis in premature newborn infants? results of a multicenter double-blind, randomized, controlled trial. J Pediatr 1997;130:103–9.

125. Darlow BA, et al. Vitamin C supplementation in very preterm infants: a randomised controlled trial. Arch Dis Child Fetal Neonatal Ed 2005;90:F117–22.

126. Wagner CL, Greer FR, American Academy of Pediatrics Section on, B., American Academy of Pediatrics Committee on, N. Prevention of rickets and vitamin D deficiency in infants, children, and adolescents. Pediatrics 2008;122:1142–52.

127. Monangi N, Slaughter JL, Dawodu A, et al. Vitamin D status of early preterm infants and the effects of vitamin d intake during hospital stay. Arch Dis Child Fetal Neonatal Ed 2014;99:F166–8.

128. Fort P, et al. A comparison of 3 vitamin d dosing regimens in extremely preterm infants: a randomized controlled trial. J Pediatr 2016;174:132–138 e131.

129. Yang Y, Li Z, Yan G, et al. Effect of different doses of vitamin d supplementation on preterm infants - an updated meta-analysis. J Matern Fetal Neonatal Med 2018;31:3065–74.

130. Golan-Tripto I, et al. The effect of vitamin d administration on vitamin d status and respiratory morbidity in late premature infants. Pediatr Pulmonol 2020;55:3080–7.

131. Carey AN, Duggan C. 50 years ago in the journal of pediatrics: vitamin e deficiency: a previously unrecognized cause of hemolytic anemia in the premature infant. J Pediatr 2017;181:162.

132. Phelps DL, Rosenbaum AL, Isenberg SJ, et al. Tocopherol efficacy and safety for preventing retinopathy of prematurity: a randomized, controlled, double-masked trial. Pediatrics 1987;79:489–500.

133. Johnson L, et al. Effect of sustained pharmacologic vitamin e levels on incidence and severity of retinopathy of prematurity: a controlled clinical trial. J Pediatr 1989;114:827–38.

134. Fish WH, Cohen M, Franzek D, et al. Effect of intramuscular vitamin E on mortality and intracranial hemorrhage in neonates of 1000 grams or less. Pediatrics 1990;85:578–84.

135. Speer ME, et al. Intraventricular hemorrhage and vitamin e in the very low-birth-weight infant: evidence for efficacy of early intramuscular vitamin E administration. Pediatrics 1984;74:1107–12.

136. Brion LP, Bell EF, Raghuveer TS. Vitamin E supplementation for prevention of morbidity and mortality in preterm infants. Cochrane Database Syst Rev 2003;4:CD003665.

137. Bell EF, et al. Serum tocopherol levels in very preterm infants after a single dose of vitamin E at birth. Pediatrics 2013;132:e1626–33.

Evidence-Based Approaches to Successful Oral Feeding in Infants with Feeding Difficulties

Kathryn A. Hasenstab, BS BME[a,b],
Sudarshan R. Jadcherla, MD, FRCPI, DCH, AGAF[a,b,c,d,e],*

KEYWORDS

- Infant • Neonate • Feeding difficulties • Dysphagia • Swallowing • Gastrostomy
- Gavage

KEY POINTS

- Evaluation of the infant, parent, and provider triad can identify and distinguish root causes of feeding difficulties as a process measure and/or a swallowing skill deficit.
- Evidence-based feeding process assessments may include clinical history and examination, 5-day feeding diary, and cue-based feeding and feeding quality scales.
- Evidence-based assessments specific to infant physiology and pathophysiology should be individualized and dependent on suspected phases (oral, pharyngo-esophageal, gastric/intestinal, cross-system regulation) of swallowing dysfunction
- Superior feeding outcomes are possible using evidence-based management approaches targeting process optimization and individualized therapies (oro-motor stimulation, manipulation of hunger and gut motility, effective comorbidity management, and education).

Abbreviations	
LOHS	length of hospital stay
NICU	neonatal intensive care unit
PMA	postmenstrual age
HRM	high resolution manometry
GERD	gastroesophageal reflux disease

[a] Innovative Infant Feeding Disorders Research Program, Nationwide Children's Hospital, 700 Children's Drive, Columbus, OH 43205, USA; [b] Center for Perinatal Research, The Research Institute at Nationwide Children's Hospital, 575 Children's Crossroads, Columbus, OH 43215, USA; [c] Division of Neonatology, Nationwide Children's Hospital, 700 Children's Drive, Columbus, OH 43205, USA; [d] Division Pediatric Gastroenterology, Hepatology and Nutrition, Department of Pediatrics, Nationwide Children's Hospital, 700 Children's Drive, Columbus, OH 43205, USA; [e] Department of Pediatrics, The Ohio State University College of Medicine, 370 W 9th Ave, Columbus, OH 43210, USA
* Corresponding author. 575 Children's Crossroads, Columbus, OH 43215.
E-mail address: Sudarshan.Jadcherla@nationwidechildrens.org

Clin Perinatol 49 (2022) 503–520
https://doi.org/10.1016/j.clp.2022.02.004
0095-5108/22/© 2022 Elsevier Inc. All rights reserved.

INTRODUCTION

Parental and provider expectations for healthy full term-born infants are independent oral feeding while keeping the length of hospital stay (LOHS) as short as possible. Mothers also expect to be discharged with their baby. However, all these expectations are hard to realize in the event of high-risk pregnancy and childbirth or on admission to the neonatal intensive care unit (NICU). Per the American Academy of Pediatrics, hospital stay is based on the mother–infant dyad to endure adequate maternal recovery, infant stability, and ability/confidence of care for both self and newborn.[1] Complicated NICU admissions and/or preterm births require additional time for airway-digestive support, maintenance of homeostasis, and for the development of safe feeding and breathing strategies for discharge. Therefore, extended stay in the NICU is expected, and is dependent on gestational age at birth, neuropathology, cardiopulmonary illness, digestive pathologies, and congenital anomalies; each of these pathologies adds to the LOHS.[2] Contrary to expectations, independent oral feeding in such high-risk neonates may not be achievable in a defined time period owing to numerous factors complicating feeding. Hence, short- or long-term nutritional support via chronic tube is increasing with prevalence up to 20% in NICU infants.[3–6] Estimated cost of gastrostomy at discharge is approximately $47,000 the first year and $180,000 over 5 years per infant.[7] Additional common surgical procedures elevating costs may include fundoplication and/or tracheostomy. Fundoplication prevalence is approximately 12% varying from 0% to 64%[8] and is commonly performed at the time of gastrostomy, but remains controversial with the lack of objective assessment. Tracheostomy may also be performed as a consequence of recurrent pneumonia and failure of aero-digestive protective mechanisms, but may also be implicated in dysfunctional swallowing mechanics and dysphagia,[9–11] while increasing parental stress and altering social interactions.[12]

Infants with feeding difficulties may present with acute symptoms such as apnea/bradycardia/desaturation, coughing/choking/gagging, arching, emesis, and irritability/crying, poor endurance, or stridor during feeding. If acute symptoms are not attended to, more troublesome and chronic symptoms may develop including failure to thrive, feeding intolerance, early satiety, pneumonia, and oral aversion. All these symptoms have the potential to negatively impact timely feeding milestones, infant nutrition, growth, and neurodevelopment. Extreme cases may result in death or severe morbidities. Managing infants with feeding difficulties is complex owing to the heterogeneity of patient-, parent-, provider-, and practice characteristics. This article will review evidence-based approaches to attain successful oral feeding milestones in infants with feeding difficulties. Specifically addressed topics are: (1) definitions including distinguishing feeding difficulties as a process measure and swallowing disorders as a skill deficit, (2) potential mechanisms and evidence-based assessments of infant feeding difficulties, and (3) and evidence-based approaches to infant feeding high-risk NICU infants.

DEFINITIONS

Although the terminology used in describing the "feeding-related problems" can be vague and not universally applied, common base definitions are important to consider in the context of infant feeding so as to apply appropriate diagnostic skills (**Box 1**). Almost all infants with swallowing disorders have feeding difficulties, but not all infants with feeding difficulties have swallowing disorders (**Fig. 1**). Therefore, it is critical for providers to distinguish between *feeding difficulties (a process measure) vs swallowing disorders (a skill deficit)* which may be assessed via thorough general, systemic and feeding-focused clinical evaluation and questioning, and/or specialized, instrumental testing if required.

Box 1
Common terminologies and definitions of infant feeding difficulties

Feeding difficulties: Troublesome symptoms or inadequate oral intake during infant feeding. This may be related to the actual act of feeding, feedings, or the feeding process.

- *Eating:* the act of ingesting nutrients
- *Feeding (used as a verb):* any aspect of the actual feeding process between the parent/caregiver and infant.
  - ⌐ Parent/provider: preparation, method of administration, and infant's feeding skills.
  - ○ Infant: Feeding Skills (See Swallowing Difficulty later in discussion)
- *Feedings (used as a noun):* refers to the nutrients offered to promote growth
- *Feeding milestones*[13]: Timely feeding targets for optimal growth and development

Milestone	Definition	On-Time Target
Trophic Feeding	Minute volumes of enteral tube feeding for gut priming: dependent on age, morbidities, and acuity level	10–20 mL/kg/d within 3 d of admission and continued for a duration of 3–5 d overall
Full Enteral Feeding	Sufficient gastrointestinal tract feeding volume via tube feeding as a primary source of nutrition	Enteral gavage feeding of at least 120 mL/kg/d by 2–4 wk of life and increasing, with less dependence on IV nutrition
First Oral Feeding	First oral offering	At least by 33–34 wk postmenstrual age based on infant cues
Full Oral Feeding	Sustained oral intake of at least 120 mL/kg/d as primary source of nutrition	By 36–38 wk postmenstrual age of at least 120 mL/kg/d and increasing
Ad lib Oral Feeding	Oral feeding whenever infant exhibits feeding readiness cues	By full-term PMA and/or at hospital discharge, typically oral intake > 150 mL/kg/d, and increasing, thus favoring positive growth trends

- *Tube feeding:* gavage, nasogastric, orogastric, transpyloric, gastrostomy
- *Swallowing difficulties:* A skill deficit during any phase of swallowing
- *Nutritive sucking:* Rhythmic oral expression (suction) and tongue compression to transport fluid bolus from the oral cavity into the pharynx
- *Swallowing:* Anterograde bolus movement from the oral cavity through the pharyngo-esophageal segment and into the stomach
- *Suck-swallow-breathe coordination:* Rhythmic brief oral sucks, pharyngeal contractions, and deglutition apneas associated with bolus clearance resulting in the absence of symptoms
- *Swallowing Phases During Infant Feeding*
  - ○ *Oral preparatory:* manipulation of fluid to form bolus, minimal in infants
  - ○ *Oral:* propulsion of bolus from tongue to produce pharyngeal swallow
  - ○ *Pharyngeal:* bolus propulsion via velo-pharyngeal and hypo/oro-pharyngeal peristalsis, glottal closure should also be present during this phase
  - ○ *Esophageal:* bolus propulsion via sequential upper esophageal sphincter relaxation, esophageal peristalsis, and lower esophageal relaxation
  - ○ *Gastric\Intestinal:* bolus propulsion via persistent gastro-duodenal contractions

POTENTIAL MECHANISMS AND EVIDENCE-BASED ASSESSMENTS OF INFANT FEEDING DIFFICULTIES
The Infant Feeding Process

Feeding (used as a verb) is a complex multi-systemic process wherein an infant is fed with nutrients to facilitate thriving at all times-during health or illness. In the breast-fed

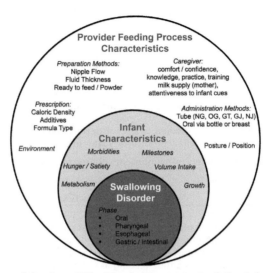

Fig. 1. Mechanisms of feeding difficulties in the context of the infant–parent–provider triad. Note the distinction between swallowing disorders (dysphagia) and other possible mechanisms that may contribute to feeding difficulties either from process problems or systemic problems in the infant. NG-nasogastric; OG- orogastric; GT-gastrostomy tube; GJ-gastro jejunal; NG-naso jejunal.

infant or breast milk-fed infant, mother plays a predominant role. In formula-fed infants, several additional provider-participants may be involved with milk preparation, sterilization of feeding-apparatus, provider's prescription of nutrients and methods, delivery methods, the act of feeding the infant based on cues, on-demand or time-scheduled, monitoring for quality cues or abnormalities, documentation of the session to maintain consistency between providers, and reporting during daily care rounds, so that progress can be made with the infant's feeding. Commonly, the direct feeding providers are either the mothers or nurses or assistants, who need to be knowledgeable about the high-risk infant's feeding capabilities and vulnerabilities, besides recognizing and aborting potential symptoms, if any. Standardizing the feeding process will minimize practice variation among the interdisciplinary providers and common accountability metrics can be the norm. Such metrics during the oral feeding phase can be (a) postmenstrual age (PMA) at 1st oral feeding, (b) PMA at full (120 mL/kg/d) and ad lib (at least 150 mL/kg/d or greater) oral feeding, and (c) LOHS.[13,14] Often, the LOHS can be affected by the practice variation and failure to seek consensus with feeding an infant with complex issues and multi-systemic symptoms. In such feeding difficulties, chronic tube feeding is the current norm, although avoidance of tube feeding is the most desired goal.

Infant feeding is a process with numerous extrinsic and intrinsic factors (**Box 2**). Extrinsic factors can be assessed and examined at the level of the parent or provider, while intrinsic factors are at the level of the individual patient; these are further described later in discussion.

1. *At parent–provider level* - The following factors may be evaluated to ensure optimal feeding so as to avoid failure to thrive: *Frequency of feeding* depends on the recognition of hunger cues and may be around 3–4-h intervals. This permits gastric emptying and prepares the stomach to be ready for the next feed. Infants often send hunger cues that are easily recognized by the mother who then provides

Box 2
Factors to consider when evaluating the infant feeding process

Practice Variability Measures

- Caregiver (nurse, mother, father, family members, consistent caretakers)
  - Feeding experience and recognition of cues and quality of feeds
  - Practices (preparation, prescription, administration, and so forth)

- Medical Provider
  - Training/experience
  - Diagnosis
    - Empiric based
    - Evidence and mechanisms based
  - Therapies
    - Nonpharmacologic (position, nipple modification, thickener, and so forth)
    - Medical (prokinetics, acid suppressive, airway management measures)
    - Surgical (gastrostomy, fundoplication, tracheostomy)

Patient Characteristics

- Physiology/pathophysiology

- Maturation

- Morbidities

- Growth patterns

- Technological dependence

- Metabolism

- Feeding and satiety

- Feeding quality

- Symptoms

- Behaviors

- Swallowing skills

Feed Characteristics

- Route
  - Gavage
    - nasogastric/orogastric/gastrostomy/gastrojejunal/nasojejunal
    - gravity/pump feeds/continuous or simulated bolus
  - Oral
    - breast/bottle

- Frequency
  - continuous/interval/ad lib or cue based
  - number of feeds per day

- Duration
  - Gavage pump-slow/fast infusion rate
  - Oral-limited (ex. 15–20 min)/infant driven (short - 5 min) or long (>45 min)

- Total fluid volume (mL/kg/day), volume intake mL

- Fluid type
  - Breastmilk/formula
    - Formula
      - Ready to feed/powder added to water
      - Standard or specialized (antiregurgitation, elemental, hypoallergenic, and so forth)

- Temperature: Room/Warm

- Viscosity

- Osmolality
- Additives (thickeners, vitamins, fortifiers, and so forth)
- Volume offered/volume taken
- Fluid caloric density
- Bottle System
  - Nipple (flow rate and other characteristics)
  - Bottle design characteristics

the feed. This is easy in the case of healthy full-term infants, but high-risk infants may not provide the hunger cues, or the cues are not easily recognizable. Furthermore, the symptoms/signs may be heterogeneous and often feeds are withheld. This problem can get more complex in those who are on medications to treat lung or neurologic diseases. A *cue-based feeding scale*[15] for high-risk infants has been developed which provides some guidance to feed orally. Infants often stop feeding on the stomach being full; however, it is not always easy to recognize that in high-risk infants. A satiety or *feeding quality scale*[15] has been developed that provides some guidance as to how the feeding session ended. Monitoring hunger and satiety cues provide some continuity with documenting progress with feeding, or lack thereof. This is also helpful in minimizing the practice variation among the feeding providers, from feed-to-feed. *Prescription of feedings and the method of feeding* is an important consideration for successful oral feeding. Often in the NICUs, the type of feed, method of feeding, and frequency of feeding need to be documented (ordered in the chart/electronic medical record) so as to permit the feeding provider (mother, nurse, or nurse assistant) to offer feeds to the infant. This simple process measure is sometimes overlooked, and there can be delays in starting oral feeds among those receiving any type of gavage-tube feeds. *Caloric density, optimal temperature, volume, and nutrient modifications* are other entities that are provider dependent. Medical providers (often the physician or advanced practice provider) may pay attention to the overall needs of the infant based on individual morbidity indicators, oxygen requirements, metabolism, and growth patterns. Often, it is a common practice to provide infants with denser and higher calorie formulas (>20 calories/oz) when volume restriction is a common feature to protect the lungs from increased liquid load (as in infants with lung disease or heart disease) or in infants with frequent feeding intolerance and emesis. The additives to milk (breast milk or base formula) may increase the viscosity, osmolality, density, and even the taste (as with the addition of medications). Thus, care is needed to identify that process that may have contributed to the feeding difficulty, so as to avoid unnecessary evaluation, because the solutions may be simple avoidance of that additive.

2. *At individual patient level* - Each infant is unique and has distinct physiologic or pathophysiological features. Therefore, personalization is needed wherein one approach may not fit all, particularly in high-risk infants. By monitoring infant growth and development within the NICU, as well as by providing attention to airway-digestive milestones and support, the physician can provide the modification of feeding opportunities and suggest adjustments as per the clinical condition. Volume consumed via the oral route, behaviors, aerodigestive symptoms, somatic and cardiorespiratory symptoms will provide signals to potential pathologies in difficult feeders.

3. *Assessment tools of the feeding process:* Useful feeding process evaluation tools may include the appropriate history of the problem, general clinical evaluation, analysis of a 5-day feeding diary for symptoms, nutrient intake methods and losses if any, growth curve trends, and systemic clinical evaluation of cardiorespiratory–neurologic–aerodigestive systems. Based on these signs/symptoms, diagnostic and management approaches can be tailored and personalized using a multi-pronged approach.

Swallowing Physiology and Dysphagia (Swallowing Disorder)

Swallowing skills or reflexes are first developed around 11 to 12 weeks' gestation[16] and are necessary for safe bolus transit during ex utero. Swallowing is a sensory-motor function involving numerous muscles and afferents and efferents from neurologic, respiratory, digestive, and cardiac systems.[17] Anatomic regions of interest include the oral cavity, pharynx, larynx, glottis, upper esophageal sphincter (UES), esophagus, and gastro-esophageal junction (GEJ) which is comprised of the diaphragm and lower esophageal sphincter (**Fig. 2**A). Nerves of interest include the

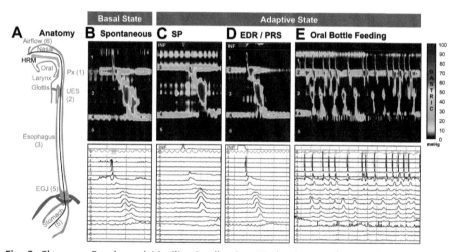

Fig. 2. Pharyngo-Esophageal Motility Swallowing Mechanisms under Basal and Adaptive Conditions in Infants. Px-pharynx; UES- upper esophageal sphincter; LES- lower esophageal sphincter; SP- secondary peristalsis; EDR-esophago-deglutition reflex; PRS- pharyngeal reflexive swallow; Inf-infusion; DA-deglutition apnea. (*A*) Swallowing Anatomy. A high-resolution manometry (HRM) catheter is placed to record motility changes (pressure, mm Hg) from the naso-pharynx to the stomach. A nasal airflow thermistor (orange) is used to detect respiratory changes (upstroke: inhalation, downstroke: exhalation) and correlates with glottal closure during brief DA with pharyngeal swallowing. Numbers indicate corresponding sections on motility during basal and adaptive states. *Top Panels (B–D):* Esophago-pressure topography (EPT) coloring takes into account pressure, time, and esophageal length. Blue indicates low pressures and purple high pressures. *Bottom Panels (B–D):* Conventional line plots reveal the same motility patterns (black *lines*) in pressure and time domains along with the respiratory signal (orange). Note that pharyngeal swallowing or primary peristalsis (characterized by pharyngeal peristalsis, UES relaxation, esophageal peristalsis, LES relaxation, and DA-gray shaded boxes) is observed during (*A*) spontaneous swallowing, (*D*) pharyngeal or esophageal stimulation (EDR or PRS depending on stimulus locus), and (*E*) infant eating. (*C*) SP (characterized by UES contraction, esophageal peristalsis, and LES relaxation) is only observed during esophageal stimulation.

glossopharyngeal nerve (IX), hypoglossal (XII), vagus nerve (X), pharyngo-esophageal nerve, superior-, inferior-, and recurrent-laryngeal nerves, and cardiac sympathetic plexuses.[17] During infant eating, coordinated cross-system regulation is needed for efficient and safe suck-swallow-breathing rhythms. Swallowing disorders (dysphagia) may occur if there is any dysfunction during oral, pharyngeal, esophageal, gastric, or intestinal phases of eating. Downstream motility dysfunctions can present as upstream problems with poor clearance and transit. Upstream problems can cause poor or delayed initiation of swallowing and clearance, thus resulting in aerodigestive symptoms. These are common scenarios in premature infants when adequate time for maturation, repair, and recovery of neuro-muscular apparatus is needed while maintaining breathing stability during bolus extraction and peristalsis. Maldevelopment, maturational delays, malfunction, and maladaptation of sensory-motor reflex pathways can present with abnormal symptoms/signs.[18–22] In the presence of developmental anomalies, any or all of these mechanisms are aberrant. Different physiologic aspects of infant eating, potential pathophysiologic or dysphagic mechanisms and evidence-based assessments associated with each function are explained later in discussion.

1. Oral Phase

Physiology and pathophysiology: Sucking functions are undertaken by the following muscles and nerves: orbicularis oris, buccinators, the medial and lateral pterygoid, masseter, temporalis, mentalis, and intrinsic muscles of tongue, via cranial nerves V, VII, XII, IX, and X of both sides. During the oral phase, the infant latches on to the nipple with both lips while pressing the tongue to the palate and pulling in the cheeks to generate a rhythmic suction pressure to extract milk from the bottle or breast. During this latch there is no leak of pressure from around the nipple normally, otherwise there is drooling. After bolus formation, lingual propulsion ensues, wherein the tongue sweeps the head of the bolus toward the pharynx. Direct consequences of absent, weak, or in-coordinated sucking reflexes with downstream clearance may include drooling, pooling, poor bolus extraction, ineffective bolus transit, and potentially aspiration.

Evidence-based assessments: The Neonatal Oral-Motor Assessment Scale (NOMAS) and revised NOMAS may be used to assess and characterize oral motor function as normal, disorganized, or dysfunctional rhythms.[23] However, a more recent study in preterm infants has shown that NOMAS was a poor predictor of feeding skills, while birth, birthweight, and initial feeding efficiency predict shorter transition and earlier acquisition of oral feeding.[24] Thus, the oral feeding scale (OFS) can also be used to evaluate infant feeding proficiency and rate of milk transfer for the identification of immature feeding skills or endurance issues.[25] Alternatively, a specialized physiology-based evaluation uses pressure transducers (for the evaluation of suction and expression mechanics) configured to a bottle nipple to assess the infant's nutritive sucking skills[26]

2. Pharyngo-Esophageal Phase

Physiology and pathophysiology: Regarding pharyngo-esophageal motility, 2 types of swallow patterns exist in infants termed as primary or secondary peristalsis (largely distinguished by pharyngeal and UES activity).[27–30] During *primary peristalsis* or pharyngeal swallowing, bolus propulsion occurs via pharyngeal peristalsis along with a brief (<2 sec) deglutition apnea (a biomarker of glottal closure), UES relaxation, esophageal peristalsis, and GEJ relaxation.[27,29,31–35] Pharyngeal swallowing may be voluntary (ie, occurs spontaneously- **Fig. 2B** or during eating- **Fig. 2E**) or involuntary/reflexive as in the case of pharyngeal or esophageal stimulation (see **Fig. 2**D). During the act of eating, coordination of the oral cavity, digestive tract, airway, or suck/swallow/breathing rhythms is also necessary to ensure safe bolus transit and proper digestion. *Secondary peristalsis* characterized by UES contraction, esophageal peristalsis, and GEJ relaxation is involuntary and only observed with esophageal stimulation (ie, gastroesophageal reflux, GER) to protect the airway and clear the esophageal contents[29,30,36] (**Fig. 2**C). Pharyngo-esophageal motility is modified by infant maturation (gestational and postnatal age) and morbidities (respiratory, neurologic, cardiac, congenital conditions, and so forth), and characteristics of stimulus (media, dose, and so forth).[2,7,22,29–32,35–47] Failure of safe bolus transit or airway protective mechanisms during pharyngeal or esophageal provocation may result in laryngeal penetration, laryngeal aspiration, coughing/choking, and/or laryngeal chemoreflex. Pathophysiologic mechanisms may be detected by deficits in sensory (response latency, thresholds) and/or motor (frequency, magnitude, duration) characteristics. Specific examples may include: increased frequency of pharyngeal swallowing indicating poor clearance or excessive secretions, absent or prolonged responses, incomplete UES or LES relaxation (achalasia), weak contractile responses, hypo- or hyper-sensitivity, dysfunctional cross-system communication, prolonged glottal closure and apnea, and bradycardic rhythms.[48,49] In infants with chronic dysphagia, esophageal, pharyngeal, and oral feeding swallowing rhythms are distinct.[2,7,50] Moreover, in dysphagic infants that have feeding failure or received a gastrostomy (vs those that attained oral feeding): (a) complete peristalsis is decreased[7], (b) the frequency/occurrence of peristaltic response is lower for pharyngeal and esophageal reflexes,[2,7] and UES contractile and LES relaxation reflexes do not advance with maturation[50] (c) sucking, swallowing (primary peristalsis), and breathing rhythms are decreased during oral feeding challenge.[2,7]

Evidence Based Assessments: Motility testing is obtained to evaluate pharyngeal and esophageal phases using high-resolution manometry or water perfusion methods.[29,30,32,35,44,46,47,51] Evaluation can be performed under varied conditions (described later in discussion) and individualized to the infant with further description of normal and abnormal responses.[48]

A. Evaluation during basal state permits the evaluation of background swallowing activity when the infant is at rest. Frequency of pharyngeal swallow (per minute) ranges from 1 to 3[31] but may be altered by the level of alertness or sleep. Lower frequency during awake states may indicate neuropathology, while higher frequency may occur due to excessive secretions, GER, and/or poor bolus clearance. Sphincter tone during basal state provides clues to skeletal (UES) and smooth muscle (LES) strength; average resting UES tone is 18 to 48 mm Hg at full-term status,[31] and average resting LES tone ranges from 5 to 20 mm Hg between 26 and 33 weeks PMA and 10–14 mm Hg between 35 and 39 weeks PMA.[34] Tone is typically decreased during sleep, but low tone may indicate hypotonicity and high tone hypertonicity. Low LES tone may indicate elevated risk for GER, and high tone is noted with poor esophageal clearance and achalasia. Low UES tone may provide poor protection against supra-esophageal GER, and high tone with poor relaxation indicates risk for poor pharyngeal clearance, achalasia, and/or aspiration.

B. Evaluation during the adaptive state is conducted during pharyngeal provocation using minute volumes (0.1–0.5 mL) of sterile water or saline to evaluate pharyngeal reflexes and chemosensitivity in response to bolus presence as in the case of descending oral bolus or supraesophageal GER.[21,32,33,35,52] Esophageal provocation testing is a controlled and monitored to evaluate esophageal reflexes and mechano-, osmo-, and chemo-receptor sensitivity using air, sterile water, and apple juice, respectively, to simulate GER.[30,34,53] An oral feeding challenge test is a 3-min oral feed undertaken to monitor rhythms of the pharynx, esophagus, and respiration along with any symptoms.[2,7,46,47]

Although motility testing gives extensive detail and may identify causal mechanisms of symptoms,[18,20,22,39] it is not widely available, especially in the infant population. *Video-fluoroscopic swallow study (VFSS)* is a widely available tool used to evaluate the oral, pharyngeal, and penetration/aspiration mechanisms, but requires radiation exposure and is highly variable in testing protocol. Attempts are underway to standardize VFSS testing methods, reporting, and interpreting methods in bottle-fed infants.[54,55] A *24-h pH-impedance* test is another tool becoming more widely available in the infant population that can rule out GER disease (GERD). Symptoms that are common to both dysphagia and GERD are able to be evaluated via symptom correlation indices and give clues to mechanisms.[19,56,57] *Endoscopy* can rule out any structural anomalies or esophagitis. An *upper gastrointestinal (UGI) series* can be useful to detect anatomic anomalies of foregut, hiatal hernia (LES and diaphragm separation), or achalasia, and UGI fluoroscopy with contrast may be useful when strictures or delayed transit is suspected.

3. Gastric/Intestinal Phase

Physiology and pathophysiology: Acid-mediated digestion begins in the stomach, with the stomach appearing normally distended after feeds. Intra-gastric presentation of feeds provides a physiologic stimulus to the stomach thus permitting gastric motility, enzymatic and mucosal functions. Important components among the motility function include: (i) receptive relaxation to accommodate an increasing volume, (ii) contraction at the lower esophageal sphincter to prevent gastroesophageal reflux while the contraction of pyloric sphincters to prevent premature release of chyme from the stomach, (iii) mixing or trituration during the gastric digestive phase, and finally (iv) co-ordination of gastrointestinal motility wherein the relaxation of pyloric sphincter occurs while intense gastric contractions occur to let the partially digested bolus to enter the duodenum for the next phase of digestion. Neonatal intestinal motility differs between fasting and fed states.[58] In infants, during fasting, the inter-digestive motility cycle is characterized by quiescent periods, nonpropagating activity, and phasic propagating activity (migrating motor complex).[59] These migrating motor complexes are decreased in preterm infants but improve with maturation.[59,60] The fed state is characterized by persistent motility activity in both term and preterm infants,[59] and may be modified by feeding methods (infusion rate) and nutrients (caloric density, concentration, osmolality, fat and fiber content, pH).[61] Inhibition of intestinal motor responses during feeding may contribute to feeding intolerance.[62] Delayed gastric emptying may also contribute to feeding intolerance. Poor gastric accommodation or gastric tone after feeds may contribute to GER, gastric residuals, and feeding intolerance.

Evidence-based assessments: UGI can be performed to evaluate the anatomic structure and function of the stomach and duodenum and is integral in the detection of pyloric stenosis, malrotation, and strictures. *Gastric antral ultrasound* or *scintigraphy* tests can be performed to determine gastric emptying. A recent study determined that the gastric emptying time in healthy formula-fed neonates averages 93 minutes ranging from 45 to 150 minutes.[63] Ultrasound can also be used for the detection of pyloric stenosis. *Intestinal motility evaluation* via manometric methods can evaluate intestinal motor function during fasting and fed states.

4. Cross-system Regulatory Functions

Physiology and pathophysiology: In addition to examining each phase as an individual function as described above, swallowing requires constant cross-

A   **B**

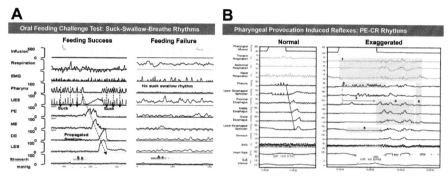

Fig. 3. Cross-System Regulation in Infants. PE-CR: (*A*) Suck-swallow breathing rhythms are coordinated in successfully oral-fed infants, compared with absent rhythms in infants with feeding failure. (*B*) Normal pharyngoesophageal cardiorespiratory (PE-CR) response to sterile water pharyngeal stimulus is characterized by multiple pharyngeal reflexive swallowing and terminal complete esophageal peristaltic clearance (blue *arrow*) with minimal impact on cardio-respiratory rhythms. During abnormal PE-CR response, pharyngoesophageal rhythms are uncoordinated, prolonged, and lacking complete esophageal peristaltic clearance (2–6) resulting in exaggerated and prolonged respiratory changes including deglutition apnea (1) and significant heart rate drop (bradycardia). ([*A*] *Adapted with permission from* Wolters Kluwer Health, Inc.: Jadcherla et al. Evaluation and management of neonatal dysphagia: impact of pharyngoesophageal motility studies and multidisciplinary feeding strategy, J Pediatr Gastroenterol Nutr, 48(2):186–92; and [*B*] From Hasenstab-Kenney, Bellodas Sanchez, Jadcherla et al. "Mechanisms of bradycardia in premature infants: Aerodigestive cardiac regularity-rhythm interactions." Physiol Rep. 2020 Jul;8(13):7.)

communication and coordination between oral, pharyngeal, esophageal, gastric, intestinal, neurologic, respiratory, and cardiac systems. An example of effective and ineffective cross-system interactions between suck-swallow-and breathing rhythms can be observed in **Fig. 3**A. Adding another level of complexity is the infant's maturational level and self-regulatory capacity. Hence, rhythms may exist but be immature or uncoordinated (**Fig. 3**B), resulting in laryngeal chemoreflex and symptoms such as apnea/bradycardia/desaturation at younger maturation or coughing/choking at older maturation.[21,22] As self-regulatory rhythms improve with maturation, interventions such as pacing techniques or feeding modifications may be needed in the meantime. It is important to note, if critical windows of opportunity (feeding milestones) are delayed or missed it is difficult for infants to learn oral feeding later skills on in life.

Evidence-based assessments: Testing to evaluate cross-system regulatory functions of an upstream swallowing function may include: VFSS,[54,55] fiberoptic endoscopic evaluation of swallowing (FEES), suck-swallow-respiratory testing,[64] and oropharyngeal esophageal scintigraphy. Downstream swallowing function may include UGI series (esophagus, stomach, intestines) and pharyngo-esophageal motility. Finally, the combination of upstream and downstream swallowing function may include pharyngo-esophageal motility concurrent with impedance and VFSS,[65] respiratory inductance plethysmography or nasal airflow thermistor,[20,39] ultrasonography,[33,66] and cardio-respiratory monitoring.[21,22] In the situation of suspected airway and vocal cord issues, otolaryngology evaluation using airway endoscopy methods or video-fluoroscopy methods may be necessary.

EVIDENCE-BASED MODELS FOR FEEDING THE NEONATAL INTENSIVE CARE UNIT INFANT: A HOLISTIC APPROACH

As the maturing neonate is in a constant state of rapid dynamic physiologic and pathophysiologic changes, optimal multidisciplinary and individualized feeding therapies (such as oro-motor stimulation, manipulation of hunger and gut motility, management of comorbidities, and anticipatory guidance based on evidence) show promise for potential feeding rehabilitation.[2,7] Using this approach, even NICU infants with severe chronic feeding difficulties were able to obtain independent oral feeding at discharge or 1-year chronologic age.[2] Development of these interdisciplinary NICU feeding management strategies can be translated to the bedside via provider and parental education and tailored to the infant's individual needs. Additionally, day-to-day practice variation within the unit can be optimized via implementation of a SIMPLE (simplified, individualized, milestone-targeted, pragmatic, longitudinal, and educational) feeding model that incorporates the infant–parent and provider triad to accelerate feeding milestones and decrease economic burden[13,14]

Additional Tailored Approaches for Consideration

Consideration of adequate time for infant maturation is a necessity, as high-risk infants do not meet the required aero-digestive-neurologic maturity at a given chronologic age. For example, infants with severe neuropathology or chronic lung disease (CLD) have delays with foregut maturation and oral feeding abilities. The exact timeline for the maturation of oro-pharyngeal skills in such a setting is not known. Therefore, consistent evidence-based personalized therapies are needed with special emphasis on morbidities as described later in discussion:

Bronchopulmonary dysplasia and chronic lung disease: Infants with *bronchopulmonary dysplasia* (BPD) or CLD have a higher risk of delayed feeding milestones or feeding failure.[20] Effective feeding management requires the stabilization of chronic disease with a focus on best nutrition to attain anabolic states and best growth rates. In infants with BPD, chest X-ray to assess chronic abnormalities that may be suggestive of aspiration or focal disease, while in extreme cases of severe BPD, control-ventilation CT scans may be needed to assess the severity and extent of the disease. Airway management methods in such infants include nasal cannula oxygen, nasal continuous positive airway pressure, and mechanical ventilation. In full-term newborn lambs on nasal respiratory support, bottle feeding has been shown to be safe even in those with tachypnea.[67] In infants with BPD, aerodigestive reflexes are similarly developed in those on noninvasive respiratory support,[20] and clinically significant aspiration pneumonia was not detected in those orally fed while on nasal continuous positive airway pressure.[68] Achieving superior feeding and growth outcomes in infants with BPD using cue-based feeding methods and SIMPLE feeding strategies under controlled conditions is possible,[14,15] but extreme caution and continuous monitoring must be followed.

Gastroesophageal reflux disease (GERD): GERD is commonly suspected as a cause of feeding difficulties in infants. Sensitivity due to bolus, acid, or nonacid components of GER may indicate esophageal sensitivities of esophageal mechano-, chemo-, or osmo-receptors, or esophageal dysmotility mechanisms.[18,30,48] A recent study has shown that infants diagnosed with GERD may develop dysphagic mechanisms despite acid suppressive therapy.[69] As there are numerous overlapping symptoms of GERD and dysphagia, underlying mechanisms should be identified and treated appropriately.[18,20,22,39,56] Evidence-based therapies are recommended rather than empiric strategies. Nonpharmacologic approaches should be considered first, even before trying any pharmacologic agents. If fundoplication is being considered, motility evaluation should be performed for the evaluation of LES tone. If LES tone is already adequate or hypertonic, fundoplication may exacerbate swallowing difficulties. It is important to note that LES tone increases with maturation, thus lowering the risk of GER in enterally fed preterm neonates.[34] Additionally, in a study of infants with acid GERD, although LES tone decreased, with maturation 71% of infants still achieved successful oral feeding at discharge with none receiving fundoplication.[69]

Apparent life-threatening events (ALTE)/brief resolved unexplained events (BRUE): Providers frequently treat infants with ALTE/ BRUE events for GERD when no other etiology is present. However, recent studies show that dysfunctional esophageal peristaltic mechanisms may play an important role, with GER mechanisms being relatively rare.[22,39] Appropriate history of when events occur (before, during, or after feeds) and diagnostic testing may be necessary to determine the true cause. Events during oral feeding may indicate poor self-regulation and the need for pacing techniques, while spontaneous events may indicate immature cardio-respiratory and pharyngo-esophageal rhythms which typically improve with maturation.

Neuropathology: Infants with neuropathology are at high risk of feeding difficulties. In infants with hypoxic-ischemic encephalopathy, esophageal peristaltic reflexes are prolonged and uncoordinated,[70] while pharyngeal reflexes are associated with decreased number of pharyngeal swallows, increased UES tone and reactivity, and LES dysregulation (mechanisms which may contribute to pooling and aspiration) which likely do not improve with maturation.[40,44] However, reflexes are improved with cooling intervention.[70] Neuropathology may warrant neural imaging to provide anticipatory guidance to parents and providers, and this is relevant as feeding course among infants at risk for cerebral palsy and neurodevelopmental delays can vary.

SUMMARY

Evaluation of infant feeding is complex and should consider not only the infant but also the management approach between the infant, parent/caregiver, and medical provider. By evaluating the feeding process in its entirety, the root cause is able to be targeted. Referral for specialized testing of swallowing function should be performed if the assessment of the feeding process indicates suspicion of swallowing disorder. Diagnostic assessment of an infant's feeding and swallowing skills should be targeted and individualized based on medical history, clinical examination, and signs/symptoms. It is important to identify anatomic versus functional deficits (oral, pharyngeal, esophageal, cross-system) using tests previously mentioned. Additionally, the utilization of an evidence-based process optimization feeding model (SIMPLE) for NICU infants may aid in achieving superior feeding outcomes and decreased economic burden.

CLINICS CARE POINTS

- Evidence-Based Feeding Diagnosis and Management Approaches in Infants with Feeding/ Swallowing Difficulties
- Diagnostic studies should identify mechanisms of feeding difficulties as process-driven or infant skills driven.
- Management approaches should target the infant/parent/provider triad and use a standardized SIMPLE approach to address feeding process issues,[13,14] and personalized feeding strategies based on infant's swallowing physiology/pathophysiology to address infant skill deficits.[2,7]

Best practices box

Oral Feeding in Infants with Feeding/Swallowing Difficulties

What is the current practice?
- Guidelines for infants with feeding/swallowing difficulties are lacking resulting in sustained feeding failure, use of non–evidence-based therapies, prolonged tube feeding, and increased morbidity and economic burden

Best Practice/Guideline/Care Path Objective(s)
- Use evidence-based diagnostic and management strategies that target the infant/parent/ provider triad
- Recognize clinically significant measures to monitor meaningful outcomes

What changes in current practice are likely to improve outcomes?
- Identify mechanisms of feeding difficulties that are process-driven and/or deficits in the infant's safe-swallowing skills
  - For process-driven feeding difficulties: Optimize feeding processes using a SIMPLE approach
  - For swallowing difficulties: Use multidisciplinary and precision-based medicine targeting physiology/pathophysiology to individualize feeding therapies which may include nutritive stimulation and manipulation of hunger and gut motility

Major Recommendations

Diagnosis
- To identify feeding process difficulties: use objective assessments and testing such as infant feeding readiness and quality scales and a 5-day feeding diary
- For suspicion of swallowing dysfunction: target testing to suspected regions of dysfunction, that is, oral, pharyngo-esophageal, gastric/intestinal, and/or cross-system regulation for the development of personalized therapies
- Clarify if swallowing difficulties are due to dysfunctional, immature, maldeveloped, or maladaptive mechanisms.

Therapies
- Standardize feeding processes via education, parent/provider participation, and compliance monitoring, while also personalizing feeding management based on infant swallowing skills.
- Effectively manage any comorbidities and encourage cautious feeding if appropriate.

Summary Statement

Deficiencies in the feeding process or infant feeding skills can be identified and targeted using multidisciplinary and individualized diagnostic and targeted management approaches.

Bibliographic Source(s):[2,7,13,14]

DISCLOSURE

The authors have nothing to disclose.

REFERENCES

1. Benitz WE, Committee on F, AAoP Newborn. Hospital stay for healthy term newborn infants. Pediatrics 2015;135(5):948–53.
2. Jadcherla SR, Peng J, Moore R, et al. Impact of personalized feeding program in 100 NICU infants: pathophysiology-based approach for better outcomes. J Pediatr Gastroenterol Nutr 2012;54(1):62–70.
3. Greene NH, Greenberg RG, O'Brien SM, et al. Variation in gastrostomy tube Placement in premature infants in the United States. Am J Perinatol 2019; 36(12):1243–9.

4. Horton J, Atwood C, Gnagi S, et al. Temporal trends of Pediatric dysphagia in Hospitalized patients. Dysphagia 2018;33(5):655–61.

5. Nassel D, Chartrand C, Dore-Bergeron MJ, et al. Very preterm infants with Technological dependence at home: impact on Resource Use and family. Neonatology 2019;115(4):363–70.

6. American Academy of Pediatrics Committee on Fetus and Newborn. Hospital discharge of the high-risk neonate. Pediatrics 2008;122(5):1119–26.

7. Jadcherla SR, Stoner E, Gupta A, et al. Evaluation and management of neonatal dysphagia: impact of pharyngoesophageal motility studies and multidisciplinary feeding strategy. J Pediatr Gastroenterol Nutr 2009;48(2):186–92.

8. Stey AM, Vinocur CD, Moss RL, et al. Hospital variation in rates of concurrent fundoplication during gastrostomy enteral access procedures. Surg Endosc 2018; 32(5):2201–11.

9. Abraham SS, Wolf EL. Swallowing physiology of toddlers with long-term tracheostomies: a preliminary study. Dysphagia 2000;15(4):206–12.

10. Norman V, Louw B, Kritzinger A. Incidence and description of dysphagia in infants and toddlers with tracheostomies: a retrospective review. Int J Pediatr Otorhinolaryngol 2007;71(7):1087–92.

11. Streppel M, Veder LL, Pullens B, et al. Swallowing problems in children with a tracheostomy tube. Int J Pediatr Otorhinolaryngol 2019;124:30–3.

12. Montagnino BA, Mauricio RV. The child with a tracheostomy and gastrostomy: parental stress and coping in the home–a pilot study. Pediatr Nurs 2004;30(5): 373–80, 401.

13. Jadcherla SR, Dail J, Malkar MB, et al. Impact of process optimization and quality improvement measures on neonatal feeding outcomes at an all-Referral neonatal intensive care Unit. JPEN J Parenter Enteral Nutr 2016;40(5):646–55.

14. Bapat R, Gulati IK, Jadcherla S. Impact of SIMPLE feeding quality improvement strategies on aerodigestive milestones and feeding outcomes in BPD infants. Hosp Pediatr 2019;9(11):859–66.

15. Davidson E, Hinton D, Ryan-Wenger N, et al. Quality improvement study of effectiveness of cue-based feeding in infants with bronchopulmonary dysplasia in the neonatal intensive care unit. J Obstet Gynecol Neonatal Nurs 2013;42(6):629–40.

16. Grassi R, Farina R, Floriani I, et al. Assessment of fetal swallowing with gray-scale and color Doppler sonography. AJR Am J Roentgenol 2005;185(5):1322–7.

17. Hasenstab KA, Jadcherla SR, et al. Gastroesophageal Reflux Disease in the Neonatal Intensive Care Unit Neonate. Clin Perinatol 2020;47(2):243–63.

18. Collins CR, Hasenstab KA, Nawaz S, et al. Mechanisms of aerodigestive symptoms in infants with varying acid reflux Index determined by esophageal manometry. J Pediatr 2019;206:240–7.

19. Jadcherla SR, Peng J, Chan CY, et al. Significance of gastroesophageal refluxate in relation to physical, chemical, and spatiotemporal characteristics in symptomatic intensive care unit neonates. Pediatr Res 2011;70(2):192–8.

20. Jadcherla SR, Hasenstab KA, Shaker R, et al. Mechanisms of cough provocation and cough resolution in neonates with bronchopulmonary dysplasia. Pediatr Res 2015;78(4):462–9.

21. Hasenstab KA, Nawaz S, Lang IM, et al. Pharyngoesophageal and cardiorespiratory interactions: potential implications for premature infants at risk of clinically significant cardiorespiratory events. Am J Physiol Gastrointest Liver Physiol 2019; 316(2):G304–12.

22. Hasenstab-Kenney KA, Bellodas Sanchez J, Prabhakar V, et al. Mechanisms of bradycardia in premature infants: aerodigestive-cardiac regulatory-rhythm interactions. Phys Rep 2020;8(13):e14495.

23. Palmer MM, Crawley K, Blanco IA. Neonatal Oral-Motor Assessment scale: a reliability study. J Perinatol 1993;13(1):28–35.

24. Bingham PM, Ashikaga T, Abbasi S. Relationship of neonatal oral motor assessment scale to feeding performance of premature infants. J Neonatal Nurs 2012; 18(1):30–6.

25. Lau C, Smith EO. A novel approach to assess oral feeding skills of preterm infants. Neonatology 2011;100(1):64–70.

26. Lau C, Alagugurusamy R, Schanler RJ, et al. Characterization of the developmental stages of sucking in preterm infants during bottle feeding. Acta Paediatr 2000;89(7):846–52.

27. Jadcherla SR, Shaker R. Esophageal and upper esophageal sphincter motor function in babies. Am J Med 2001;111(Suppl 8A):64S–8S.

28. Jadcherla SR. Manometric evaluation of esophageal-protective reflexes in infants and children. Am J Med 2003;115(Suppl 3A):157S–60S.

29. Jadcherla SR, Duong HQ, Hoffmann RG, et al. Esophageal body and upper esophageal sphincter motor responses to esophageal provocation during maturation in preterm newborns. J Pediatr 2003;143(1):31–8.

30. Jadcherla SR, Hoffmann RG, Shaker R. Effect of maturation of the magnitude of mechanosensitive and chemosensitive reflexes in the premature human esophagus. J Pediatr 2006;149(1):77–82.

31. Jadcherla SR, Duong HQ, Hofmann C, et al. Characteristics of upper oesophageal sphincter and oesophageal body during maturation in healthy human neonates compared with adults. Neurogastroenterol Motil 2005;17(5):663–70.

32. Jadcherla SR, Gupta A, Stoner E, et al. Pharyngeal swallowing: defining pharyngeal and upper esophageal sphincter relationships in human neonates. J Pediatr 2007;151(6):597–603.

33. Jadcherla SR, Gupta A, Wang M, et al. Definition and implications of novel pharyngo-glottal reflex in human infants using concurrent manometry ultrasonography. Am J Gastroenterol 2009;104(10):2572–82.

34. Pena EM, Parks VN, Peng J, et al. Lower esophageal sphincter relaxation reflex kinetics: effects of peristaltic reflexes and maturation in human premature neonates. Am J Physiol Gastrointest Liver Physiol 2010;299(6):G1386–95.

35. Hasenstab KA, Sitaram S, Lang IM, et al. Maturation Modulates pharyngeal-stimulus Provoked pharyngeal and respiratory rhythms in human infants. Dysphagia 2018;33(1):63–75.

36. Gupta A, Gulati P, Kim W, et al. Effect of postnatal maturation on the mechanisms of esophageal propulsion in preterm human neonates: primary and secondary peristalsis. Am J Gastroenterol 2009;104(2):411–9.

37. Jadcherla SR, Wang M, Vijayapal AS, et al. Impact of prematurity and comorbidities on feeding milestones in neonates: a retrospective study. J Perinatol 2010;30(3):201–8.

38. Jadcherla SR, Chan CY, Fernandez S, et al. Maturation of upstream and downstream esophageal reflexes in human premature neonates: the role of sleep and awake states. Am J Physiol Gastrointest Liver Physiol 2013;305(9):G649–58.

39. Hasenstab KA, Jadcherla SR. Respiratory events in infants presenting with apparent life threatening events: is there an explanation from esophageal motility? J Pediatr 2014;165(2):250–255 e251.

40. Gulati IK, Shubert TR, Sitaram S, et al. Effects of birth asphyxia on the modulation of pharyngeal provocation-induced adaptive reflexes. Am J Physiol Gastrointest Liver Physiol 2015;309(8):G662–9.

41. Jadcherla SR, Shubert TR, Gulati IK, et al. Upper and lower esophageal sphincter kinetics are modified during maturation: effect of pharyngeal stimulus in premature infants. Pediatr Res 2015;77(1–1):99–106.

42. Jadcherla SR, Shubert TR, Malkar MB, et al. Gestational and postnatal modulation of esophageal sphincter reflexes in human premature neonates. Pediatr Res 2015;78(5):540–6.

43. Jadcherla SR, Hasenstab KA, Sitaram S, et al. Effect of nasal noninvasive respiratory support methods on pharyngeal provocation-induced aerodigestive reflexes in infants. Am J Physiol Gastrointest Liver Physiol 2016;310(11):G1006–14.

44. Jensen PS, Gulati IK, Shubert TR, et al. Pharyngeal stimulus-induced reflexes are impaired in infants with perinatal asphyxia: Does maturation modify? Neurogastroenterol Motil 2017;29(7).

45. Hart BJ, Viswanathan S, Jadcherla SR. Persistent feeding difficulties among infants with fetal opioid exposure: mechanisms and clinical reasoning. J Matern Fetal Neonatal Med 2018;1–7.

46. Jadcherla SR, Prabhakar V, Hasenstab KA, et al. Defining pharyngeal contractile integral during high-resolution manometry in neonates: a neuromotor marker of pharyngeal vigor. Pediatr Res 2018;84(3):341–7.

47. Prabhakar V, Hasenstab KA, Osborn E, et al. Pharyngeal contractile and regulatory characteristics are distinct during nutritive oral stimulus in preterm-born infants: implications for clinical and research applications. Neurogastroenterol Motil 2019;31(8):1–7.

48.. Sultana Z, Hasenstab KA, Jadcherla SR. Pharyngo-esophageal motility reflex mechanisms in the human neonate: Importance of integrative cross-systems physiology. Am J Physiol Gastrointest Liver Physiol 2021;321(2):G139–48.

49. Hasenstab KA, Jadcherla SR. Gastroesophageal reflux disease in the neonatal intensive care Unit neonate: Controversies, current Understanding, and Future Directions. Clin Perinatol 2020;47(2):243–63.

50. Swiader N, Hasenstab KA, Yildiz VO, et al. Characterization of esophageal and sphincter reflexes across maturation in dysphagic infants with oral feeding success vs infants requiring gastrostomy. Dysphagia 2021;37(1):148–57.

51. Shubert TR, Sitaram S, Jadcherla SR. Effects of pacifier and taste on swallowing, esophageal motility, transit, and respiratory rhythm in human neonates. Neurogastroenterol Motil 2016;28(4):532–42.

52. Davies AM, Koenig JS, Thach BT. Upper airway chemoreflex responses to saline and water in preterm infants. J Appl Phys (1985) 1988;64(4):1412–20.

53. Jadcherla SR, Hasenstab KA, Gulati IK, et al. Impact of feeding strategies with acid suppression on esophageal reflexes in human neonates with gastroesophageal reflux disease: a Single-Blinded Randomized clinical trial. Clin Transl Gastroenterol 2020;11(11):e00249.

54. Lefton-Greif MA, McGrattan KE, Carson KA, et al. First Steps towards development of an instrument for the Reproducible Quantification of oropharyngeal swallow physiology in bottle-fed children. Dysphagia 2018;33(1):76–82.

55. Martin-Harris B, Carson KA, Pinto JM, et al. BaByVFSSImP((c)) A novel Measurement tool for Videofluoroscopic assessment of swallowing Impairment in bottle-fed babies: Establishing a standard. Dysphagia 2020;35(1):90–8.

56. Jadcherla SR, Sultana Z, Hasenstab-Kenney KA, et al. Differentiating esophageal sensitivity phenotypes using pH-impedance in intensive care unit infants referred for gastroesophageal reflux symptoms. Pediatr Res 2021;89(3):636–44.

57. Jadcherla SR, Gupta A, Fernandez S, et al. Spatiotemporal characteristics of acid refluxate and relationship to symptoms in premature and term infants with chronic lung disease. Am J Gastroenterol 2008;103(3):720–8.

58. Amarnath RP, Berseth CL, Malagelada JR, et al. Postnatal maturation of small intestinal motility in preterm and term infants. Neurogastroenterol Motil 1989;1(2):138–43.

59. Berseth CL. Neonatal small intestinal motility: motor responses to feeding in term and preterm infants. J Pediatr 1990;117(5):777–82.

60. Berseth CL. Gestational evolution of small intestine motility in preterm and term infants. J Pediatr 1989;115(4):646–51.

61. Jadcherla SR, Berseth CL. Acute and chronic intestinal motor activity responses to two infant formulas. Pediatrics 1995;96(2 Pt 1):331–5.

62. Jadcherla SR, Berseth CL. Antroduodenal motility and feeding outcome among neonatal extracorporeal membrane oxygenation survivors. J Pediatr Gastroenterol Nutr 2005;41(3):347–50.

63. Lee JJ, Price JC, Duren A, et al. Ultrasound evaluation of gastric emptying time in healthy term neonates after formula feeding. Anesthesiology 2021;134(6):845–51.

64. Lau C, Smith EO, Schanler RJ. Coordination of suck-swallow and swallow respiration in preterm infants. Acta Paediatr 2003;92(6):721–7.

65. Rommel N, Selleslagh M, Hoffman I, et al. Objective assessment of swallow function in children with suspected aspiration using pharyngeal automated impedance manometry. J Pediatr Gastroenterol Nutr 2014;58(6):789–94.

66. Jadcherla SR, Gupta A, Coley BD, et al. Esophago-glottal closure reflex in human infants: a novel reflex elicited with concurrent manometry and ultrasonography. Am J Gastroenterol 2007;102(10):2286–93.

67. Alain C, Samson N, Nadeau C, et al. Nasal respiratory support and tachypnea and oral feeding in full-term newborn lambs. J Appl Phys (1985) 2021;130(5):1436–47.

68. Hanin M, Nuthakki S, Malkar MB, et al. Safety and Efficacy of oral feeding in infants with BPD on nasal CPAP. Dysphagia 2015;30(2):121–7.

69. Jadcherla S, Hasenstab K, Gulati I, et al. Impact of feeding strategies with acid suppression on esophageal reflexes in human neonates with gastroesophageal reflux disease: a Single-Blinded Randomized clinical trial. Clin Translational Gastroenterol 2020;11(11):e00249.

70. Hill CD, Jadcherla SR. Esophageal mechanosensitive mechanisms are impaired in neonates with hypoxic-ischemic encephalopathy. J Pediatr 2013;162(5):976–82.

Short Bowel Syndrome and Dysmotility

Muralidhar H. Premkumar, MBBS, DCH, DNB, MRCPCH, MS

KEYWORDS

- SBS • Short gut • Intestinal failure • Hypomotility • Hypermotility
- Promotility agents • Prokinetics • Antidiarrheal agents

KEY POINTS

- The mortality following short bowel syndrome (SBS) has vastly improved in neonates, but the morbidity remains high.
- Clinical challenges secondary to dysmotility constitute a significant cause of morbidity in infants with SBS.
- The tests to diagnose dysmotility in infants with SBS are limited.
- Limited choices, poor safety profile, and lack of evidence are barriers in medical therapy of dysmotility in SBS.
- Surgical techniques to treat dysmotility in SBS are restricted to only those who fail medical therapy and intestinal rehabilitation, and carry significant risks.

INTRODUCTION

Intestinal failure is defined as the anatomic or functional loss of the intestine resulting in an inability to digest and absorb enteral nutrients, resulting in prolonged dependence on parenteral nutrition.[1] Short bowel syndrome (SBS) denotes situations whereby there is anatomic loss of intestinal length leading to intestinal failure. Functional intestinal length less than 200 cm is defined as SBS in adults.[2] However, in children, the length of the small bowel varies with the age of the subject.[3,4] Rickham defined SBS in infants as residual bowel length of less than 30% of the small intestines.[5] The causes of SBS in neonates include conditions such as necrotizing enterocolitis, gastroschisis, atresia, volvulus, and omphalocele.[6]

The prevalence of SBS is variable. North American studies have shown a prevalence of 24.5 cases per 100,000 births.[7] The incidence in low birth weight infants was 7 per 1000, with a higher prevalence of 11 per 1000 in extremely low birth weight infants.[6] Recent data demonstrate vastly improved survival of over 90% but this is accompanied by high morbidity.[8] Most of the morbidity arises from feeding

Associate Professor, Division of Neonatology, Department of Pediatrics, Baylor College of Medicine, Texas Children's Hospital, 6621 Fannin, Suite 6104, Houston, TX 77030, USA
E-mail address: premkuma@bcm.edu

Clin Perinatol 49 (2022) 521–536
https://doi.org/10.1016/j.clp.2022.02.013   **perinatology.theclinics.com**
0095-5108/22/© 2022 Elsevier Inc. All rights reserved.

Abbreviations	
LILT	Longitudinal intestinal lengthening technique
MMC	Migrating motor complexes
SCFA	Short-chain fatty acids
STEP	Serial transverse enteroplasty

intolerance due to either hypomotility or hypermotility.[9] The dysmotility in surgical SBS in infants is poorly characterized due to a lack of specific definitions. Signs and symptoms of hypomotility include feeding intolerance, increased gastric output, bilious and nonbilious emesis, gastric and intestinal dilatation, and abdominal distension. Hypermotility is usually noticed as feeding intolerance, increased ostomy output, steatorrhea, and diarrhea. Signs and symptoms of dysmotility are exhibited in 43% of complicated gastroschisis and nearly 50% of infants with atresia.[10] A much lower proportion of infants with necrotizing enterocolitis (11%–23%) demonstrate dysmotility.[11–13]

PHYSIOLOGIC BASIS OF THE MOTILITY OF THE GASTROINTESTINAL TRACT
Neural Control

The central nervous system, enteric nervous system, neurotransmitters, and chemoreceptors
The central nervous system and enteric nervous system provide both the sensory (afferent) and motor (efferent) neurons to the gut. The parasympathetic preganglionic fibers in the vagus nerve and the sympathetic postganglionic fibers in the splanchnic nerve carry the sensory neurons. The motor innervation of the gastrointestinal tract is supplied by the autonomic nervous system with contributions from both the parasympathetic and the sympathetic divisions.[14,15]

The enteric nervous system is far more extensive compared with the central nervous system and is made up of the myenteric Auerbach plexus and the submucosal Meissner plexus. Auerbach plexus is involved in dilatation and contraction, whereas the Meissner plexus is involved with the secretory function.[16] The innervation of the gastrointestinal tract also involves several neurotransmitters such as acetylcholine and substance P, which are excitatory, promoting contraction, and nitric oxide, vasoactive intestinal polypeptide, and adenosine triphosphate that are inhibitory and encourage relaxation. The gastrointestinal tract is also regulated by the endocrine and paracrine mediators such as gastrin, gastric inhibitory polypeptide, secretin, cholecystokinin, and pancreatic polypeptide.[17,18]

The gastrointestinal system from the esophagus to the rectum is abundant in a variety of chemoreceptors that mediate functions such as motility and secretion. The esophagus has both dopaminergic and serotoninergic receptors. The stomach, duodenum, small bowel, and colon have dopaminergic, serotonin, motilin, and opioid receptors. Motilin receptors are present in the stomach and the duodenum, while the colon is rich in opioid receptors.[17,19–22]

MOTILITY OF THE GASTROINTESTINAL TRACT

Swallowing and distension secondary to the presence of food stimulate contractions in the body of the esophagus propagating in an aboral manner. A swallow-related relaxation of the lower esophageal sphincter allows the movement of food into the stomach. The stomach functions as 2 separate myoelectric regions: a proximal portion including fundus and third of corpus, functioning mainly as a storage organ; a distal portion including remaining corpus, antrum, and pylorus with a role in the mechanical breakdown of food. The gastric slow waves occur at a frequency of 3 cycles/min. These waves are less frequent in preterm infants but gradually increase with age. Solid consistency of the diet, an increase in caloric density, and long-chain triglycerides delay gastric emptying.

The small intestine is a long tubular structure with several muscular layers arranged in different configurations contributing to its ability to break down food and move unabsorbed food forward. The muscular layers consist of a muscular mucosa, a thin submucosal layer, a thick circumferentially arranged, and an outer thinner longitudinally arranged layer of muscles. The interstitial cells of Cajal provide the communication between the circular and the longitudinal muscles.

Gastrointestinal contractions are regulated by both myogenic and neural control. The interstitial cells of Cajal initiate slow-wave membrane potentials around the circumference of the intestine. The changes in the resting membrane potential in the smooth muscles below the threshold required for contractions are called slow waves. These membrane potentials do not cause muscle contraction traveling down the intestine. Excitatory input from mechanical, sensory, and chemical receptors results in depolarization to a threshold potential causing a release of acetylcholine and influx of calcium, generating a spike potential. The calcium binds with calmodulin, further allowing binding of actin and myosin, generating a contraction.

During fasting, migrating band of contractions called migrating motor complexes (MMC), also known as interdigestive motor complexes, migrate aborally in clusters through the antrum and intestines in a cyclical pattern. Four phases of MMC are described (**Fig. 1**). During phase 1, called the quiescent stage, no action potentials are present. During phase 2, irregular contractions involving both segmenting and peristaltic movements are seen. Regular, intense contractions with maximal amplitude resulting from action potentials superimposing on the slow wave are seen during phase 3, followed by a short contractile activity during phase 4. The MMC functions as a housekeeper, sweeping the contents of the intestine forward, thereby preventing stasis and bacterial overgrowth.[23]

The periodicity of MMC is controlled primarily by the enteric nervous system with some contribution from the central nervous system. Nutrition interrupts MMC and initiates irregular segmental muscle contractions of the fed state, facilitating the churning of the chyme, helping digestion. Fat content in the food slows the frequency and reduces the amplitude of the muscular activity much more than the carbohydrates and protein.[24,25] Unlike the small intestine, the colon is in a state of continuous digestion; hence interdigestive patterns such as MMC are not observed. The movement of colonic content is mainly through high-amplitude propagated contractions and partially through segmental contractions.

PATHOLOGIC BASIS OF MOTILITY DISORDERS IN SHORT BOWEL SYNDROME

The histopathology of gastrointestinal conditions such as necrotizing enterocolitis, gastroschisis, and atresia reflect both the acute and chronic postinflammatory changes. The observations in intestinal specimens of infants with necrotizing enterocolitis include postinflammatory necrosis, postischemic changes, and vascular degeneration. There is also increased collagen deposition contributing to fibrotic changes distributed across all layers. Pathologic specimens obtained from the proximal end of intestinal atresia show the segmental absence of muscular layers and replacement with fibrotic tissue with a decrease in the number and intensity of the

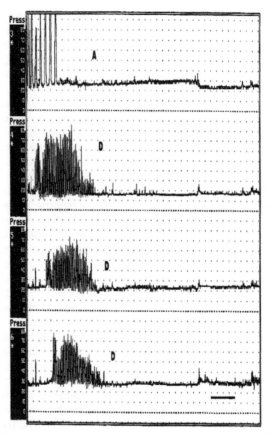

Fig. 1. A typical migrating motor complex during fasting in a human subject. The recording was obtained with intraluminal miniature pressure transducers spaced 8 cm apart in the antrum *(A)* and duodenum *(D)*. High-amplitude contractions are distally propagated (Scale bar = 2 mn) From Broussard DL. Gastrointestinal motility in the neonate. Clin Perinatol. 1995 Mar; 22:39.

ganglion cells. In the distal atretic part, the lack of both muscular layers and neural ganglion cells and distortion to the architecture of the ganglia of the myenteric plexus has been described.[26,27]

The mechanisms of hypermotility are not well understood. In a normal subject, exposure of the ileum to the lipid content in nutrition stimulates the release of neurotensin, enteroglucagon, and neuropeptide YY which initiates a negative feedback loop resulting in slowing of intestinal motility. This is often referred to as 'ileal brake.[28] Loss of the terminal portions of the ileum results in loss of the ileal brake, leading to perturbations in the MMC. This results in increased propagative then segmental contractions leading to increased motility, a shorter gastrointestinal transit, malabsorption, and diarrhea.[29]

INVESTIGATIONS OF MOTILITY DISORDERS IN SHORT BOWEL SYNDROME

Studies that have been used in dysmotility in SBS include antroduodenal manometry, gastric-emptying scintigraphy, and upper gastrointestinal contrast studies.[30] In antroduodenal manometry, stomach and duodenal motility are evaluated by measuring intraluminal pressures achieved either by a water perfused catheter system or a solid-state catheter. The lumen obliterating contractions activate the pressure transducers on the catheter providing data regarding the gastric and duodenal motility.[31] The contractions are assessed during three phases: the fasting or interdigestive phase, the feeding phase, and a provocative testing phase, whereby the response is evaluated following a promotility agent.[32] In one study by Takahashi and colleagues, the authors used manometry to study intestinal dilatation and dysmotility.[30] The mean duration and frequency of phase 3 contractions were typical for their age. However, the mean contraction amplitude of phase 2 and 3 contractions was low for their age. The authors surmised that the low contraction amplitude was the major contributor to the dilated bowel loop and the loss of function.

Gastric scintigraphy assesses the clearance of a radioisotope-labeled meal from the stomach by measuring the gamma rays. The gastric count by scintigraphy correlates with the amount of feed in the stomach without the need for complex geometric assumptions. Unlike breath testing, this test is not dependent on the absorptive function and pulmonary function. Though scintigraphy is often considered the gold standard to assess gastric emptying, intolerance and emesis are often barriers. Scintigraphy also requires transport to the radiology unit out of the intensive care or a portable gamma-ray unit. The limitations posed by the small size of the pediatric subject and the lack of normative data lead to wide variation in the interpretation and diminish the utility of these studies.[32–34]

Gastrointestinal contrast studies do not provide an accurate assessment of gastrointestinal motility. Firstly, the consistency of the enteral feed and its interaction with the gastrointestinal tract is different from that of the contrast agent. Also, the endocrine, paracrine, neurotransmitter talk that emanates from the interaction of the nutritional content with the gastrointestinal tract is different and often absent with contrast medium. However, the actual value of a contrast study lies in its ability to differentiate a mechanical from a functional obstruction.

TREATMENT OF MOTILITY DISORDERS IN SHORT BOWEL SYNDROME

The motility challenges in infants with SBS can be due to either hypomotility or hypermotility. The medical therapies and surgical techniques described in the treatment of these conditions are listed in **Table 1**.

MEDICAL THERAPIES IN HYPOMOTILITY STATES IN SHORT BOWEL SYNDROME
Promotility Agents

Promotility agents or prokinetics induce coordinated mobility facilitating forward propulsion of intestinal contents. The promotility agents should not be used in the presence of gastrointestinal obstruction or narrowing. The promotility agents mentioned later in discussion are described based on the mechanism of action on the receptors in the gastrointestinal tract.

Antidopaminergic agents
The dopaminergic receptors are extensively located in the stomach and duodenum. The dopaminergic-D2 receptor agonist/antagonist increases the tone of the lower esophageal sphincter and relaxes the gastric fundus, and improves the coordination of the antroduodenum and pyloric relaxation. This coordinated effort results in improved gastric emptying and intestinal transit. As the dopaminergic receptor representation in the small bowel and colon is relatively small, it has little action on the colon.[19,35]

Table 1
List of medical therapies and surgical techniques in the treatment of hypomotility and hypermotility states in SBS

	For Hypomotility Issues	For Hypermotility Issues
Medical therapies	Promotility agents: a. Antidopaminergic agents b. Serotoninergic agents c. Motilin agonist	Antidiarrheal/antimotility agents: a. Absorbents b. Opioid agonists c. Sequestering agents
Surgical techniques	Autologous Intestinal Reconstruction a. Simple reconstructive surgeries. (Tapering, Resection) b. Longitudinal Intestinal Lengthening Technique (LILT) c. Serial Transverse Enteroplasty (STEP)	a. Antiperistaltic intestinal segment b. Isoperistaltic interposition of the colon c. Intestinal valves/sphincters

Domperidone acts as a mixed agonist/antagonist on peripheral D2 receptors.[35] Metoclopramide's mechanism of action includes D2 receptor antagonistic activity, along with serotonergic activity at serotonin 3 and 4 receptors. Domperidone has been found to be helpful in adult patients with gastroparesis but is less commonly studied in children with SBS.[36] Domperidone is not currently available in the United States. Habituation and decreased response to prolonged use is a disadvantage of this medication. The use of metoclopramide is restricted by the undesired side effect of extrapyramidal reactions such as tardive dyskinesia. Tardive dyskinesia is a late-onset extrapyramidal reaction that can result in a severe irreversible movement disorder involving torticollis, thrusting of the tongue, bulbar speech, oculogyric crisis, involuntary movements of limbs and face, dyspnea, and trismus. There is no specific treatment of tardive dyskinesia apart from the cessation of metoclopramide. Intravenous or intramuscular diphenhydramine hydrochloride can provide resolution in some cases. Neonates and infants are at higher risk for extrapyramidal reactions due to suboptimal clearing of metoclopramide due to immature hepatic and renal clearing mechanisms. Food and Drug Administration leaflet recommends the restriction of the use of metoclopramide to adults and not to extend beyond 12 weeks. In a randomized, double-blind trial of metoclopramide in infants for the resolution of gastroesophageal reflux subjects were treated with metoclopramide at the dose of 0.1 mg/kg four times a day or a placebo for a week. Metoclopramide use did not alter the gastric emptying time as measured by scintigraphy but reduced the amount of time spent with a pH of less than 4.[37]

Levosulpiride is a newer antidopaminergic medication that has D2 receptor antagonistic and serotonin-4 receptor agonist properties with resultant promotility effects in the stomach and small bowel. It is thought to be as effective as metoclopramide and domperidone, but the concerns with central nervous system action remain.[38,39]

Serotonergic agents

Serotonergic receptors are extensively located in the gastrointestinal tract along the esophagus, stomach, duodenum, jejunum, and colon. The serotonergic agents initiate action potentials, resulting in smooth muscle contractions with the release of acetylcholine.[17] Cisapride is a serotonergic drug that was used as a prokinetic medication before being discontinued due to safety reasons. Cisapride is an agonist in serotonin 4 and an antagonist in serotonin 3 receptors. Based on the distribution of the receptors, it induces prokinetic activity in the distal esophagus, antral-duodenal contractions, and coordination, jejunal motility, thereby decreasing both gastric and intestinal transit time.[40] Due to complications of cardiac arrhythmia, sudden death, the use of cisapride was stopped in the United States.[17] Since its discontinuation in 2000 though, newer serotonergic agonists have been studied, although concerns regarding cardiac arrhythmia remain in the newer analogs, and data regarding their use in children with SBS is lacking.

Motilin agonists

Motilin is a hormone secreted by the entero-endocrine (M) cells of the upper gastro-intestinal tract during the fasting state and plays a vital role in the motility of the gastrointestinal tract by promoting the MMC.[41,42] The motilin receptors are more abundant in the upper gastrointestinal tract and hence stimulate gastric and small intestine motility. Motilin is mainly secreted in the fasting states, and its levels decrease with the ingestion of food. Erythromycin, clarithromycin, amoxicillin-clavulanate are some of the motilin receptor agonists, collectively called motilides. Erythromycin activates the G protein-coupled motilin receptors resulting in concentration-dependent contractions of the stomach. These erythromycin-induced phase 3 MMC contractions then result in improved gastrointestinal transit.[41,42] In a recent meta-analysis, the use of erythromycin and clarithromycin in preterm low birth weight infants, was studied. Nineteen studies with erythromycin and 2 studies with clarithromycin were eligible.[43] The use of erythromycin in preterm infants was associated with improved feeding tolerance; however, it was found to be of low to very low-quality evidence. Similar studies of the use of erythromycin in infants with SBS are scarce. In one study, erythromycin was compared with placebo in infants with uncomplicated gastroschisis with the outcome of achieving enteral autonomy. Erythromycin was administered at the dose of 3 mg/kg four times daily. This study failed to show any benefits with the use of erythromycin in improved feeding tolerance in infants with uncomplicated gastroschisis.[44] As doses of 5 to 12.5 mg/kg/dose every 6 hours have been described, in our institute, we use 5 to 10 mg/kg/dose every 6 hours.

Apart from the effect on the motilin receptors, amoxicillin-clavulanate is thought to interact with the gamma-aminobutyric acid receptor in the myenteric plexus. In a study performed in 6 healthy subjects treated with amoxicillin-clavulanate in both fasting and fed states, duodenojejunal manometry showed an increase in duration and strength of propagated contractions.[45] In another study, amoxicillin-clavulanate in 20 patients undergoing antroduodenal manometry induced phase 3 MMC in the fasting state but not fed state.[46] In a recent case-control retrospective cohort study, the use of amoxicillin-clavulanate was associated with higher tolerated enteral feeding volumes and smaller gastric residuals in children who were admitted to a pediatric intensive care unit.[47] The more potent prokinetic effects in the duodenum and jejunum makes amoxicillin-clavulanate a better prokinetic than erythromycin in the opinion of many clinicians. As a prokinetic, we use amoxicillin-clavulanate in the dosage of 10 to 20 mg/kg/dose every 12 hours. However, the evidence to support the use of amoxicillin-clavulanate in infants with SBS is weaker than that of erythromycin. Undesirable effects of macrolides include an impact on the gut microbiota due to their antibiotic actions.

MEDICAL THERAPIES IN HYPERMOTILITY STATES IN SHORT BOWEL SYNDROME
Antidiarrheal Medications

Infants and children with SBS often suffer from hypermotility disorders, which can manifest with malabsorption, diarrhea, and or increased ostomy output. In such conditions, several agents are used to slow down gastrointestinal transit. As these agents slow the gastrointestinal transit without enhancing the absorption, caution should be exercised and is best avoided in patients with intestinal bacterial overgrowth.

Absorbent drugs

Absorbents include dietary fibers such as guar gum and pectin. Dietary fiber can be of soluble and insoluble varieties. Both the soluble and the insoluble forms osmotically absorb water and slow the gastrointestinal transit by altering the stool consistency. Also, dietary fiber is passed on to the colon in an undigested form, whereby it is acted on by the intestinal bacteria liberating short-chain fatty acids (SCFA). SCFA serve as metabolic fuel to the enterocytes in the colon, supporting their proliferation and growth.[48] Pectin and guar gum are examples of dietary fiber used in the management of diarrhea. The description of the use of pectin in children with SBS is scant. In a case report by Finkel and colleagues, a three-year-old child with SBS was supplemented with pectin. They reported a reduction in the stool output, increased gastrointestinal transit time, along with an increase in positive nitrogen balance.[49]

Guar gum is a soluble form of dietary fiber that on reaching the colon, is acted on by the bacteria liberating SCFA. In a double-blind, randomized control study involving 126 infants with acute diarrhea, the supplementation of partially hydrolyzed guar gum in oral rehydration solution reduced diarrhea, and increased stool output suggesting increased gastrointestinal transit time.[48]

Opioid agents

Opioids act on the mu-opioid receptor of the gastrointestinal tract as a partial agonist. Loperamide is a phenyl piperidine derivative with structural similarity to other opioid receptor agonists such as diphenoxylate.[50] Loperamide has good gastrointestinal absorption but is metabolized by cytochrome P450 (CYP450) and crosses the blood–brain barrier minimally. Due to these properties, it lacks the analgesic property but has local effects on the gastrointestinal system. Loperamide decreases the peristalsis of the gut by increasing the tone of the intestines, increasing the nonpropulsive activity of the longitudinal muscles, and decreasing the secretion of, and increasing the absorption of, gastrointestinal fluid secretions. Drug interactions with CYP450 inhibitors (such as erythromycin) and hepatic impairment might result in a prolongation of the duration of its action. Undesirable effects include ileus, constipation, and drowsiness.[50,51]

In a double-blind, randomized cross-over trial, loperamide, diphenoxylate, and codeine were compared in 30 adult subjects with chronic diarrhea. It was noted that the antidiarrheal action was the strongest with loperamide (3 times that of diphenoxylate, and 50 times that of codeine) while also having the fewest central nervous system effects.[52] Similar studies comparing opioid agonists in SBS are scarce.[53,54] In one double-blind cross-over study, the efficacy of loperamide was compared with diphenoxylate in adult subjects who had diarrhea following intestinal resection due to Crohn's disease. Loperamide was associated with better stool consistency, lower stool frequency and was preferred by the subjects.[54]

Sequestering agents

In SBS, the process of absorption of bile salts is interrupted due to the resection of the terminal ileum, a reduced mucosal surface, and faster transit times. Bile salts are instead delivered to the colon, inducing a process of osmotic and secretory diarrhea. The inability of the liver to compensate for the loss of bile acid caused by malabsorption results in fat malabsorption and loss of fat-soluble vitamins.[55] Sequestering agents such as cholestyramine bind to bile acids and mitigate watery diarrhea. In addition, cholestyramine also partially interrupts the enterohepatic circulation and increases the synthesis of bile salts by using the endogenous cholesterol via 7-α-hydroxylation.[56]

Surgical Techniques in Hypomotility States in Short Bowel Syndrome

Autologous intestinal reconstruction

Hypomotility in surgical SBS is often due to a result of dilatation of the small bowel, thereby affecting the peristalsis leading to delayed transit of contents in the small bowel. This often leads to the stagnation of intestinal content and bacterial overgrowth, thereby worsening intestinal dilatation and motility. Autologous Intestinal Reconstruction surgeries are aimed at restoring the size of the intestinal lumen toward normal ranges without affecting the length of the bowel. Surgery should only be considered after supportive and medical interventions have failed to resolve or control the symptoms and when the adaptation of the intestines has stabilized and the tolerance to enteral nutrition has plateaued. Simple bowel reconstruction techniques involve tapering or resection of the dilated portions of the intestine. In the tapering procedure, the intestinal lumen is folded inwards along the antimesenteric border. In simple resection, a triangular piece of the dilated intestines along the antimesenteric border is resected. Two specific, more complicated autologous intestinal reconstruction techniques which are worth mentioning are longitudinal intestinal lengthening technique (LILT) and serial transverse enteroplasty (STEP).

Longitudinal intestinal lengthening technique. In this technique, the dilated bowel is transected longitudinally into two halves which are then converted into smaller cylindrical structures by suturing their free ends (**Fig. 2**). These newly created intestinal tubes are then anastomosed end-to-end in an isoperistaltic manner to establish continuity. This restores the lumen closer to standard diameter facilitating better contractile function. In this technique, the surgeon separates the 2 layers of the mesentery along the avascular plane and transects the dilated bowel along with the 2 points on the mesenteric and the antimesenteric border.[57] For better results, the bowel should be enlarged to at least twice the standard diameter before this procedure and should not have a primary hypomotility disorder.[58] Sometimes, the dilated bowel is artificially induced by obstructing the proximal stoma in a controlled manner over a period of several months.

Serial transverse enteroplasty. Similar to LILT, the goal of this procedure is to normalize the dilated lumen into a narrower normal caliber lumen while improving the length of the intestines. In this procedure, the dilated bowel is partially transected alternatingly on the opposite borders (mesenteric and anti-mesenteric) in a zig-zag pattern fashioning a narrower and longer lumen of the small bowel (**Fig. 3**).[57] A newer modification of the STEP procedure is the Spiral Intestinal Lengthening and Tailoring, whereby continuous spiral transections are performed between the mesenteric and antimesenteric borders, which are then stretched, and the edges are sutured continuously.

Experience with the STEP procedure has been reassuring, with enteral autonomy occurring in more than 45%. A recent meta-analysis showed a significant improvement (more than 81%) in enteral tolerance in children who underwent this procedure.[59] In comparison, both STEP and LILT procedures have similar outcomes. The STEP procedure is thought to be less complicated and relatively easier to perform, with fewer restrictions on the length of the residual bowel. However, both LILT and STEP

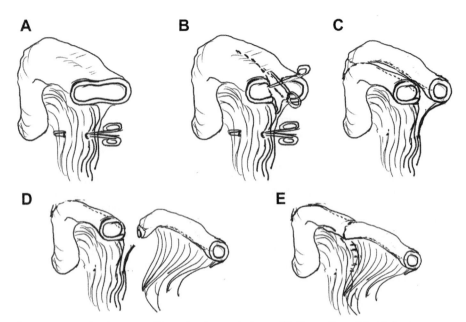

Fig. 2. Longitudinal intestinal lengthening technique: (*A*) Blunt dissection of the mesentery along the avascular plane; (*B*) transection of dilated bowel along mesenteric and antimesenteric plane; (*C*) Surgical creation of 2 smaller caliber lumen intestinal loops; (*D, E*) Resection and isoperistaltic anastomosis of the surgically created loops.

procedures have a considerable risk for both short and long-term complications, including recurrence of dilatation, subsequent bacterial overgrowth, and postoperative narrowing and obstruction. The need for transplantation (LILT 26%, STEP 16%) and mortality (LILT 30%, STEP 14%) are also significant.[60,61] Of note, STEP can be

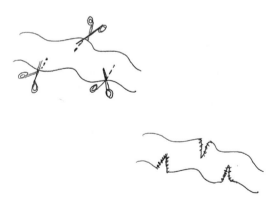

Fig. 3. Serial transverse enteroplasty: The dilated bowel is partially transected alternatingly on the opposite borders (mesenteric and anti-mesenteric) in a zig-zag pattern fashioning a narrower and longer lumen of the small bowel.

repeated to surgically treat recurrent dilatations, while LILT is limited by the inability to repeat the procedure.

Surgical Techniques in Hypermotility States in Short Bowel Syndrome

The following surgical methods are attempted in conditions with reduced gastrointestinal transit time due to hypermotility not responsive to either medical or supportive management. Dysmotility is a contraindication to these techniques.

Antiperistaltic intestinal segment

In this technique, a small segment of the small bowel or colon is retrieved and reverse-anastomosed in an antiperistaltic orientation. This implantation is usually conducted in the terminal parts of the small bowel. This segment functions as a physiologic brake and increases the gastrointestinal transit time. Reports of this technique in infants are sparse. In one account, an infant with 10 cm jejunum following necrotizing enterocolitis underwent this procedure and was successfully weaned off of parenteral nutrition within 3 years.[62] Studies conducted in adults have suggested that improvement in the absorption of nutrients leads to reduced dependence on parenteral nutrition.[63]

Isoperistaltic interposition of colon

In this technique, a segment of the colon is anastomosed in isoperistaltic orientation. The differences in the motility pattern between the colon and the small bowel are thought to prolong the gastrointestinal transit time. It is observed that the transposed segment of the colon can participate in water and electrolytes absorption. Adaptive changes in the transplanted colon are also noted over time which might result in improved nutrient absorption. Limited reporting of this procedure in children highlights success in SBS.[64,65]

Valves and sphincters

Artificial narrowing of the intestines is surgically designed to delay gastrointestinal transit and improve absorption. These valves are placed in the distal part of the small bowel. Sometimes such valves are also created to artificially induce the dilatation of the bowel to perform an autologous intestinal lengthening procedure at a later date. Performed in the distal bowel, it can function similar to the ileocecal valve.[65,66]

Future Directions

With the improved survival of infants with SBS, dysmotility-associated morbidities are expected to increase in severity and chronicity. Dysmotility is a major morbidity in infants with SBS, impairing feeding tolerance, and prolonging dependence on parenteral nutrition. Currently, there is a minimal choice of medical therapies to address gastrointestinal dysmotility in infants with SBS. Their use is impeded by unproven efficacy and concerning adverse effect profiles. In the absence of similar studies in newborn infants, supporting data are extrapolated from children of older age groups and adults. Research is needed in the development of newer therapies with an improved safety profile and better efficacy that will mitigate the effects of dysmotility. One of the reasons for the lack of evidence-based data is the rarity of the diagnosis, making it impossible for single-institution studies to generate good quality evidence. While we wait for the gold standard multicenter randomized control trial, tertiary intestinal rehabilitation centers should combine their data to develop the next best evidence to support the use of medical therapies and surgical techniques in the treatment of dysmotility in SBS.

BEST PRACTICES

What is the current practice for disorders of motility in short bowel syndrome?

Congenital causes of SBS (gastroschisis, atresia) are more likely to have motility disorders than the post-natal causes of SBS (Necrotizing enterocolitis, spontaneous intestinal perforation). Treatment of motility disorders should be tailored considering the etiology of SBS, the history of surgical repair, and the anatomy of the residual gastrointestinal tract. The ability to diagnose motility disorders in infants is impeded by the limitations of the small size of the patient and the lack of normative data.

What changes in current practice are likely to improve outcomes?

- Improved studies to understand the pathogenesis of dysmotility in SBS in infants.
- Better evidence base to support existing treatment strategies and development of newer therapies in the treatment of motility disorders in SBS in infants.
- Harness the potential of consortiums of tertiary intestinal rehabilitation centers to develop and strengthen management strategies for motility disorders of infants with SBS.

Major Recommendations?

Hypomotility disorders in patients with SBS:

- Promotility agents should be considered only after concerns for mechanical obstruction have been alleviated.
- Gastrointestinal contrast studies can differentiate mechanical from functional obstruction but are not reliable tests to assess gastrointestinal motility.
- Gastric scintigraphy can be considered in patients suspected of delayed gastric emptying.
- Motilin agonists (Erythromycin and Amoxicillin-clavulanate) are the commonly used promotility agents with a comparatively better safety profile. (Low certainty evidence, weak recommendation)
- Surgical techniques (LILT and STEP) should be considered only after failure of medical management.

Hypermotility disorders in patients with SBS:

- Adsorbents (dietary fibers) and opioid agents can be valuable in treating SBS patients with hypermotility. (Very low certainly evidence, weak recommendation)

Summary statement:

Disorders of motility are a significant cause of morbidity in SBS.

- The management is challenging due to limitations with currently avalable diagnostic and therapeutic options. Additional studies are needed to improve the evidence for now available diagnostics, and medical and surgical therapies for motility disorders of SBS. Bibliographic Sources: Data from references[10–13, 43–47,48–51,59–61].

DISCLOSURE

M.H. Premkumar is a consultant to Fresenius Kabi Inc.

REFERENCES

1. Pironi L. Definitions of intestinal failure and the short bowel syndrome. Best Pract Res Clin Gastroenterol 2016;30(2):173–85.
2. Nightingale J, Woodward JM, Small B, Nutrition Committee of the British Society of G. Guidelines for management of patients with a short bowel. Gut 2006; 55(Suppl 4):iv1–12.

3. Struljs MC, Diamond IR, de Silva N, et al. Establishing norms for intestinal length in children. J Pediatr Surg 2009;44(5):933–8.
4. Touloukian RJ, Smith GJ. Normal intestinal length in preterm infants. J Pediatr Surg 1983;18(6):720–3.
5. Rickham PP. Massive small intestinal resection in newborn infants. Hunterian lecture delivered at the Royal College of surgeons of England on 13th April 1967. Ann R Coll Surg Engl Dec 1967;41(6):480–92.
6. Cole CR, Hansen NI, Higgins RD, et al. Very low birth weight preterm infants with surgical short bowel syndrome: incidence, morbidity and mortality, and growth outcomes at 18 to 22 months. Pediatrics 2008;122(3):e573–82.
7. Wales PW, de Silva N, Kim J, et al. Neonatal short bowel syndrome: population-based estimates of incidence and mortality rates. J Pediatr Surg 2004;39(5): 690–5.
8. Fatemizadeh R, Gollins L, Hagan J, et al. In neonatal-onset surgical short bowel syndrome survival is high, and enteral autonomy is related to residual bowel length. JPEN J Parenter Enteral Nutr 2021. https://doi.org/10.1002/jpen.2124.
9. Smazal AL, Massieu LA, Gollins L, et al. Small proportion of low-birth-weight infants with ostomy and intestinal failure due to short-bowel syndrome achieve enteral autonomy prior to reanastomosis. JPEN J Parenter Enteral Nutr 2021; 45(2):331–8.
10. Phillips JD, Raval MV, Redden C, et al. Gastroschisis, atresia, dysmotility: surgical treatment strategies for a distinct clinical entity. J Pediatr Surg 2008;43(12): 2208–12.
11. Ganapathy V, Hay JW, Kim JH, et al. Long term healthcare costs of infants who survived neonatal necrotizing enterocolitis: a retrospective longitudinal study among infants enrolled in Texas Medicaid. BMC Pediatr 2013;13:127.
12. Ladd AP, Rescorla FJ, West KW, et al. Long-term follow-up after bowel resection for necrotizing enterocolitis: factors affecting outcome. J Pediatr Surg 1998;33(7): 967–72.
13. Bazacliu C, Neu J. Necrotizing enterocolitis: long term complications. Curr Pediatr Rev 2019;15(2):115–24.
14. Altschuler SM, Bao XM, Bieger D, et al. Viscerotopic representation of the upper alimentary tract in the rat: sensory ganglia and nuclei of the solitary and spinal trigeminal tracts. J Comp Neurol 1989;283(2):248–68.
15. Kalia M, Sullivan JM. Brainstem projections of sensory and motor components of the vagus nerve in the rat. J Comp Neurol 1982;211(3):248–65.
16. Wood JD. Intrinsic neural control of intestinal motility. Annu Rev Physiol 1981;43: 33–51.
17. Beattie DT, Smith JA. Serotonin pharmacology in the gastrointestinal tract: a review. Naunyn Schmiedebergs Arch Pharmacol 2008;377(3):181–203.
18. Shah V, Lyford G, Gores G, et al. Nitric oxide in gastrointestinal health and disease. Gastroenterology 2004;126(3):903–13.
19. Glavin GB, Szabo S. Dopamine in gastrointestinal disease. Dig Dis Sci 1990; 35(9):1153–61.
20. Holzer P. New approaches to the treatment of opioid-induced constipation. Eur Rev Med Pharmacol Sci 2008;12(Suppl 1):119–27.
21. Takeshita E, Matsuura B, Dong M, et al. Molecular characterization and distribution of motilin family receptors in the human gastrointestinal tract. J Gastroenterol 2006;41(3):223–30.
22. Chen CY, Tsai CY. Ghrelin and motilin in the gastrointestinal system. Curr Pharm Des 2012;18(31):4755–65.

23. Vantrappen G, Janssens J, Hellemans J, et al. The interdigestive motor complex of normal subjects and patients with bacterial overgrowth of the small intestine. J Clin Invest 1977;59(6):1158–66.

24. Berseth CL. Gestational evolution of small intestine motility in preterm and term infants. J Pediatr 1989;115(4):646–51.

25. Bisset WM, Watt JB, Rivers RP, et al. Ontogeny of fasting small intestinal motor activity in the human infant. Gut 1988;29(4):483–8.

26. Ozguner IF, Savas C, Ozguner M, et al. Intestinal atresia with segmental musculature and neural defect. J Pediatr Surg 2005;40(8):1232–7.

27. Ramachandran P, Vincent P, Ganesh S, et al. Morphological abnormalities in the innervation of the atretic segment of bowel in neonates with intestinal atresia. Pediatr Surg Int 2007;23(12):1183–6.

28. Spiller RC, Trotman IF, Higgins BE, et al. The ileal brake–inhibition of jejunal motility after ileal fat perfusion in man. Gut 1984;25(4):365–74.

29. Van Citters GW, Lin HC. Ileal brake: neuropeptidergic control of intestinal transit. Curr Gastroenterol Rep 2006;8(5):367–73.

30. Takahashi A, Tomomasa T, Suzuki N, et al. The relationship between disturbed transit and dilated bowel, and manometric findings of dilated bowel in patients with duodenal atresia and stenosis. J Pediatr Surg 1997;32(8):1157–60.

31. Patcharatrakul T, Gonlachanvit S. Technique of functional and motility test: how to perform antroduodenal manometry. J Neurogastroenterol Motil 2013;19(3):395–404.

32. Alexander JL, Mutyala R. Understanding gastrointestinal motility studies in pediatrics. Curr Probl Pediatr Adolesc Health Care 2020;50(8):100843.

33. Abell TL, Camilleri M, Donohoe K, et al. Consensus recommendations for gastric emptying scintigraphy: a joint report of the American neurogastroenterology and motility Society and the Society of Nuclear Medicine. Am J Gastroenterol 2008;103(3):753–63.

34. Ng TSC, Putta N, Kwatra NS, et al. Pediatric solid gastric emptying scintigraphy: normative value guidelines and nonstandard meal alternatives. Am J Gastroenterol 2020;115(11):1830–9.

35. Barone JA. Domperidone: a peripherally acting dopamine2-receptor antagonist. Ann Pharmacother 1999;33(4):429–40.

36. Patterson D, Abell T, Rothstein R, et al. A double-blind multicenter comparison of domperidone and metoclopramide in the treatment of diabetic patients with symptoms of gastroparesis. Am J Gastroenterol 1999;94(5):1230–4.

37. Tolia V, Calhoun J, Kuhns L, et al. Randomized, prospective double-blind trial of metoclopramide and placebo for gastroesophageal reflux in infants. J Pediatr 1989;115(1):141–5.

38. Mearin F, Rodrigo L, Perez-Mota A, et al. Levosulpiride and cisapride in the treatment of dysmotility-like functional dyspepsia: a randomized, double-masked trial. Clin Gastroenterol Hepatol 2004;2(4):301–8.

39. Mansi C, Borro P, Giacomini M, et al. Comparative effects of levosulpiride and cisapride on gastric emptying and symptoms in patients with functional dyspepsia and gastroparesis. Aliment Pharmacol Ther 2000;14(5):561–9.

40. Costedio MM, Hyman N, Mawe GM. Serotonin and its role in colonic function and in gastrointestinal disorders. Dis Colon Rectum 2007;50(3):376–88.

41. Al-Missri MZ, Jialal I. Physiology, Motilin. In: StatPearls [Internet]. Treasure Island (FL): StatPearls Publishing; January, 2022. PMID: 31424893.

42. Kato S, Takahashi A, Shindo M, et al. Characterization of the gastric motility response to human motilin and erythromycin in human motilin receptor-expressing transgenic mice. PLoS One 2019;14(2):e0205939.

43. Basu S, Smith S. Macrolides for the prevention and treatment of feeding intolerance in preterm low birth weight infants: a systematic review and meta-analysis. Eur J Pediatr 2021;180(2):353–78.

44. Curry JI, Lander AD, Stringer MD, et al, Committee BMR. A multicenter, randomized, double-blind, placebo-controlled trial of the prokinetic agent erythromycin in the postoperative recovery of infants with gastroschisis. J Pediatr Surg 2004; 39(4):565–9.

45. Caron F, Ducrotte P, Lerebours E, et al. Effects of amoxicillin-clavulanate combination on the motility of the small intestine in human beings. Antimicrob Agents Chemother 1991;35(6):1085–8.

46. Gomez R, Fernandez S, Aspirot A, et al. Effect of amoxicillin/clavulanate on gastrointestinal motility in children. J Pediatr Gastroenterol Nutr 2012;54(6): 780–4.

47. Chiusolo F, Capriati T, Erba I, et al. Management of enteral nutrition in the pediatric intensive care unit: prokinetic effects of amoxicillin/clavulanate in real life conditions. Pediatr Gastroenterol Hepatol Nutr 2020;23(6):521–30.

48. Alam NH, Ashraf H, Kamruzzaman M, et al. Efficacy of partially hydrolyzed guar gum (PHGG) supplemented modified oral rehydration solution in the treatment of severely malnourished children with watery diarrhoea: a randomised double-blind controlled trial. J Health Popul Nutr 2015;34:3.

49. Finkel Y, Brown G, Smith HL, et al. The effects of a pectin-supplemented elemental diet in a boy with short gut syndrome. Acta Paediatr Scand 1990; 79(10):983–6.

50. Baker DE. Loperamide: a pharmacological review. Rev Gastroenterol Disord 2007;7(Suppl 3):S11–8.

51. Daly JW, Harper J. Loperamide: novel effects on capacitative calcium influx. Cell Mol Life Sci 2000;57(1):149–57.

52. Palmer KR, Corbett CL, Holdsworth CD. Double-blind cross-over study comparing loperamide, codeine and diphenoxylate in the treatment of chronic diarrhea. Gastroenterology 1980;79(6):1272–5.

53. King RF, Norton T, Hill GL. A double-blind crossover study of the effect of loperamide hydrochloride and codeine phosphate on ileostomy output. Aust N Z J Surg 1982;52(2):121–4.

54. Bergman L, Djarv L. A comparative study of loperamide and diphenoxylate in the treatment of chronic diarrhoea caused by intestinal resection. Ann Clin Res 1981; 13(6):402–5.

55. Sinha L, Liston R, Testa HJ, et al. Idiopathic bile acid malabsorption: qualitative and quantitative clinical features and response to cholestyramine. Aliment Pharmacol Ther 1998;12(9):839–44.

56. Riaz S, John S. Cholestyramine Resin. In: StatPearls [Internet]. Treasure Island (FL): StatPearls Publishing; Jan, 2022. PMID: 30475562.

57. Pakarinen MP. Autologous intestinal reconstruction surgery as part of comprehensive management of intestinal failure. Pediatr Surg Int 2015;31(5):453–64.

58. Bianchi A. Intestinal loop lengthening–a technique for increasing small intestinal length. J Pediatr Surg 1980;15(2):145–51.

59. Fernandes MA, Usatin D, Allen IE, et al. Improved enteral tolerance following step procedure: systematic literature review and meta-analysis. Pediatr Surg Int 2016; 32(10):921–6.

60. Frongia G, Kessler M, Weih S, et al. Comparison of LILT and STEP procedures in children with short bowel syndrome – a systematic review of the literature. J Pediatr Surg 2013;48(8):1794–805.

61. Sudan D, Thompson J, Botha J, et al. Comparison of intestinal lengthening procedures for patients with short bowel syndrome. Ann Surg 2007;246(4):593–601 [discussion: 601-4].

62. Trinkle JK, Bryant LR. Reversed colon segment in an infant with massive small bowel resection: a case report. J Ky Med Assoc 1967;65(11):1090–1091 passim.

63. Beyer-Berjot L, Joly F, Maggiori L, et al. Segmental reversal of the small bowel can end permanent parenteral nutrition dependency: an experience of 38 adults with short bowel syndrome. Ann Surg 2012;256(5):739–44 [discussion: 744-5].

64. Glick PL, de Lorimier AA, Adzick NS, et al. Colon interposition: an adjuvant operation for short-gut syndrome. J Pediatr Surg 1984;19(6):719–25.

65. Hollwarth ME. Surgical strategies in short bowel syndrome. Pediatr Surg Int 2017; 33(4):413–9.

66. Ricotta J, Zuidema GD, Gadacz TR, et al. Construction of an ileocecal valve and its role in massive resection of the small intestine. Surg Gynecol Obstet 1981; 152(3):310–4.

Malabsorption Syndromes and Food Intolerance

Jonathan Medernach, DO, Jeremy P. Middleton, MD*

KEYWORDS

- Malabsorption • Feeding intolerance • Cow's milk protein allergy
- Food protein-induced disorders • Secretory diarrhea • Osmotic diarrhea
- Congenital diarrhea

KEY POINTS

- Feeding intolerance in preterm and term neonates is common with several possible causes.
- Food protein-induced disorders can mimic signs and symptoms of more sinister problems such as necrotizing enterocolitis.
- Laboratory testing for food protein-induced disorders is nonspecific, and oral food challenge is the gold standard for diagnosis if it can be performed safely.
- A key diagnostic tool for a malabsorption syndrome is the cessation of diarrhea during the fasting state.
- Although laboratory and histopathologic evaluation can guide the clinician when evaluating newborns for malabsorption syndromes, molecular genetic testing is often necessary to provide a specific diagnosis.

INTRODUCTION

Optimization of nutrition in preterm infants is imperative and carries implications for long-term outcomes. Unfortunately, there are many obstacles to ensuring optimal growth in premature infants including infection, immaturity of the gastrointestinal tract, and medication side effects. It can be difficult to distinguish what is preventing feeding advancement or tolerance because many of the clinical signs and symptoms are similar. Much attention is paid to feeding intolerance in the neonatal intensive care unit (NICU) not only because of its consequences on growth and development but also because it may indicate necrotizing enterocolitis (NEC), which can cause significant morbidity and mortality in premature neonates.[1] Diagnostic challenges arise when neonates have persistent or recurrent feeding intolerance that is not due to NEC. Two specific problems that can both mimic the symptoms of NEC and prevent adequate nutrition are malabsorption syndromes and food intolerance. The following

Department of Pediatrics, Division of Pediatric Gastroenterology, Hepatology, and Nutrition. University of Virginia Children's Hospital, University of Virginia, Charlottesville, VA, USA
* Corresponding author.
E-mail address: jpm8k@virginia.edu

Clin Perinatol 49 (2022) 537–555
https://doi.org/10.1016/j.clp.2022.02.015
0095-5108/22/© 2022 Elsevier Inc. All rights reserved.

article discusses the role of food intolerance and malabsorption as causes of feeding intolerance in the NICU.

DEFINITIONS

The terminology describing an abnormal response to food intake can be quite confusing and is often used incorrectly. A food hypersensitivity is any adverse reaction to food that is not psychologically driven.[2] Food hypersensitivity can be further broken down into that which is immune-mediated (food allergy) versus that which is not (food intolerance). Food intolerance is very common, affecting up to 20% of the population, often causing a variety of nonspecific gastrointestinal (GI) complaints ranging from bloating and diarrhea to abdominal pain and constipation.[3] There are a variety of culprits that lead to food intolerance. Causes of GI symptoms include chemicals such as salicylates and caffeine or specific components in food such as wheat in those with nonceliac gluten intolerance, fructans in those with irritable bowel syndrome, and lactose in individuals with lactase-nonpersistence.[3] Food allergy is immune-mediated and is further delineated as immunoglobulin E (IgE)-mediated, non-IgE-mediated, or mixed.[4] Although food intolerance is frequently evaluated and treated in the general pediatrician's office, it is rarely encountered in the NICU. That being said, the term "feeding intolerance" is often used in the NICU to describe the inability to advance enteral nutrition. Because most of the adverse reactions to "food" in the NICU is actually a non-IgE-mediated food allergy, the term food protein-induced GI disease will be used.

The primary function of the GI tract is food assimilation. This is accomplished by digestion of food into small enough components to be absorbed across the small intestine epithelium and then transported into the systemic circulation. When there is a problem with food assimilation, the term malabsorption is often used in the clinical setting independent of whether the problem lies in digestion, absorption, or transport.

CLINICAL SIGNS AND SYMPTOMS OF MALABSORPTION AND FOOD PROTEIN-INDUCED GASTROINTESTINAL DISEASE

Both food protein-induced GI disease and malabsorption cause similar symptoms of feeding intolerance in the NICU. There is no universally accepted definition of feeding intolerance. Concept analysis describing feeding intolerance as "the inability to digest enteral feedings presented as gastric residual volumes of more than 50%, abdominal distension or emesis or both, and the disruption of the patient's feeding plan" is nonspecific and does not include any lower GI symptoms such as diarrhea or rectal bleeding that may preclude delivering adequate nutrition.[5] Upper GI symptoms can include regurgitation, increased gastric residuals, oral avoidance, vomiting, and abdominal distention. Lower GI symptoms include changes in stool frequency and consistency as well as presence of blood. There are a variety of extraintestinal problems that may lead to feeding intolerance such sepsis, congenital heart defects, inborn errors of metabolism, endocrinopathies, and abnormalities of the nervous system, but a complete review of these etiologies is outside the scope of this article. The following algorithm is offered to help best determine GI causes of feeding intolerance in neonates (**Fig. 1**). When feeding intolerance leads to nonbloody diarrhea, further delineation of the cause can be accomplished by following our proposed evaluation algorithm (**Fig. 2**).

FOOD PROTEIN-INDUCED GASTROINTESTINAL DISEASE

In neonates, food protein-induced GI disease is due to an immune-meditated reaction to certain proteins in breastmilk or formula. It can lead to a variety of symptoms

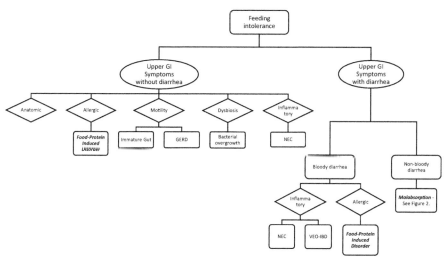

Fig. 1. Differential diagnosis of feeding intolerance in preterm neonates. gastroesophageal reflux (GERD); necrotizing enterocolitis (NEC); very-early onset inflammatory bowel disease (VEO-IBD).

including fussiness, rectal bleeding, intermittent abdominal distention, increased gastric residuals, and/or vomiting. It can be further characterized as IgE-mediated, non-IgE-mediated, or mixed.[4] Neonates with allergic disease much more frequently suffer from a non-IgE-mediated process that has historically been referred to as cow's milk protein allergy. To better describe the inflammatory condition of this process, it is recommended that these conditions be referred to as food protein-induced disorders.

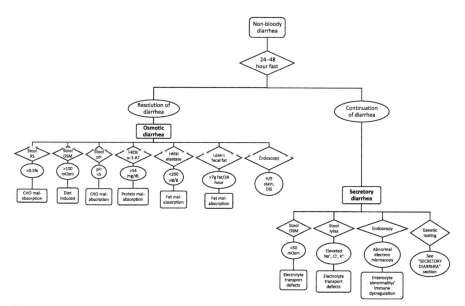

Fig. 2. Diagnostic approach of neonates with nonbloody diarrhea. carbohydrate (CHO); disaccharidase (DIS) analysis; hematoxylin and eosin (H&E); osmolality (OSM); reducing substances (RS); α-1-antrypsin (α-1-AT).

Depending on the location of the inflammatory response, these disorders include food protein-induced allergic proctocolitis (FPIAP), food protein-induced enteropathy, or food protein-induced enterocolitis syndrome (FPIES).

The pathophysiology of these disorders remains poorly understood, although much attention has been paid to these conditions during the past 2 decades. Without a large systemic IgE response, mucosal IgE has been suggested to play a role.[6] Specifically in children with FPIES, there seems to be a T-cell-mediated inflammatory response leading to increased levels of intestinal interferon gamma (IFN-γ) and decreased levels of transforming growth factor beta (TGF-β).[7,8] The pathophysiology of FPIAP is least understood, although it does lead to a profound eosinophilic colitis.

Food protein-induced allergic proctocolitis is the most common non-IgE-mediated food allergy syndrome. Mostly described in term infants up to 6 months of age, it is estimated this condition affects 2% to 3% of infants.[9] It is most frequently seen in nursing infants but can also be seen in children fed with cow's milk or soy-based formulas. Symptoms are typically mild, composed of streaks or flecks of blood and mucus in and on the stools but grossly bloody stools can be quite frightening to the family and provider alike.[10] Affected infants may have elevated total IgE, peripheral eosinophilia, and elevated fecal calprotectin levels; however, serum IgE radioallergosorbent (RAST) and skin prick tests to common foods are typically negative.[11] Treatment in breastfed children is maternal elimination of the presumed offending agents, most often cow's milk protein, soy, egg, and corn.[12] In bottlefed infants, it is recommended they transition to an extensively hydrolyzed formula; however, 5% of children will require an amino acid formula.[13] Most children will grow out of this condition by 12 months of age, and reintroduction of food can be accomplished at home without medical supervision. Although most infants present with FPIAP after discharge from the nursery or NICU, there are case reports of term and preterm infants having symptoms within the first several days of life.[14,15]

Food protein-induced enterocolitis syndrome is a condition that can affect children at any time after birth up to 1 year old. It is much less common than FPIAP, occurring in less than 1% of infants.[16,17] Children can present with a variety of symptoms including lethargy, severe diarrhea, bloody stools, acute edema, and even shock. FPIES is very uncommon in exclusively breastfed infants, and if they do develop symptoms, it is usually after the introduction of solid foods containing cow's milk, soy, rice, and/or oats.[10] Although some children may develop hypoalbuminemia, metabolic acidosis and methemoglobinemia, total IgE, eosinophilia, and serum IgE RAST testing are usually unrevealing. Treatment is elimination of the offending foodstuffs. During acute attacks, treatment is composed of supportive care, and there are several case series suggesting parenteral administration of 5-hydroxytryptamine (5-HT3) antagonists may be beneficial.[18] Most children outgrow this condition by 3 to 5 years of age. A clinically supervised oral food challenge is recommended when reintroduction of the offending food item is considered. International guidelines now exist that describe FPIES and propose specific diagnostic criteria separating FPIES into acute and chronic syndromes.[19] Although this can be a challenging diagnosis to make in infants and young children, it is even more difficult to make in term and preterm neonates.

Despite efforts to fully categorize non-IgE-mediated food protein-induced disorders, there remain phenotypes that lie outside of these definitions. With this in mind, the European Society of Pediatric Gastroenterology, Hepatology and Nutrition continues to use the terminology cow's milk protein allergy (CMPA). A position article was written to help practitioners define best practice diagnosis and treatment algorithms.[9] Part of the dilemma is that disorders besides non-IgE-mediated food protein sensitivities may improve with the elimination of cow's milk protein from the infant's diet. Fussiness and frequent regurgitation or vomiting has been attributed to CMPA; however, there remains significant debate regarding the overlap of gastroesophageal reflux disease and CMPA.[20] Cow's milk protein allergy has been associated with delayed gastric emptying and abnormal electrogastrography[21] and can lead to antral hypertrophy with foveolar hyperplasia as well as hypertrophic gastropathy.[22,23] One group has even categorized neonatal CMPA into 4 types based on the presence or absence of vomiting and bloody stools.[24] Although there was no difference in peripheral eosinophilia, total IgE, or milk-specific IgE, the authors suggest that each group cluster may have different mechanisms of pathophysiology.

Despite a lack of understanding of the mechanisms causing food protein-induced disorders, guidelines exist to help clinicians evaluate and treat term neonates and infants.[9] Unfortunately, what is understood about these disorders in preterm neonates largely comes from case reports and case series (**Table 1**). A variety of clinical manifestations have been described including vomiting, abdominal distention, lethargy, hypothermia, increased gastric residuals, diarrhea, bloody stools, and ascites. In the NICU, many of these are alarm symptoms for NEC, and in fact, immune response to cow's milk protein has been suggested as a possible cause for NEC.[25] Preterm infants with NEC not only have mononuclear cells that are sensitized to cow's milk protein but their cytokine profiles in response to β-lactoglobulin and casein are temporally related to active NEC.[25] Some authors posit that premature infants with symptoms attributed to recurrent NEC are actually experiencing food protein-induced disorders and have shown clinical improvement when infants are transitioned to formulas containing extensively hydrolyzed protein or amino acids.[26–28]

Even when a clinician has a high level of clinical suspicion that a premature infant has a food protein-induced disorder, specific testing remains elusive. In infants with FPIAP, only 40% have peripheral eosinophilia[29] and despite reports of IgE sensitization, consensus statements recommend against allergy testing.[30] There is emerging data on the use of fecal calprotectin to identify FPIAP in term infants,[11] but this is less helpful in premature infants with symptoms similar to NEC, which also is associated with elevated fecal calprotectin levels.[31] In a small series of 10 premature infants with food protein-induced symptoms, 70% had a positive atopy patch test,[32] although larger studies in term infants reveal conflicting results.[33] Although endoscopic evaluation with biopsy may identify eosinophilic infiltration in infants with food protein-induced disorders, endoscopy is an invasive procedure that should not be performed on infants with a possible diagnosis of NEC.[34] Oral food challenge remains the standard for definitively diagnosing food-protein disorders.[9] Unfortunately, reintroduction of the offending protein can be challenging due to the severity of symptoms in the premature infant and clinicians often choose to label a child as having a food protein-induced disorder without confirmatory food challenges.

PHYSIOLOGY OF DIGESTION

To better understand malabsorption syndromes, it is important to understand the normal physiology of the digestive processes within the small intestine because the overwhelming majority of nutrient absorption occurs there. The small intestine has an incredible absorptive capacity because of an enormous surface area often quoted to be the size of a tennis court in adults.[35] Digestion is the chemical breakdown of food by enzymes secreted from the mouth, stomach, and pancreas. The final steps of digestion occur at the brush border of enterocytes where nutrients are absorbed.[36] The absorption of nutrients into enterocytes varies depending on the type of nutrient and occurs via passive diffusion, facilitated diffusion, or active transport. Once

Table 1
Food protein-induced disorders described in premature infants

Author	Study Description	Gestational Age/Age of Symptoms	Clinical Features	Evaluation	Treatment
Powell[33]	Case report of 2 patients (1 premature)	32 wk/15 d old	Bloody diarrhea, lethargy, hypothermia	Laboratories: leukocytosis, stool eosinophils, abnormal oral food challenge	Hydrolyzed formula (Nutramigen®)
Faber et al[14]	Case report of single patient	33 wk/1 d old	Hematochezia, diarrhea	Laboratories: acidosis, eosinophilia, anemia, positive IgE cow's milk Biopsy: increased eosinophils, lymphoid aggregates	Amino acid formula (Neocate®)
Srinivasan et al[34]	Case report of single patient	26 wk/17 d old	Recurrent abdominal distention, bloody stools, lethargy	Laboratories: eosinophilia AXR: diffuse dilated bowel and pneumatosis	Amino acid formula (Neocate®)
Preto et al[35]	Case report of single patient	28 wk/17 d old	Recurrent abdominal distention, vomiting	Laboratories: eosinophilia, positive IgE α-globulin and β-globulin, negative IgE casein	Breast milk and extensively hydrolyzed whey formula
Covielloet et al[36]	Case report of 2 patients (twins)	30 wk/10 d old	Lethargy, vomiting, abdominal distention, bloody stools, feeding intolerance	Laboratories: eosinophilia, positive IgE α-globulin and β-globulin	Amino acid formula (Neocate®)

Study	Design	Age	Clinical presentation	Laboratory/Imaging	Treatment
Nakasone et al[37]	Case report of a single patient	25 wk/20 d old	Abdominal distention, respiratory distress, edema, ascites	Laboratories: hypoalbuminemia, lymphocyte stimulation test negative for hydrolyzed formula, human-α-lactalbumin, bovine-κ-casein but positive for soy formula and bovine-lactoferrin AXR: dilated bowel without pneumatosis U/S: ascites	Donor breast milk
Lefestey et al[27]	Case Series of 5 infants	26–35 wk/2–73 d old	Abdominal distention, increased gastric residuals, bloody stools, vomiting—3 patients with relapsing symptoms	Laboratories: normal CRP, eosinophilia (40%), hypoalbuminemia (60%) AXR: pneumatosis (100%)	Hydrolyzed or amino acid formula
Jang et al[38]	Case series of 4 infants	30 wk/1–43 d old	Bloody stools	Laboratories: eosinophilia (mean 320) endoscopy: erythema, ulceration, nodular hyperplasia eosinophilic infiltrate	Hydrolyzed formula, amino acid formula or maternal elimination of cow's milk, eggs, nuts, soybeans, fish, wheat
Cordova et al[26]	Retrospective study of all premature infants requiring multiple courses of parenteral nutrition requiring hydrolyzed or amino acid formula—14 patients	Unknown/unknown	Abdominal distention, increased gastric residuals, vomiting, bloody stools (36%)	Unknown	Discharge formula: Hydrolyzed (43%), amino acid (57%)

(continued on next page)

Table 1
(continued)

Author	Study Description	Gestational Age/Age of Symptoms	Clinical Features	Evaluation	Treatment
Miyazawi et al[25]	Survey of Japanese NICUs	Mean gestational age 36.9 wk (25.3–42)/7 d (0–67 d)	Vomiting, bloody stools, abdominal distention, increased gastric residuals, growth failure, shock, rash	Laboratories: IgE milk allergens (positive 55%); lymphocyte stimulation test (positive 84%); fecal eosinophils (positive 75%); peripheral eosinophilia (50%)	Unknown
Morita et al[39]	Retrospective study of premature infants with ICD-9 code for milk allergy—12 patients (0.5% of all admissions over 6 y)	Mean gestational age 31 wk (25–36)/23 d (4–49 d)	Vomiting, bloody stools, feeding difficulty, abdominal distention, gastric hemorrhage, apnea	Laboratories: peripheral eosinophilia, IgE milk (9%); fecal eosinophils (100%)	Hydrolyzed formula

carbohydrates, proteins, and medium chain fats have been absorbed into the enterocyte, they are secreted directly into the portal venous blood, whereas long chain fats are repackaged into chylomicrons and then secreted into lacteals.

Carbohydrate Digestion and Absorption

More than 90% of the carbohydrate calories in human breast milk come from the disaccharide, lactose. There are small amounts of galactose oligosaccharides in human breast milk, but these amounts account for very little energy, and their composition varies depending on maternal factors.[37] Lactose is also the primary carbohydrate in cow's milk based formulas, as opposed to soy formula, where the primary carbohydrate is glucose polymers.[38] Digestion of carbohydrates starts in the mouth with the secretion of salivary α-amylase, which is deactivated in the stomach due to the high acidity. Most of the carbohydrate digestion occurs in the small intestine via pancreatic α-amylase and intestinal glucoamylase. The interior α-1,4-glycoside bonds of amylose are broken down by pancreatic amylase, but the carbohydrates are not yet small enough to be absorbed.[36]

At the level of the brush border, 4 disaccharidases (maltase, isomaltase, sucrase, and lactase) further hydrolyze disaccharides and oligosaccharides.[39] Sucrase and isomaltase form a compound molecule, which breaks down α-dextrins, maltotriose, and maltose into glucose. Sucrase hydrolyzes sucrose into glucose and fructose, in addition to hydrolyzing α-dextrins, maltotriose, and maltose into glucose. Lactase hydrolyzes lactose into glucose and galactose. In healthy infants, there is an abundance of disaccharidases, and so the rate-limiting step is glucose absorption, rather than the digestion of the carbohydrates to glucose. In normal conditions, most of sugar digestion and absorption occurs in the proximal jejunum.[36]

The monosaccharides (glucose, galactose, fructose) are absorbed into enterocytes both passively and actively. Fructose is transported into the enterocyte via facilitated diffusion using the fructose transporter, type 5 (GLUT-5 transporter). Glucose and galactose enter the enterocyte via secondary active transport using the sodium-glucose (SGLT-1) cotransport system. This is an ATP-dependent Na^+ cotransporter that uses the extracellular to intracellular Na^+ gradient to energize the transport of glucose and galactose into the cell. Once monosaccharides are within enterocytes, they are transported to the intercellular space via the Na^+ independent GLUT-2 transporter on the basolateral surface of enterocytes.[36]

Protein Digestion and Absorption

The protein levels in breast milk vary depending on whether the infant is born preterm or term. Preterm breast milk tends to have more protein. During the first month, the protein content decreases regardless of the gestational age of the infant.[37] The protein components of breast milk and cow's milk formula are similar, although the ratio of casein to whey in formula can vary, whereas in breast milk, it is 60% whey.[40] In soy-based formulas, the nature of the protein necessitates supplementation with methionine, taurine, and carnitine.[38] Unlike carbohydrate digestion, which begins in the mouth, proteins are first broken down in the stomach by pepsin. Pepsin is secreted as pepsinogen by chief cells and then activated by the high acidity environment of the stomach.[36] Once the gastric contents enter the small intestine, the alkaline environment inactivates pepsin.

As food enters the small intestine, the pancreas releases several different proteases that can be classified as either endopeptidases or exopeptidases. Endopeptidases (trypsin, chymotrypsin, and elastase) hydrolyze the internal peptide bonds of proteins and exopeptidases (Carboxypeptidase A and B) hydrolyze the external peptide bonds of proteins.[36] Similar to pepsin, these peptidases are released in an inactivated form and are then activated by a substrate. The major pancreatic peptidase is trypsin, which is secreted as trypsinogen and then activated by enterokinase located at the enterocyte brush border. Once activated, trypsin can work autocatalytically to activate other pancreatic peptidases. The peptidases break down ingested proteins into peptides of various sizes and free amino acids.[36]

Protein digestion results in approximately 40% free amino acids and 60% peptides between 2 to 6 amino acid residues.[36] Amino acids are transported into the enterocyte via both active transport and facilitated diffusion. As with monosaccharide transport, active transport of amino acids and peptides relies on Na^+ cotransporters. The transporter for individual amino acids is related to its polarity and charge. Small peptides are absorbed in different locations of the jejunum as compared with free amino acids. Once in the cell, peptides are broken down into amino acids in the cytoplasm and then transported into the portal circulation.[36]

Fat Digestion and Absorption

Similar to protein, the fat content in preterm breast milk is somewhat higher than that of mothers who deliver infants at term. The fat content in breast milk varies greatly depending on the timing during the feed. Hindmilk can contain up to 3 times as much fat as foremilk.[41] The fat content in breast milk also fluctuates by the time of day, with afternoon and evening feedings having the highest fat content.[42] Most fat in breast milk is long chain triglycerides with the major fatty acids of palmitic, stearic, oleic, and linoleic acid.[43] Breast milk also contains a moderate amount of medium chain triglycerides and small amounts of short and very long chain triglycerides.

Digestion of fat starts in the stomach where fat is emulsified into smaller droplets that can be hydrolyzed by lingual and gastric lipases as well as lipases in breast milk.[44] Pancreatic lipase hydrolyzes triglycerides by breaking the ester bonds, which releases free fatty acids and monoglycerides. Phospholipase A_2 is a proenzyme that is activated by trypsin and hydrolyzes phospholipids creating lysophospholipid and free fatty acids. The third enzyme involved in lipolysis is cholesterol esterase, which hydrolyzes all 3 ester linkages in triglycerides and also hydrolyzes the ester bonds in vitamins A, D, and E.[36] Free fatty acids, monoglycerides, and bile salts combine to form mixed micelles, which are then absorbed into the enterocyte by diffusion. It is important to note that short-chain and medium-chain fatty acids can diffuse directly into the cell without forming micelles because of their higher solubility in aqueous solutions.[36] In the enterocyte, triglycerides are reassembled and combined with cholesterol and apoproteins to form chylomicrons, which then enter the lacteal. Medium-chain fatty acids are directly absorbed into the portal blood.

Understanding the normal function of the GI tract can help us understand why an infant might be experiencing diarrhea. Malabsorption syndromes can occur when there is a problem with the digestion, absorption, or transport of carbohydrate, fat, or protein. When this occurs, these substrates travel through the GI tract unaltered or broken down by gut flora, which can lead to a more rapid transit by either fermentation of carbohydrates by bacteria or because of alteration in regulatory mechanisms.[45] Malabsorption leads to an osmotic diarrhea that will cease with the elimination of the substrate during a fasting state. This is in contrast to secretory or inflammatory diarrhea, which persists despite fasting.

OSMOTIC DIARRHEA

The evaluation of intractable, nonbloody diarrhea in an otherwise stable patient with reliable IV access should start with a 24 to 48 hour fasting period (see **Fig. 2**). During this time, the infant should be on dextrose-containing fluids with an adequate glucose infusion rate to maintain euglycemia. If there is resolution of diarrhea during a fasting state, then the cause of the diarrhea is likely osmotic. The following section reviews testing that can help uncover specific malabsorption processes.

Carbohydrates

More so than protein or fat absorption issues, carbohydrate malabsorption is the main culprit for nonbloody diarrhea in neonates with malabsorption syndromes either as an isolated deficiency or as part of pancreatic insufficiency. Infants suffering from carbohydrate malabsorption typically experience watery and acidic diarrhea. Carbohydrate malabsorption most typically results from deficiencies in brush border enzymes. In addition to diarrhea, bacterial fermentation of malabsorbed carbohydrates can lead to abdominal distension and cramping.[36] The malabsorbed sugars are fermented by anaerobic bacteria producing short chain fatty acids, which produces acid stools with pH < 5.[46] Stool reducing substances measure the reducing sugars glucose, galactose, and fructose which should not be present in significant amounts in stool. A positive test of greater than 0.5% indicates the child is likely experiencing monosaccharide malabsorption.[47] A stool osmotic gap can be calculated as 290 mOsm/kg − 2 × (stool Na^+ + stool K^+).[48] Osmotic diarrhea tends to have a high osmotic gap; greater than 100 mOsm secondary to the unabsorbed carbohydrate contributing to a higher osmolality (OSM).[49] Although invasive, esophagogastroduodenoscopy with biopsy and disaccharidase quantification can definitively diagnose specific disaccharide deficiencies. In studies of patients with disaccharidase deficiency, up to half had normal histology.[50]

Congenital lactase deficiency is an extremely rare autosomal recessive disorder. Affected infants lack the enzyme necessary to digest lactose.[51] As a result, affected infants typically experience severe watery diarrhea immediately after birth and suffer from growth failure and dehydration as well as other symptoms typical of carbohydrate malabsorption.[52] Because lactose is the principal carbohydrate in both breast milk and cow's milk-based formulas, patients will need to be fed a soy formula, protein hydrolysate, or amino acid based formula, all of which are lactose-free.[52]

Although there are other disaccharidase deficiencies, these patients typically present after weaning from breast milk or lactose-containing formulas. Congenital sucrase-isomaltase deficiency has a high prevalence in the Inuit population, up to 10%. In this population, there has been a homozygous frame shift mutation identified as the cause for enzyme deficiency.[53] Overall, there have been at least 25 gene mutations identified.[54] Symptoms can be nonspecific and indistinguishable from congenital lactase deficiency, except for the timing of the diarrhea. It is possible that children with sucrose-isomaltase deficiency may have signs of malabsorption if formulas with sucrose or polycose are introduced early. The treatment of sucrase-isomaltase deficiency is a lactose-containing or carbohydrate-free formula.[53] Enzyme replacement therapy, sacrosidase, is also available for patients who do not respond to sucrose-free diet alone.[54]

Protein and Lipid

Isolated protein malabsorption is very uncommon and typically associated with pancreatic insufficiency. Although there are abnormalities in specific peptidases, they are not clinically significant. Congenital enterokinase deficiency is an autosomal recessive disorder causing a decrease in protease activity, enterokinase. Without enterokinase, there is not activation of trypsinogen resulting in inactivity of all pancreatic enzymes, which leads to diarrhea and hypoproteinemia.[55]

There are many reasons for fat malabsorption in the neonate. Although adults are extremely efficient at absorbing fat, neonates are less so secondary to smaller bile-acid pools, decreased lipolysis efficiency, and less bioavailable fat in formula.[56] Although it can present as nonbloody diarrhea, steatorrhea in infants is usually less oily and can often be more bulky than watery.[57] Fat malabsorption can arise from issues related to lipolysis, inability to activate pancreatic enzymes, issues related to micelle formation, inadequate pancreatic enzymes, or abnormal transport into circulation.[58] Often profound osmotic diarrhea seen in fat malabsorption syndrome comes from the concurrent carbohydrate malabsorption in children with pancreatic insufficiency.

Exocrine pancreatic insufficiency (EPI) is a common cause of fat malabsorption in premature and term infants. EPI most typically occurs in infants because the pancreas cannot produce and/or excrete the enzymes necessary for fat digestion. The gold standard for diagnosing EPI is a secretin stimulation test. A tube is inserted into the duodenum and pancreatic secretions are collected for enzyme analysis after a dose of secretin is administered intravenously. This test is very invasive, and there are no standard protocols for infants and young children.[59] Fecal elastase has been used as an alternative means of assessing exocrine pancreatic function because elastase is secreted by the pancreas and is not degraded in the intestines.[60] The sensitivity and specificity of fecal elastase testing varies widely depending on the study cited. There is some degree of variation from serial stool samples, so it is recommended to collect stool on multiple days.[61] Care should also be taken when there is diarrhea or known bowel inflammation because this can result in false-negative fecal elastase results.[60] A timed quantitative fecal fat collection is the gold standard for indirect testing of exocrine pancreatic function; however, this typically requires a 72-hour stool collection.[59]

Cystic fibrosis (CF) is the most common cause of EPI in infants and children. Cystic fibrosis is an autosomal recessive disorder caused by mutations of the cystic fibrosis transmembrane conductance regulator (CFTR) which is a chloride channel. In absorptive tissues such as sweat ducts, CFTR primarily absorbs chloride, which explains why the concentration of chloride is elevated in people suffering from CF. In contrast, in secretory tissues such as pancreatic ducts, CFTR primarily secretes chloride into the lumen. Because of decreased chloride secretion into the pancreatic ducts, there is a marked diminution in the volume of pancreatic ductular secretion producing small duct obstruction, leading to autodigestion of the pancreas and ultimately EPI.[60] Approximately 85% of patients with CF suffer from EPI and is typically present at birth.[62] Affected patients typically experience poor weight gain often without diarrhea or other major GI symptoms. Treatment should be focused on maintaining adequate nutrition to promote growth, supplementing fat-soluble vitamins (A, D, E, K), and the use of pancreatic enzyme replacement therapy.[62]

Shwachman-Diamond syndrome is the second most common cause of EPI in infants and young children. This is an autosomal recessive disorder that results in bone marrow failure and EPI. Pancreatic dysfunction typically occurs within the first 6 to 12 months of life.[63] Treatment is similar to CF, focusing on nutrition and vitamin optimization. Other rare causes of EPI are Johanson-Blizzard syndrome, which causes a variety of endocrinopathies as well as fatty replacement of the pancreas or Pearson syndrome, which causes bone marrow suppression and pancreatic fibrosis.[58]

SECRETORY DIARRHEA

Compared with osmotic diarrhea, secretory diarrhea in premature or term infants is rare but should be included on the differential diagnosis, especially if there is persistent diarrhea during a 48-hour fast. This section will cover 3 major mechanisms that lead to secretory diarrhea: electrolyte transport defects, enterocyte abnormalities, and immune dysregulation.

ELECTROLYTE TRANSPORT DEFECTS

Stool osmolality (OSM) can be extremely helpful when an electrolyte transport defect is suspected. Although this testing is nonspecific, it can direct clinicians to do further work-up for congenital sodium or chloride diarrhea. With electrolyte transport defects, a large amount of NaCl is excreted in the stool resulting in a low osmotic gap, typically less than 50 mOsm.[47] Typically aggressive electrolyte replacement is necessary as these conditions can be associated with life-threatening metabolic derangements.

Congenital Sodium Diarrhea

It is difficult to estimate the incidence of congenital sodium diarrhea (CSD) because there have only been a handful of reported cases. Case reports implicate multiple genes leading to excessive stool sodium losses causing severe hyponatremia and metabolic acidosis.[64] Clinical features vary depending on the gene involved. All patients with solute carrier family 9 member A3 (SLC9A3) gene mutation, which causes dysregulation of the Na^+/H^+ antiporter in the small bowel, have been found to have polyhydramnios and intestinal dilation on prenatal ultrasound.[65] Serine Peptidase Inhibitor (SPINT2) mutations leading to altered serine protease activity result in a syndrome of choanal atresia, hypertelorism, and corneal erosions.[66] Based on case series, treatment of both these disorders with either intravenous or oral sodium supplementation is necessary. While some infants seem to outgrow the diarrhea as they get older, others have lifelong difficulties with diarrhea. Due to large sodium losses, growth needs to be followed closely since sodium is an essential nutrient for optimal neonatal growth.[67,68]

Congenital Chloride Diarrhea

Unlike CSD, only one gene has been identified as the cause of congenital chloride diarrhea (CCD). SLC26A3 is a Cl^-/HCO_3 anion exchanger in the enterocyte plasma membrane.[69] This defect causes increased secretion of chloride and excessive retention of bicarbonate resulting in hyperchloremic metabolic alkalosis.[64] Once again, newborns typically present with polyhydramnios and profuse, potentially life-threatening watery diarrhea. Infants tend to have favorable outcomes with aggressive replacement of Cl^- with either NaCl or KCl. In a small retrospective study, affected patients had lifelong persistent diarrhea. They may also develop renal disease, intestinal inflammation, and inguinal hernias. Congenital chloride diarrhea is one of the causes of a false-positive sweat chloride test.[70]

ENTEROCYTE ABNORMALITIES

When the cause of persistent watery diarrhea remains uncertain, tissue samples can be obtained via upper endoscopy. Typically, tissue samples are stained with hematoxylin and eosin, which allow for visualization of overall cell structure using light microscopy.[71] However, there are certain enterocyte abnormalities that cannot be detected with standard tissue sample preparation and light microscopy, and electron microscopy is needed to identify ultrastructural abnormalities of enterocytes.

Microvillous Inclusion Disease

There are 2 forms of microvillous inclusion disease (MVID), both causing a secretory diarrhea. Early onset MVID begins immediately after birth and has a worse outcome as compared with late onset, which typically begins at 3 to 4 months of life.[64] Mutations in the myosin-Vb (MYO5B) gene are currently the only identified defects linked to MVID. MYO5B deficiency is hypothesized to result in abnormal trafficking of enterocyte vacuoles, which leads to intracellular aggregation of vacuoles containing microvilli.[72] Electron microscopy demonstrates inclusions and vesicles on the apical side of the enterocyte as well as villous and microvillous atrophy.[73] In case reports examining outcomes of patients with early onset MVID, all but one required long-term parenteral nutrition or small bowel transplant.[72]

Congenital Tufting Enteropathy

Similar to MVID, congenital tufting enteropathy (CTE) has a high rate of morbidity and mortality. Under normal conditions, epithelial cell adhesion molecule (EpCAM) mediates cell–cell interactions. Gene mutations in EpCAM result in crypt-villi disorganization.[64,74] Mutations encoding SPINT2 are associated with a syndromic form of CTE, which is characterized by ocular abnormalities, choanal atresia, and atresia of skin and bone.[75] Electron microscopy is required to make this diagnosis and demonstrates villous atrophy, crypt hyperplasia, and focal epithelial tufts.[74] Treatment is focused on nutritional support and patients typically require lifelong parenteral nutrition.[74,76]

Immune Dysregulation

There are a variety of disorders of immune regulation that can result in chronic diarrhea and feeding intolerance. In most cases, the diarrhea is the result of immune-mediated destruction or distortion of enterocytes, which causes malabsorption and/or an inflammatory diarrhea. Immune dysregulation, polyendocrinopathy, enteropathy, X-linked syndrome results from mutations in the forkhead box P3 (FOXP3) gene. Patients typically present in the first 3 months of life with diarrhea, dermatitis, diabetes mellitus, thyroiditis, and hemolytic anemia. Diagnosis is made with genetic testing. There can be villous blunting on duodenal biopsy, but this is a nonspecific finding. The disease course is lethal unless treated with immunosuppression and bone marrow transplant.[64,77] Common variable immune deficiency is an autosomal recessive disorder that results from mutations in the inducible T cell costimulator (ICOS) gene.[47] Villous blunting and lymphonodular hyperplasia can be seen on biopsy. Antienterocyte antibodies can also be present, indicating an autoimmune component.[78,79] X-linked agammaglobulinemia is another disorder of the immune system, which is incredibly rare but a cause of secretory diarrhea.[79] If there are nonspecific biopsy findings as mentioned above and suspicion for secretory diarrhea, immunologic and genetic testing should be considered.

SUMMARY

Inability to advance feeds or symptoms of feeding intolerance and diarrhea are commonly encountered symptoms in the NICU and can lead to inadequate nutrition support. The differential diagnosis of these symptoms is vast and can carry with it a high morbidity and mortality. The lack of current recommendations for a standardized evaluation of these symptoms can delay diagnosis and have negative implications for the neonate. This article highlights food protein-intolerance and malabsorption syndromes as possible causes of feeding intolerance in the NICU. The provided algorithms can serve as a guide for clinicians to better standardize clinical decision-making in these challenging patients.

Best practice

What is the current practice?

Malabsorption and food intolerance in neonates

Best practice/guidelines/care path objectives
- Early recognition of feeding intolerance and initiating appropriate diagnostic evaluation
- Provide algorithms to aid in the correct diagnosis of feeding intolerance and diarrhea
- Interpretation of laboratories and additional testing to arrive at proper diagnosis
- Early implementation of appropriate treatment to optimize growth and development

What changes in current practice are likely to improve outcomes?

- Algorithms proposing standardized processes for evaluating and diagnosing feeding intolerance and diarrhea in neonates

- Less invasive and highly specific testing that is readily available to promptly diagnose malabsorption causes

Major recommendations

- Classify feeding intolerance based on upper GI symptoms with or without diarrhea

- Upper GI symptoms with associated diarrhea require further testing to evaluate for an osmotic or secretory cause

- Use stool and serum laboratories, intestinal biopsies, and genetic testing as confirmatory testing based on algorithms provided above

- Implement appropriate nutritional and supplemental interventions quickly to prevent issues with growth and development

- Monitor for disease complications and understand when further evaluation is needed

Summary statement

When infants have ongoing feeding intolerance, clinicians should consider food protein-induced disorders and malabsorption early in the symptom course using proposed algorithms to confirm the diagnosis and implement proper treatment.

Data from Refs.[8–12,17–19,41–43,48–50,53,54]

DISCLOSURE

Neither author has relevant financial relationships with commercial interests.

REFERENCES

1. Fitzgibbons SC, Ching Y, Yu D, et al. Mortality of necrotizing enterocolitis expressed by birth weight categories. J Pediatr Surg 2009;44(6):1072–5 [discussion: 1075-1076].
2. Tuck CJ, Biesiekierski JR, Schmid-Grendelmeier P, et al. Food intolerances. Nutrients 2019;11(7):E1684.
3. Lomer MCE. Review article: the aetiology, diagnosis, mechanisms and clinical evidence for food intolerance. Aliment Pharmacol Ther 2015;41(3):262–75.
4. NIAID-Sponsored Expert Panel, Boyce JA, Assa'ad A, Burks AW, et al. Guidelines for the diagnosis and management of food allergy in the United States: report of the NIAID-sponsored expert panel. J Allergy Clin Immunol 2010;126(6 Suppl): S1–58.

5. Moore TA, Wilson ME. Feeding intolerance: a concept analysis. Adv Neonatal Care 2011;11(3):149–54.

6. Lin XP, Magnusson J, Ahlstedt S, et al. Local allergic reaction in food-hypersensitive adults despite a lack of systemic food-specific IgE. J Allergy Clin Immunol 2002;109(5):879–87.

7. Caubet J-C, Nowak-Węgrzyn A. Current understanding of the immune mechanisms of food protein-induced enterocolitis syndrome. Expert Rev Clin Immunol 2011;7(3):317–27.

8. Chung HL, Hwang JB, Park JJ, et al. Expression of transforming growth factor beta1, transforming growth factor type I and II receptors, and TNF-alpha in the mucosa of the small intestine in infants with food protein-induced enterocolitis syndrome. J Allergy Clin Immunol 2002;109(1):150–4.

9. Koletzko S, Niggemann B, Arato A, et al. Diagnostic approach and management of cow's-milk protein allergy in infants and children: ESPGHAN GI Committee Practical Guidelines. J Pediatr Gastroenterol Nutr 2012;55(2):221–9.

10. Nowak-Węgrzyn A. Food protein-induced enterocolitis syndrome and allergic proctocolitis. Allergy Asthma Proc 2015;36(3):172–84.

11. Beşer OF, Sancak S, Erkan T, et al. Can fecal calprotectin level be used as a markers of inflammation in the diagnosis and follow-up of cow's milk protein allergy? Allergy Asthma Immunol Res 2014;6(1):33–8.

12. Lake AM. Food-induced eosinophilic proctocolitis. J Pediatr Gastroenterol Nutr 2000;30(Suppl):S58–60.

13. American Academy of Pediatrics. Committee on Nutrition. Hypoallergenic infant formulas. Pediatrics 2000;106(2 Pt 1):346–9.

14. Kumar D, Repucci A, Wyatt-Ashmead J, et al. Allergic colitis presenting in the first day of life: report of three cases. J Pediatr Gastroenterol Nutr 2000;31(2):195–7.

15. Faber MR, Rieu P, Semmekrot BA, et al. Allergic colitis presenting within the first hours of premature life: clinical observations. Acta Paediatr 2007;94(10):1514–5.

16. Mehr S, Frith K, Barnes EH, et al, FPIES Study Group. Food protein-induced enterocolitis syndrome in Australia: a population-based study, 2012-2014. J Allergy Clin Immunol 2017;140(5):1323–30.

17. Mehr S, Kakakios A, Frith K, et al. Food protein-induced enterocolitis syndrome: 16-year experience. Pediatrics 2009;123(3):e459–64.

18. Miceli Sopo S, Battista A, Greco M, et al. Ondansetron for food protein-induced enterocolitis syndrome. Int Arch Allergy Immunol 2014;164(2):137–9.

19. Nowak-Węgrzyn A, Chehade M, Groetch ME, et al. International consensus guidelines for the diagnosis and management of food protein–induced enterocolitis syndrome: executive summary—Workgroup report of the adverse reactions to foods Committee, American Academy of Allergy, Asthma & Immunology. J Allergy Clin Immunol 2017;139(4):1111–26.e4.

20. Vandenplas Y, Gottrand F, Veereman-Wauters G, et al. Gastrointestinal manifestations of cow's milk protein allergy and gastrointestinal motility: cow's milk protein allergy and gastrointestinal motility. Acta Paediatr 2012;101(11):1105–9.

21. Ravelli AM, Tobanelli P, Volpi S, et al. Vomiting and gastric motility in infants with cow's milk allergy. J Pediatr Gastroenterol Nutr 2001;32(1):6.

22. Fishbein M, Kirschner BS, Gonzales-Vallina R, et al. Menetrier's disease associated with formula protein allergy and small intestinal injury in an infant. Gastroenterology 1992;103(5):1664–8.

23. Morinville V, Bernard C, Forget S. Foveolar hyperplasia secondary to cow's milk protein hypersensitivity presenting with clinical features of pyloric stenosis. J Pediatr Surg 2004;39(1):E29–31.

24. Nomura I, Morita H, Hosokawa S, et al. Four distinct subtypes of non–IgE-mediated gastrointestinal food allergies in neonates and infants, distinguished by their initial symptoms. J Allergy Clin Immunol 2011;127(3):685–8.e8.

25. Abdelhamid AE, Chuang S-L, Hayes P, et al. Evolution of in vitro cow's milk protein–specific inflammatory and regulatory cytokine responses in preterm infants with necrotising enterocolitis. J Pediatr Gastroenterol Nutr 2013;56(1):5–11.

26. Miyazawa T, Itabashi K, Imai T. Retrospective multicenter survey on food-related symptoms suggestive of cow's milk allergy in NICU neonates. Allergol Int 2013; 62(1):85–90.

27. Cordova J, Sriram S, Patton T, et al. Manifestations of cow's-milk protein intolerance in preterm infants. J Pediatr Gastroenterol Nutr 2016;62(1):140–4.

28. Lenfestey MW, de la Cruz D, Neu J. Food protein–induced enterocolitis instead of necrotizing enterocolitis? a neonatal intensive care unit case series. J Pediatr 2018;200:270–3.

29. Lozinsky AC, Morais MB de. Eosinophilic colitis in infants. J Pediatr (Rio J) 2014; 90(1):16–21.

30. Meyer R, Chebar Lozinsky A, Fleischer DM, et al. Diagnosis and management of Non-IgE gastrointestinal allergies in breastfed infants—an EAACI Position Paper. Allergy 2020;75(1):14–32.

31. Aydemir O, Aydemir C, Sarikabadayi YU, et al. Fecal calprotectin levels are increased in infants with necrotizing enterocolitis. J Maternal Fetal Neonatal Med 2012;25(11):2237–41.

32. Dupont C, Soulaines P, Lapillonne A, et al. Atopy patch test for early diagnosis of cow's milk allergy in preterm infants. J Pediatr Gastroenterol Nutr 2010;50(4): 463–4.

33. Nocerino R, Granata V, Di Costanzo M, et al. Atopy patch tests are useful to predict oral tolerance in children with gastrointestinal symptoms related to non-IgE-mediated cow's milk allergy. Allergy 2013;68(2):246–8.

34. Mezoff EA, Williams KC, Erdman SH. Gastrointestinal endoscopy in the neonate. Clin Perinatol 2020;47(2):413–22.

35. Helander HF, Fändriks L. Surface area of the digestive tract - revisited. Scand J Gastroenterol 2014;49(6):681–9.

36. Johnson. Gastrointestinal Physiology 7th Edition.; 2006.

37. Ballard O, Morrow AL. Human milk composition. Pediatr Clin North Am 2013; 60(1):49–74.

38. Verduci E, D'Elios S, Cerrato L, et al. Cow's milk substitutes for children: nutritional aspects of milk from different mammalian species, special formula and plant-based beverages. Nutrients 2019;11(8). https://doi.org/10.3390/nu11081739.

39. Ament ME. Malabsorption syndromes in infancy and childhood. J Pediatr 1972; 81(4):685–97.

40. Jenness R. The composition of human milk. Semin Perinatol 1979;3(3):225–39.

41. Saarela T, Kokkonen J, Koivisto M. Macronutrient and energy contents of human milk fractions during the first six months of lactation. Acta Paediatr 2005;94(9): 1176–81.

42. Kent JC, Mitoulas LR, Cregan MD, et al. Volume and frequency of breastfeedings and fat content of breast milk throughout the day. Pediatrics 2006;117(3): e387–95.

43. Jensen RG, Hagerty MM, McMahon KE. Lipids of human milk and infant formulas: a review. Am J Clin Nutr 1978;31(6):990–1016.

44. Armand M, Pasquier B, André M, et al. Digestion and absorption of 2 fat emulsions with different droplet sizes in the human digestive tract. Am J Clin Nutr 1999;70(6):1096–106.
45. Keller J, Layer P. The pathophysiology of malabsorption. Viszeralmedizin 2014; 30(3):150–4.
46. Holtug K, Clausen MR, Hove H, et al. The colon in carbohydrate malabsorption: short-chain fatty acids, pH, and osmotic diarrhoea. Scand J Gastroenterol 1992; 27(7):545–52.
47. Elkadri AA. Congenital diarrheal syndromes. Clin Perinatol 2020;47(1):87–104.
48. Eherer AJ, Fordtran JS. Fecal osmotic gap and pH in experimental diarrhea of various causes. Gastroenterology 1992;103(2):545–51.
49. Castro-Rodríguez JA, Salazar-Lindo E, León-Barúa R. Differentiation of osmotic and secretory diarrhoea by stool carbohydrate and osmolar gap measurements. Arch Dis Child 1997;77(3):201–5.
50. Cohen SA, Oloyede H, Gold BD, et al. Clinical characteristics of disaccharidase deficiencies among children undergoing upper endoscopy. J Pediatr Gastroenterol Nutr 2018;66(Suppl 3):S56–60.
51. Wanes D, Husein DM, Naim HY. Congenital lactase deficiency: mutations, functional and biochemical implications, and future perspectives. Nutrients 2019; 11(2):461.
52. Savilahti E, Launiala K, Kuitunen P. Congenital lactase deficiency. A clinical study on 16 patients. Arch Dis Child 1983;58(4):246–52.
53. Marcadier JL, Boland M, Scott CR, et al. Congenital sucrase–isomaltase deficiency: identification of a common Inuit founder mutation. CMAJ 2015;187(2): 102–7.
54. Treem WR. Clinical aspects and treatment of congenital sucrase-isomaltase deficiency. J Pediatr Gastroenterol Nutr 2012;55(Supplement 2):S7–13.
55. Wang L, Zhang D, Fan C, et al. Novel compound heterozygous TMPRSS15 gene variants cause enterokinase deficiency. Front Genet 2020;11:538778.
56. Verkade HJ, Hoving EB, Muskiet FA, et al. Fat absorption in neonates: comparison of long-chain-fatty-acid and triglyceride compositions of formula, feces, and blood. Am J Clin Nutr 1991;53(3):643–51.
57. Okajima K, Nagaya K, Azuma H, et al. Biliary atresia and stool: its consistency and fat content, another potentially useful clinical information. Eur J Gastroenterol Hepatol 2016;28(1):118.
58. Wylie R, Hyams JS, Kay M. Pediatric gastrointestinal and liver diseases. 3rd edition. Elsevier, Inc; 2020.
59. Vanga RR, Tansel A, Sidiq S, et al. Diagnostic performance of measurement of fecal elastase-1 in detection of exocrine pancreatic insufficiency: systematic review and meta-analysis. Clin Gastroenterol Hepatol 2018;16(8):1220–8.e4.
60. Daftary A, Acton J, Heubi J, et al. Fecal elastase-1: utility in pancreatic function in cystic fibrosis. J Cystic Fibrosis 2006;5(2):71–6.
61. Wali PD, Loveridge-Lenza B, He Z, et al. Comparison of fecal elastase-1 and pancreatic function testing in children. J Pediatr Gastroenterol Nutr 2012;54(2): 277–80.
62. Singh VK, Schwarzenberg SJ. Pancreatic insufficiency in cystic fibrosis. J Cystic Fibrosis 2017;16:S70–8.
63. Nelson AS, Myers KC. Diagnosis, treatment, and molecular pathology of Shwachman-Diamond Syndrome. Hematol Oncol Clin North Am 2018;32(4): 687–700.

64. Berni Canani R, Terrin G, Cardillo G, et al. Congenital diarrheal disorders: improved understanding of gene defects is leading to advances in intestinal physiology and clinical management. J Pediatr Gastroenterol Nutr 2010;50(4): 360–6.
65. Dimitrov G, Bamberger S, Navard C, et al. Congenital sodium diarrhea by mutation of the SLC9A3 gene. Eur J Med Genet 2019;62(10):103712.
66. Heinz-Erian P, Müller T, Krabichler B, et al. Mutations in SPINT2 cause a syndromic form of congenital sodium diarrhea. Am J Hum Genet 2009;84(2):188–96.
67. Haycock GB. The influence of sodium on growth in infancy. Pediatr Nephrol 1993; 7(6):871–5.
68. Janecke AR, Heinz-Erian P, Yin J, et al. Reduced sodium/proton exchanger NHE3 activity causes congenital sodium diarrhea. Hum Mol Genet 2015;24(23): 6614–23.
69. Kere J, Höglund P. Inherited disorders of ion transport in the intestine. Curr Opin Genet Dev 2000;10(3):306–9.
70. Hihnala S, Höglund P, Lammi L, et al. Long-term clinical outcome in patients with congenital chloride diarrhea. J Pediatr Gastroenterol Nutr 2006;42(4):369–75.
71. Feldman AT, Wolfe D. Tissue processing and hematoxylin and eosin staining. In: Day CE, editor. Histopathology: methods and protocols. Methods in molecular biology. Springer; 2014. p. 31–43.
72. Müller T, Hess MW, Schiefermeier N, et al. MYO5B mutations cause microvillus inclusion disease and disrupt epithelial cell polarity. Nat Genet 2008;40(10): 1163–5.
73. Iancu TC, Mahajnah M, Manov I, et al. Microvillous inclusion disease: ultrastructural variability. Ultrastruct Pathol 2007;31(3):173–88.
74. Das B, Sivagnanam M. Congenital tufting enteropathy: biology, pathogenesis and mechanisms. JCM 2020;10(1):19.
75. Salomon J, Goulet O, Canioni D, et al. Genetic characterization of congenital tufting enteropathy: epcam associated phenotype and involvement of SPINT2 in the syndromic form. Hum Genet 2014;133(3):299–310.
76. Carter BA, Cohran VC, Cole CR, et al. Outcomes from a 12-week, open-label, multicenter clinical trial of teduglutide in pediatric short bowel syndrome. J Pediatr 2017;181:102–11.e5.
77. Baud O, Goulet O, Canioni D, et al. Treatment of the immune dysregulation, polyendocrinopathy, enteropathy, x-linked syndrome (IPEX) by allogeneic bone marrow transplantation. N Engl J Med 2001;344(23):1758–62.
78. Cunningham-Rundles C. Common variable immune deficiency: dissection of the variable. Immunological Rev 2019;287(1):145–61.
79. Washington K, Stenzel TT, Buckley RH, et al. Gastrointestinal pathology in patients with common variable immunodeficiency and x-linked agammaglobulinemia. Am J Surg Pathol 1996;20(10):1240–52.

Nutritional Management of Short Bowel Syndrome

Muralidhar H. Premkumar, MBBS, DCH, DNB, MRCPCH, MS[a],[*],[1],
Amuchou Soraisham, MBBS, MD, DNB, DM, FRCPC[b],[1], Nitasha Bagga, MBBS, DNB[c],
L. Adriana Massieu, RD, LD, CNSC[d], Akhil Maheshwari, MD[e]

KEYWORDS

- Breast milk • Enteral nutrition • Growth • Intestinal failure • Nutrition
- Parenteral nutrition • Short bowel syndrome • Short gut

KEY POINTS

- Short bowel syndrome (SBS) is a relatively uncommon but a major source of prolonged morbidity in infants with long-term dependence on parenteral nutrition is high.
- Therapeutic strategies should focus on initiating enteral feeds as soon as bowel function recovers. Breast milk, when available, should be the first choice of enteral feeds.
- Newer generation intravenous lipid emulsions can be an important component of the clinical management and can help prevent and treat intestinal failure-associated liver disease.
- Specialized multidisciplinary care and standardized nutritional regimens are needed to improve the clinical outcomes in SBS.

INTRODUCTION

Intestinal failure (IF) is characterized by an inability to digest and absorb nutrients resulting in dependence on parenteral nutrition (PN) due to loss of functional gut mass.[1],[2]

IF in newborn infants can result from the loss of absorptive surface, mucosal dysfunction states, or dysmotility, as shown in **Box 1**. IF following an anatomic loss of intestines is called short bowel syndrome (SBS).[1],[3],[4] In a recent study from North America, gastroschisis and necrotizing enterocolitis (NEC) accounted for 16% and 26% of all cases of IF.[5],[6] Paradoxically, the improvement in the care and survival of

[a] Division of Neonatology, Department of Pediatrics, Baylor College of Medicine, Texas Children's Hospital, 6621 Fannin, Suite 6104, Houston, TX 77030, USA; [b] Department of Pediatrics, Cumming School of Medicine, University of Calgary, Calgary, Alberta, Canada; [c] Department of Neonatology, Rainbow Children's Hospital, Hyderabad, India; [d] Department of Clinical Nutrition Services, Texas Children's Hospital, Houston, TX, USA; [e] Global Newborn Society (https://www.globalnewbornsociety.org/), Clarksville, MD, USA
[1] Both authors contributed equally to this article.
* Corresponding author.
E-mail address: premkuma@bcm.edu

Clin Perinatol 49 (2022) 557–572
https://doi.org/10.1016/j.clp.2022.02.016
0095-5108/22/© 2022 Elsevier Inc. All rights reserved.

Abbreviations	
EN	Enteral nutrition
IF	Intestinal failure
IFALD	Intestinal failure-associated liver disease
ILE	Intravenous lipid emulsions
MCT	Medium-chain triglycerides
MFR	Mucous fistula refeeding
NEC	Necrotizing enterocolitis
PN	Parenteral nutrition
RCT	Randomized controlled trial
SIBO	Small intestinal bacterial overgrowth
SBS	Short bowel syndrome

extremely premature infants and those with gastrointestinal conditions that were previously considered to be uniformly lethal has increased the incidence of SBS.[6,7] A Canadian Collaborative Study showed SBS incidence at 3.5 per 1000 in preterm infants compared with an overall incidence of 0.25 per 1000 live births.[8] In the United States, the incidence of SBS was 7 per 1000 in very low birth weight infants, and 11 per 1000 in extremely low birth weight infants.[9]

CLINICAL MANIFESTATIONS IN SHORT BOWEL SYNDROME

The loss of absorptive surface due to reduced length of the intestine reduces contact time with the mucosa, compromising digestion and absorption, leading to malabsorption. The loss of a specific part of the gut determines the clinical manifestations by the particular deficiencies of the nutrients absorbed. The pattern of nutrient absorption native to the parts of the gastrointestinal tract is shown in **Fig. 1**.[4]

The gastric dysfunction in SBS manifests primarily in either dysmotility or hypersecretion, resulting in increased gastric output. Hypersecretion is often attributed to the

---

Box 1
Causes of intestinal failure in newborn infants

- Loss of absorptive surface (Short Bowel Syndrome)
  - Prenatal causes:
    - Gastroschisis
    - Intestinal atresia
    - Midgut volvulus
    - Omphalocele
  - Postnatal causes:
    - Necrotizing enterocolitis
    - Midgut volvulus
    - Vascular thrombosis
    - Spontaneous intestinal perforation
    - Intussusception

- Loss of mucosal function
  - Congenital enteropathy
    - Microvillus inclusion disease
    - Intestinal epithelial dysplasia
  - Postinfectious diarrhea

- Loss of motility
  - Extensive Hirschsprung disease
  - Chronic intestinal pseudo-obstruction

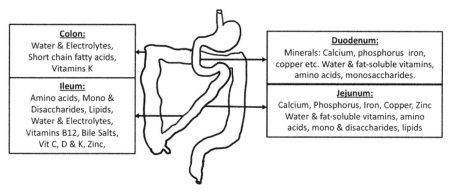

Fig. 1. Absorption of nutrients in various parts of the gastrointestinal tract.

absence of a hormone called peptide YY secreted by the ileum on contact with nutrients, initiating a negative feedback loop suppressing gastric and duodenal secretion.[10,11] In addition, the loss of exocrine pancreatic function results in malabsorption of nutrients and pancreatic insufficiency.[12] Dilatation of the intestines due to decreased motility, obstruction, and blind loops result in stasis of intraluminal contents, thus promoting bacterial overgrowth.[13] This is often exacerbated by medications such as H_2-blockers, proton pump inhibitors, and opioids. Symptoms include abdominal distention, watery stools, and lactic acidosis. Apart from these direct effects, complications such as intestinal failure-associated liver disease (IFALD), bloodstream infections, oral-aversion, growth failure, and neurodevelopmental delays manifest as consequences of SBS.

Intestinal Adaptation

Intestinal adaptation is a sequence of histologic, biochemical, and physiologic changes that set in as early as 2 to 3 days following surgery and continue throughout rehabilitation.[14,15] This is marked by compensatory changes in mucosal and muscular layers of the intestines. Enterocyte proliferation, lengthening of villi, and deepening of crypt result in both linear and circumferential growth of the intestines thus increasing the surface area by several-fold. Mediators such as insulin-like growth factors, growth hormone, glucagon-like peptides , neurotensin, and peptide YY promote this process. Exposure of intestinal mucosa to enteral feeds prompts the release of hormonal mediators, facilitating a trophic effect fostering intestinal adaptation. These anatomic and physiologic changes gradually restore digestion and absorption in the remaining intestines. The ileum has a higher ability to demonstrate intestinal adaptation compared with the jejunum.[16] The recovery process following the surgical events that result in SBS can be broadly categorized into 3 stages, as shown in **Table 1**. The acute phase of intestinal adaptation that follows immediately after a surgical event lasts from days to a few weeks and is characterized by ileus, high gastrointestinal output, and fluid-electrolyte imbalances. This is followed by the subacute phase extending over weeks to months, during which bowel function gradually returns; ileus resolves to result in decreased gastrointestinal secretions, stable fluid electrolyte status, enabling the initiation of enteral feeds. Finally, the chronic phase is observed over several months to years based on the extent of the primary loss of bowel. During the subacute and chronic phases, enteral nutrition (EN) is initiated and advanced as tolerated with concurrent weaning of PN.

Table 1
Stages of recovery, clinical concerns, and management of short bowel syndrome

Stages of SBS	Acute	Subacute	Chronic
Duration	Days – weeks	Weeks – months	Months – years
Clinical features	Ileus, Increased gastrointestinal output, Fluid and electrolyte imbalances	Decreasing gastrointestinal output IFALD SIBO Infection	Dysmotility SIBO IFALD Infection Oral aversion Growth difficulties
Management	Fluid and electrolyte replacement Optimal PN	Stabilization of PN Initiation of EN Prevent infections Prevent IFALD	Advance EN Wean PN Establish oral feeds Intestinal lengthening Organ transplantation

Abbreviations: EN, enteral nutrition; IFALD, intestinal failure associated liver disease; PN, parenteral nutrition; SBS, short bowel syndrome; SIBO, small intestinal bacterial overgrowth.

THE GOALS OF INTESTINAL REHABILITATION

The ultimate purpose of intestinal rehabilitation is to provide a morbidity-free near-normal life expectancy with appropriate growth and neurodevelopment. The goals of the intestinal rehabilitation are enumerated in **Box 2**. Although enteral autonomy is an important goal, the focus should be on providing an optimal combination of enteral and PN that supports the appropriate growth and neurodevelopmental outcomes. Enteral autonomy is achieved when the demands for adequate nutrition are supported entirely by EN with complete freedom from PN.[17,18] Independence from PN for more than 3 to 12 months with appropriate growth parameters offer a more meaningful definition of enteral autonomy.[19–21]

NUTRITIONAL STRATEGIES OF SHORT BOWEL SYNDROME

a. Correction of gastrointestinal fluid and electrolyte losses

Gastroparesis, gastric hypersecretion, intestinal ileus, and hypermotility are various causes of increased gastrointestinal losses in SBS. Gastroparesis is treated with pro-motility medications, such as erythromycin. Erythromycin acts on the motilin receptors

---

Box 2
Goals of intestinal rehabilitation

- Support nutritional needs
  - Replace nutrients based on gastrointestinal losses
  - Meet nutritional needs with parenteral and enteral nutrition
  - Prevent nutrient deficiencies
- Avoid Complications
  - Parenteral nutrition (PN)-related cholestasis, bloodstream infections
- The transition from PN to all EN
- Transition to all oral feeds
- Promote appropriate developmental milestones

by promoting the type 3 migrating motor complexes, propagating the luminal content down the intestines.[22,23] Gastric hypersecretion is often due to the loss of the inhibitory loop from the terminal ileum transmitted through peptide YY.[11,24] H_2-blockers and proton pump inhibitors may provide some benefit in treating gastric hypersecretion.[25–27]

The fluid losses from the gastrointestinal tract should be closely monitored as they are a source of dehydration and electrolyte derangement. Fluid losses equal to or slightly greater than physiologic secretions do not require any intervention. The volume of output greater than accounted by the normal physiologic secretions (20–30 mL/kg/d) are replaced either half or full volume (0.5 or 1 mL 0.9% normal saline replacement for every 1 mL of gastrointestinal output). Higher volumes (eg, >30–40 mL/kg/d) can cause fluid and electrolyte imbalance and are repleted at frequent intervals at full volume with close monitoring of fluid and electrolyte status.

b. Parenteral nutrition

Parenteral nutrition is the main mode of nutrition delivery from the time of diagnosis of SBS until enteral autonomy is achieved. The recommended goals for energy and protein delivered through PN are given in **Table 2**. These goals can be achieved with a combination of glucose, proteins, and lipids delivery. A glucose infusion rate of 11 to 12 mg/kg/min is often achieved with maximum rates as high as 14 mg/kg/min.[28]

Deficiencies of micronutrients in infants with SBS are common but underreported.[29,30] In a retrospective study of 178 children with IF, deficiencies of multiple micronutrients were noted during the transition from PN to EN and following enteral autonomy.[29] The duration of PN was a strong predictor of micronutrient deficiencies. After the transition to EN, 70% of subjects had at least one vitamin deficiency, and 77% of subjects had at least one mineral deficiency, with the most common deficiencies being vitamin D (68%), zinc (67%), and iron (37%).[30]

The recommendations for maintenance needs for micronutrients in PN are given in **Table 2**. Because copper and manganese are primarily regulated by biliary excretion, these minerals are often restricted in infants on long term-PN and cholestasis. However, copper and zinc are deficient despite providing maintenance levels on infants

Table 2
Recommended energy, protein, and micronutrient maintenance needs for parenteral nutrition

	Preterm Infants	Term Infants
Energy (kcal/kg/d)	90–120[33]	85%–90% of predicted from standard equation[a]
Protein (g/kg/d)	3.2–4	2–3
Zinc (µg/kg/d)	400	250[b]
Copper (µg/kg/d)	20	20
Manganese (µg/kg/d)	1	1
Selenium (µg/kg/d)	1.5–4.5	2
Chromium (µg/kg/d)	0.05–0.3	0.2

[a] 0 to 3 mo (Daily Reference Intake): Estimated energy requirements (EER) = [89 × wt. (kg) − 100] + 175 kcal (EER = kcal/d).
[b] Term infants require 250 mcg/kg/d of zinc initially; 50 mcg/kg/d is recommended when greater than 3 mo of age.
Data from Refs.[34–36]

with ostomies, especially while transitioning off PN[31] and require extra supplementation with close monitoring of laboratory values. In the United States, PN solutions are usually devoid of iron due to issues with compatibility and anaphylaxis. For this reason, iron is often supplemented as 25 to 50 mg/mo as a separate intravenous infusion.[32] Periodic surveillance of micronutrient status is strongly recommended in infants with short bowel syndrome to deliver appropriate amounts.

c. Intravenous lipid emulsions (ILE)

Appropriate provision of ILE is crucial for preventing essential fatty acid deficiency and IFALD. Essential fatty acid deficiency can be prevented and treated with a minimum of 1% to 2% calories from linoleic acid, provided by 0.5 to 1 g/kg/d of 100% soybean oil-based ILE (Intralipid© [Sigma-Aldrich, Inc., St. Louis, Missouri]).[37] Intestinal failure-associated liver disease (IFALD) is a state of hepatic dysfunction seen in IF and diagnosed with elevations of conjugated bilirubin greater than 2 mg/dL ($\sim$34 mmol/L).[38] IFALD is seen in as many as 22% to 30% of infants with IF on long-term PN.[39,40] Particularly, the use of 100% soybean oil-based ILE has been associated with IFALD in children and adults.[28,41] This is ascribed to the proinflammatory profile due to the high content of ω-6 fatty acids and stigmasterol in 100% soybean oil-based lipid ILE. Stigmasterol, a phytosterol, antagonizes the farnesoid X receptor, potentiating hepatocellular damage.[42] Lipid minimization strategies have been developed to prevent IFALD, following the emergence of a dose-dependent relationship of 100% soybean-based ILE with liver injury.[41,43,44] Under lipid minimization, the dose of 100% soybean-based ILE is restricted to 1 to 1.5 g/kg daily or 2 times a week.[45] This practice has been proven ineffective in randomized control trials (RCTs) and carries a high risk of essential fatty acid deficiency.[46,47] Newer generation lipid emulsions carry a more favorable anti-inflammatory profile with higher proportions of ω-3 fatty acids, higher vitamin E content, and lower stigmasterol content. Examples include multi-oil-based ILE (SMOF© [Fresenius Kabi, Bad Homburg, Germany]) and 100% fish oil-based ILE (Omegaven© [Fresenius Kabi, Bad Homburg, Germany]). The comparative biochemical characteristics of the different ILE are shown in **Table 3**. The effectiveness of 100% fish oil-based in the resolution of IFALD has been demonstrated in several retrospective and prospective cohort studies.[48–50] In a recent pair-matched analysis, infants with cholestasis who received 100% fish oil-based ILE, in comparison to 100% soybean oil-based ILE, showed higher rates of resolution of cholestasis (65% vs 16%) and lower rates of liver transplantation (4% vs 12%). A recent meta-analysis showed a modest effect of fish oil-containing lipid ILE on both the prevention and treatment of IFALD.[51,52] The European Society for Pediatric Gastroenterology Hepatology and Nutrition meta-analysis suggested that in infants who received ILE for more than 4 weeks, infants who received multicomponent fish oil-based ILE had slower elevations of conjugated bilirubin.[53] Despite the low to very low quality of evidence to support the use of newer generation ILE, the use of 100% fish oil-based ILE in the treatment of and the use of multi-oil-based ILE in the prevention of IFALD is recommended.

d. Enteral nutrition

Enteral feeding promotes the process of intestinal adaptation, improves feeding tolerance, and reduces central venous catheter duration, thereby decreasing the risk of catheter-related bloodstream infections and IFALD. There is very little consensus on the choice of initial feeds, route of feeds (oral vs enteric drip), and duration (continuous vs bolus) of feeds. In the absence of high-quality evidence, current practices are restricted to data from observational studies.

Table 3
Characteristics of intravenous lipid emulsions used in the United States

	Intralipid©	SMOF©	Omegaven©
Composition (Oil Source)			
Soybean	100%	30%	0
Coconut (Medium-chain triglyceride, MCT)	0	30%	0
Olive	0	25%	0
Fish	0	15%	100%
Biochemical Composition			
Phytosterols (mg/L)	348	48	0
α-tocopherol (mg/L)	38	200	150–296
Fatty acids (%)			
Linoleic acid (18:2) ω-6	53	37.2	4.4
Arachidonic acid(20:4) ω-6	0.1	1	2.1
α-Linolenic acid(18:3) ω-3	8	4.7	1.8
Eicosapentaenoic acid, EPA(20:5) ω-3	0	4.7	19.2
Docosahexaenoic acid, DHA (22:6) ω-3	0	4.4	12.1
ω-6:ω-3 ratio	7:1	2.5:1	1:8

Adapted from Hojsak I, Colomb V, Braegger C, Bronsky J, Campoy C, Domellöf M, Embleton N, Fidler Mis N, Hulst JM, Indrio F, Lapillonne A, Mihatsch W, Molgaard C, van Goudoever J, Fewtrell M; ESPGHAN Committee on Nutrition. ESPGHAN Committee on Nutrition Position Paper. Intravenous Lipid Emulsions and Risk of Hepatotoxicity in Infants and Children: a Systematic Review and Meta-analysis. J Pediatr Gastroenterol Nutr. 2016 May;62(5):776-92.

i. Type of EN: Breast milk, when available, should be the first choice of feed in infants with SBS because it possesses protective and trophic factors, providing beneficial effects on digestion, immunity, and the gut microbiome.[54] Breast milk, despite containing lactose, relatively low content of medium-chain triglycerides (MCTs), and complex proteins, is well tolerated in infants with SBS. When breast milk is not available, the current evidence supports an amino acid formula. In a clinical study involving 32 subjects with SBS, infants who received either breast milk or amino acid-based formula had shorter durations of PN.[55] Hydrolyzed formula has also been recommended as an alternative option.[56] An MCT-containing formula is preferred in infants with cholestasis, because MCTs do not require emulsification and esterification. MCTs can be converted into fatty acids and directly transported to the liver through the portal circulation even in pancreatic deficiency states.[57] However, long-chain triglycerides in the diet are important sources of essential fatty acids linoleic and α-linolenic acid.

ii. Mode of EN: When feeds are introduced after bowel function returns in SBS, small volume feeds are often given continuously. Continuous feeds have been shown to saturate the luminal receptors, thereby optimizing the transporters, resulting in better intestinal adaptation.[58,59] Continuous feeds are usually given as orogastric, nasogastric tube, or gastrostomy feeding. In instances of increased gastric output or emesis, transpyloric feeds are given. The disadvantages of continuous feeds include loss of fat-derived calories due to adherence of fats to the walls of the feeding tube.[60,61] Continuous feeding is also not physiologic. It is associated with alterations in gastrointestinal motility, loss of hunger, and restrictions on mobility. In comparison, bolus feeding provides periods of fasting and better amino acid and insulin levels postfeeding.[62] Bolus feeds have also been shown to result in a better gut motility and adaptation.[63] A combination of continuous feeds during the night and bolus feeds during the day offers a balance of meeting nutritional demands and mobility.

At our center, we typically wait for the recovery of bowel function and then cautiously reinitiate a trial of gastric feeds (**Fig. 2**). If there is some feeding intolerance with recurrent emesis and gastric distension due to gastric hypomotility, transpyloric or jejunal feeds is attempted. In scenarios with feeding intolerance that is challenging to treat, such as ultrashort bowel syndrome (<20–30 cm of residual bowel length), enteral feeds are provided continuously (0.5–1 mL/h or 5–10 mL/kg/d). Feed advancements are made once every 2 to 4 days by increasing the infusion rate or converting to bolus feeds while closely monitoring the stoma or stool output. Stoma or stool output of 20 to 30 mL/kg/d is tolerated as long as weight gain is optimal and electrolyte balance is maintained. If the stool output is more than 30 mL/kg/d, feed advancements should be held, or feeds should be decreased until an improvement in stool output is noted. Fortification of enteral feeds is considered when substantial amounts are tolerated to meet the growth requirements.

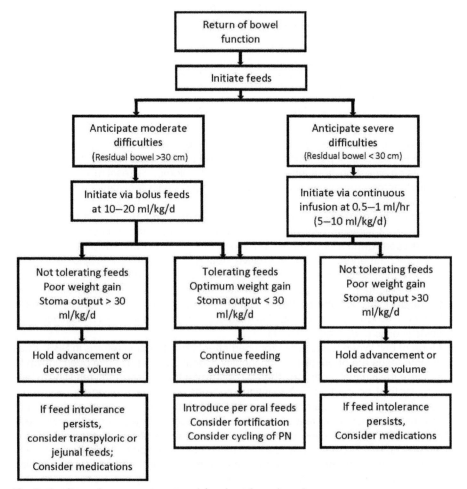

Fig. 2. Feeding advancement protocol for short bowel syndrome.

Table 4 Recommended energy and protein goals for enteral nutrition[32,33,59–61]		
	Preterm Infants	Term Infants
Energy (kcal/kg/d)	110–135	See equation below[a]
Protein (g/kg/d)	3.5–4.5	1.5 (healthy) 2–3 (critical illness)

[a] 0 to 3 mo (Daily Reference Intake): Estimated Energy Requirements (EER) = [89 × wt. (kg) – 100] + 175 kcal (EER = kcal/d).

As the infant demonstrates cues to feed by mouth, per oral feeds are attempted in small quantities. Early introduction of oral feeding reduces the chances of oral aversion and promotes safe suck–swallow cycle skills. Oral feeding also stimulates gall bladder contraction and release of luminal and pancreatic hormones, which promote digestion and gastrointestinal motility.[64]

The recommended energy and protein goals for complete EN in infants are given in **Table 4**. Although enteral autonomy is the ultimate goal, this should not be achieved at the expense of appropriate growth. The goals of nutritional support in infants with SBS must be tailored to promote appropriate growth parameters as measured by weight, head circumference, and length.

SUPPORTIVE STRATEGIES IN THE MANAGEMENT OF SHORT BOWEL SYNDROME
a. Mucous fistula refeeding

Mucus fistula refeeding (MFR) involves collecting proximal ostomy effluent and reinfusing it into the distal mucus fistula to mimic the physiologic transit of nutrients and stimulate digestion and absorption. In infants with ostomies, the likelihood of achieving sustained enteral autonomy without MFR is very challenging and hence low.[18] The MFR exposes the otherwise unused portion of the intestines and colon to enteral feeds, thereby stimulating and sustaining intestinal adaptation. The beneficial effects of MFR include an increase in weight gain, decreased electrolyte imbalance, decreased dependence on PN, and lower peak conjugated bilirubin levels.[65–67] More research is required to better define the short-term and long-term outcomes associated with MFR.

b. Cycling of parenteral nutrition

Once a steady metabolic state has been stabilized with a combination of parenteral and EN in infants with SBS, cycling of PN should be initiated.[68] Cycling PN has been shown to decrease the risk of hyperglycemia, hyperinsulinemia, hepatic steatosis, and IFALD.[64,69] However, the evidence to support the cycling of PN in the prevention of IFALD is weak. In a RCT, preterm infants who received cycling of PN did not demonstrate a reduction in IFALD.[70] Importantly, cycling of PN during the day encourages mobility, likely promoting neurodevelopment and improving quality of life.

c. Multidisciplinary care

Highly specialized multidisciplinary care of infants with SBS in a tertiary center has been shown to augment the likelihood of achieving enteral autonomy.[19,55,71] Multidisciplinary care brings together expertise from various specialties such as neonatology, surgery, gastroenterology, nursing, nutrition, pharmacy, and family support. Standardization of feeding regimens, medical therapies, surgical techniques, and nursing has improved survival and decreased morbidity. In a study conducted in Canada, the outcomes in SBS improved after the institution of multidisciplinary care. Multidisciplinary care involved standardization of feeding protocols, prophylactic antibiotics, lipid minimization, and the use of newer lipid emulsions. Following the adoption of multidisciplinary care, reduced mortality, improved rates of enteral autonomy, and reduced PN duration was observed.[71]

d. Medications

Advancement and tolerance of enteral feeds are often hindered by dysmotility, hypergastrinemia, and small intestinal bacterial overgrowth (SIBO). Hypergastrinemia and hypersecretion that can manifest with high gastric output and feeding intolerance have been shown to respond to H_2-blockers and proton pump inhibitors.[26,27] Gastroparesis and hypomotility of the small intestines have been treated with promotility agents such as erythromycin and amoxicillin-clavulanate, which act on the motilin receptors in the gastrointestinal tract and augment motility.[22,72] However, the evidence to support the use of these agents is of very low quality. In the only RCT, erythromycin failed to show significant benefits in patients with gastroschisis compared with placebo.[22] Amoxicillin-clavulanate acts on the duodenum and jejunum. Although there are very few studies of amoxicillin-clavulanate in infants with an intact gastrointestinal system,[73] there are no studies in infants with SBS. The antidopaminergic medications such as domperidone and metoclopramide, serotoninergic agents such as cisapride are used with caution due to their unfavorable side effects, including tardive dyskinesia and cardiac arrhythmia, respectively.[74,75] Opioid medications such as loperamide and diphenoxylate are used to decrease rapid intestinal transit in children and adults with SBS. SIBO is a common complication of SBS, exacerbated by hypomotility and stasis due to abnormal anatomy. Antibacterial agents such as metronidazole, amoxicillin-clavulanate, and trimethoprim-sulfamethoxazole are often used to treat SIBO.[76]

e. Probiotics

Probiotics are live microorganisms that present a beneficial effect on the host. In animal models with SBS, probiotics have increased villus length, crypt depth, and enterocyte count in the jejunum but not the ileum.[77] In rat models of SBS, *Saccharomyces boulardii* has been demonstrated to reduce bacterial translocation along with trophic effects on the mucosa.[78] In human subjects with SBS, reports of bacteremia with *Lactobacillus* GG strains present in the probiotic supplements have been described in two infants with SBS advising caution.[79] In another case series, four subjects with short bowel syndrome and central venous catheter developed *S. boulardii* fungemia following the treatment with probiotics containing these strains.[80] In a recent systematic review, the benefits of probiotics in infants and children with SBS were found to be inconsistent. Also, the adverse effects of lactobacillus bacteremia and lactic acidosis were observed. This leads us to conclude that the current data are insufficient to support the use of probiotics in infants and children with SBS.[81] In a small RCT of 18 children with SBS, lactobacillus probiotics did not result in a predictable change to the fecal microbiota or overall growth compared with placebo.[82]

Future directions

The advances in the past two decades in the nutritional management of SBS have improved outcomes tremendously. Survival rates are high, and the rates of intestinal and liver transplants are low. Although the mortality is low, morbidity remains high, stressing the need for improvements in the care of infants with SBS. Because residual bowel length is a crucial variable on the outcomes of infants with SBS, advances in surgical techniques resulting in retaining longer bowel lengths are needed. Although newer generation ILE has vastly improved the outcomes of infants with SBS, the search for the ideal ILE is not over.[83] Current development of the newer generation of ILE includes further depletion of phytosterols, enhancing antioxidant properties, and optimizing the ω3:ω6 ratio. The hope is to generate an ILE with the optimal balance of fatty acids, with reduced oxidative stress and an anti-inflammatory profile that promotes a better long-term neurodevelopmental outcome. The use of intestinal growth modulators such as Glucagon-like peptide 2 has not been adequately studied, particularly in infancy and can potentially improve outcomes significantly. In a 12-week long open-label study, infants and children who received teduglutide showed a reduction in PN volume, and an increase in tolerated enteral feed volume with no serious adverse effects.[84] In a recent study, teduglutide treatment resulted in clinically meaningful reductions in PN support in pediatric patients during 24 weeks of treatment.[85] The use of probiotics in infants with SBS deserves further study, notwithstanding the reports of bacteremia. The beneficial effects observed in preventing NEC and in animal models of SBS raise the possibility of similarly improved infant outcomes. The current treatment strategies are mainly experience-based rather than evidence-based. Hence, there is an urgent need to generate an evidence base to support the current practices of intestinal rehabilitation.

Best practices box

Best practice
- Initiation of enteral feeds soon after the return of bowel function
- Effective utilization of intravenous lipid emulsions (ILE) to prevent and treat intestinal failure-associated liver disease (IFALD)
- Interventions to minimize the risk of central line-associated bloodstream infections
- Highly specialized multidisciplinary care at an experienced center

What changes in current practice are likely to improve outcomes?
- Surgical strategies to maximize the length of the residual bowel and restoration of bowel function in short bowel syndrome (SBS)
- Next-generation ILE that are effective in the prevention and treatment of IFALD
- Develop evidence-based nutritional strategies, thus promoting standardization of practice
- Utilization of medications that promote the safe mucosal growth and function of intestines in SBS

Major Recommendations:
- Breast milk, if available, and elemental formula in the absence of breast milk as the choice of enteral nutrition (low-certainty evidence; strong recommendation)
- Multicomponent fish oil-containing ILE for the prevention of IFALD (very low-certainty evidence; weak recommendation)
- A 100% fish oil ILE for the treatment of IFALD (very low-certainty evidence; strong recommendation)
- Specialized multidisciplinary care in tertiary care centers (very low-certainty evidence; strong recommendation)

Summary Statement:
Aggressive and standardization of enteral nutritional strategies; hepatoprotective parenteral nutrition; protection from infection(s), and concomitant, close neurodevelopmental follow-up with appropriate, and timely interventions have improved the outcomes of infants with short bowel syndrome (SBS). There is a need for the continued development of evidence-based nutritional practices for the management of SBS and safe intravenous lipid emulsions that can help prevent/minimize intestinal failure-associated liver disease while supporting appropriate neurodevelopment.

Data from references [19,51–55,71]

DISCLOSURE

M.H. Premkumar is a consultant to Fresenius Kabi inc.

REFERENCES

1. Goulet O, Ruemmele F, Lacaille F, et al. Irreversible intestinal failure. J Pediatr Gastroenterol Nutr 2004;38(3):250–69.
2. Pironi L. Definitions of intestinal failure and the short bowel syndrome. Best Pract Res Clin Gastroenterol 2016;30(2):173–85.
3. Rickham PP. Massive small intestinal resection in newborn infants. Hunterian Lecture delivered at the royal college of Surgeons of england on 13th april 1967. Ann R Coll Surg Engl 1967;41(6):480–92.
4. Duggan CP, Jaksic T. Pediatric intestinal failure. N Engl J Med 2017;377(7): 666–75.
5. Squires RH, Duggan C, Teitelbaum DH, et al. Natural history of pediatric intestinal failure: initial report from the Pediatric Intestinal Failure Consortium. J Pediatr 2012;161(4):723–728 e2.
6. Han SM, Hong CR, Knell J, et al. Trends in incidence and outcomes of necrotizing enterocolitis over the last 12years: a multicenter cohort analysis. J Pediatr Surg 2020;55(6):998–1001.
7. Jones AM, Isenburg J, Salemi JL, et al. Increasing prevalence of gastroschisis– 14 states, 1995-2012. MMWR Morb Mortal Wkly Rep 2016;65(2):23–6.
8. Wales PW, de Silva N, Kim J, et al. Neonatal short bowel syndrome: population-based estimates of incidence and mortality rates. J Pediatr Surg 2004;39(5): 690–5.
9. Cole CR, Hansen NI, Higgins RD, et al, Eunice Kennedy Shriver NNRN. Very low birth weight preterm infants with surgical short bowel syndrome: incidence, morbidity and mortality, and growth outcomes at 18 to 22 months. Pediatrics 2008;122(3):e573–82.
10. Spiller RCB, S R, Silk DBA, et al. The ileal brake - a compensatory slowing of jejunal transit following ileal fat infusion in man. Clin Sci (London) 1983;64:53.
11. Van Citters GW, Lin HC. Ileal brake: neuropeptidergic control of intestinal transit. Curr Gastroenterol Rep 2006;8(5):367–73.
12. McClean P, Weaver LT. Ontogeny of human pancreatic exocrine function. Arch Dis Child 1993;68(1 Spec No):62–5.
13. Rao SSC, Bhagatwala J. Small intestinal bacterial overgrowth: clinical features and therapeutic management. Clin Transl Gastroenterol 2019;10(10):e00078.
14. Thiesen A, Drozdowski L, Iordache C, et al. Adaptation following intestinal resection: mechanisms and signals. Best Pract Res Clin Gastroenterol 2003;17(6): 981–95.
15. Cisler JJ, Buchman AL. Intestinal adaptation in short bowel syndrome. J Investig Med 2005;53(8):402–13.
16. Dowling RH, Booth CC. Structural and functional changes following small intestinal resection in the rat. Clin Sci 1967;32(1):139–49.
17. Maas C, Franz AR, von Krogh S, et al. Growth and morbidity of extremely preterm infants after early full enteral nutrition. Arch Dis Child Fetal Neonatal Ed 2018; 103(1):F79–81.
18. Smazal AL, Massieu LA, Gollins L, et al. Small proportion of low-birth-weight infants with ostomy and intestinal failure due to short-bowel syndrome achieve enteral autonomy prior to reanastomosis. JPEN J Parenter Enteral Nutr 2021; 45(2):331–8.

19. Belza C, Fitzgerald K, de Silva N, et al. Predicting intestinal adaptation in pediatric intestinal failure: a retrospective cohort study. Ann Surg 2019;269(5):988–93.
20. Fatemizadeh R, Gollins L, Hagan J, et al. In neonatal-onset surgical short bowel syndrome survival is high, and enteral autonomy is related to residual bowel length. JPEN J Parenter Enteral Nutr 2021. https://doi.org/10.1002/jpen.2124.
21. Fallon EM, Mitchell PD, Nehra D, et al. Neonates with short bowel syndrome: an optimistic future for parenteral nutrition independence. JAMA Surg 2014;149(7): 663–70.
22. Curry JI, Lander AD, Stringer MD, et al. A multicenter, randomized, double-blind, placebo-controlled trial of the prokinetic agent erythromycin in the postoperative recovery of infants with gastroschisis. J Pediatr Surg 2004;39(4):565–9.
23. Kato S, Takahashi A, Shindo M, et al. Characterization of the gastric motility response to human motilin and erythromycin in human motilin receptor-expressing transgenic mice. PLoS One 2019;14(2):e0205939.
24. Spiller RC, Trotman IF, Higgins BE, et al. The ileal brake–inhibition of jejunal motility after ileal fat perfusion in man. Gut 1984;25(4):365–74.
25. American Gastroenterological A. American Gastroenterological Association medical position statement: short bowel syndrome and intestinal transplantation. Gastroenterology 2003;124(4):1105–10.
26. Cortot A, Fleming CR, Malagelada JR. Improved nutrient absorption after cimetidine in short-bowel syndrome with gastric hypersecretion. N Engl J Med 1979; 300(2):79–80.
27. Jeppesen PB, Staun M, Tjellesen L, et al. Effect of intravenous ranitidine and omeprazole on intestinal absorption of water, sodium, and macronutrients in patients with intestinal resection. Gut 1998;43(6):763–9.
28. Gura K, Premkumar MH, Calkins KL, et al. Intravenous fish oil monotherapy as a source of calories and fatty acids promotes age-appropriate growth in pediatric patients with intestinal failure-associated liver disease. J Pediatr 2020;219: 98–105 e4.
29. Ubesie AC, Kocoshis SA, Mezoff AG, et al. Multiple micronutrient deficiencies among patients with intestinal failure during and after transition to enteral nutrition. J Pediatr 2013;163(6):1692–6.
30. Yang CF, Duro D, Zurakowski D, et al. High prevalence of multiple micronutrient deficiencies in children with intestinal failure: a longitudinal study. J Pediatr 2011; 159(1):39–44 e1.
31. Balay KS, Hawthorne KM, Hicks PD, et al. Low zinc status and absorption exist in infants with jejunostomies or ileostomies which persists after intestinal repair. Nutrients 2012;4(9):1273 81.
32. Vanek VW, Borum P, Buchman A, et al. A.S.P.E.N. position paper: recommendations for changes in commercially available parenteral multivitamin and multi-trace element products. Nutr Clin Pract 2012;27(4):440–91.
33. Joosten K, Embleton N, Yan W, et al, nutrition ESPGHAN/ESPEN/ESPR/CSPEN working group on pediatric parenteral nutrition. ESPGHAN/ESPEN/ESPR/CSPEN guidelines on pediatric parenteral nutrition: Energy. Clin Nutr 2018;37(6 Pt B): 2309–14.
34. Kleinman RE, Greer FR. Feeding the infant. In: Kleinman RE, editor. Pediatric nutrition. American Academy of Pediatrics; 2019. p. 113–62.
35. Mehta NM, Compher C, Directors ASPENBo. A.S.P.E.N. Clinical Guidelines: nutrition support of the critically ill child. JPEN J Parenter Enteral Nutr 2009;33(3): 260–76.

36. Kleinman RE, Greer FR. Feeding the infant. In: Kleinman RE, Greer FR, editors. Pediatric nutrition. American Academy of Pediatrics; 2019. p. 683–4.

37. Meurling S, Roos KA. Liver changes in rats on continuous and intermittent parenteral nutrition with and without fat (Intralipid 20%). Acta Chir Scand 1981;147(6): 475–80.

38. Lacaille F, Gupte G, Colomb V, et al. Intestinal failure-associated liver disease: a position paper of the ESPGHAN working group of intestinal failure and intestinal transplantation. J Pediatr Gastroenterol Nutr 2015;60(2):272–83.

39. Christensen RD, Henry E, Wiedmeier SE, et al. Identifying patients, on the first day of life, at high-risk of developing parenteral nutrition-associated liver disease. J Perinatol 2007;27(5):284–90.

40. Diamanti A, Basso MS, Castro M, et al. Prevalence of life-threatening complications in pediatric patients affected by intestinal failure. Transplant Proc 2007; 39(5):1632–3.

41. Cavicchi M, Beau P, Crenn P, et al. Prevalence of liver disease and contributing factors in patients receiving home parenteral nutrition for permanent intestinal failure. Ann Intern Med 2000;132(7):525–32.

42. Carter BA, Taylor OA, Prendergast DR, et al. Stigmasterol, a soy lipid-derived phytosterol, is an antagonist of the bile acid nuclear receptor FXR. Pediatr Res 2007;62(3):301–6.

43. Allardyce DB. Cholestasis caused by lipid emulsions. Surg Gynecol Obstet 1982; 154(5):641–7.

44. Colomb V, Jobert-Giraud A, Lacaille F, et al. Role of lipid emulsions in cholestasis associated with long-term parenteral nutrition in children. JPEN J Parenter Enteral Nutr 2000;24(6):345–50.

45. Cober MP, Killu G, Brattain A, et al. Intravenous fat emulsions reduction for patients with parenteral nutrition-associated liver disease. J Pediatr 2012;160(3): 421–7.

46. Calkins KL, Havranek T, Kelley-Quon LI, et al. Low-dose parenteral soybean oil for the prevention of parenteral nutrition-associated liver disease in neonates with gastrointestinal disorders. JPEN J Parenter Enteral Nutr 2017;41(3):404–11.

47. Levit OL, Calkins KL, Gibson LC, et al. Low-dose intravenous soybean oil emulsion for prevention of cholestasis in preterm neonates. JPEN J Parenter Enteral Nutr 2016;40(3):374–82.

48. Gura KM, Duggan CP, Collier SB, et al. Reversal of parenteral nutrition-associated liver disease in two infants with short bowel syndrome using parenteral fish oil: implications for future management. Pediatrics 2006;118(1): e197–201.

49. Gura KM, Premkumar MH, Calkins KL, et al. Fish oil emulsion reduces liver injury and liver transplantation in children with intestinal failure-associated liver disease: a multicenter Integrated study. J Pediatr 2021;230:46–54 e2.

50. Premkumar MH, Carter BA, Hawthorne KM, et al. High rates of resolution of cholestasis in parenteral nutrition-associated liver disease with fish oil-based lipid emulsion monotherapy. J Pediatr 2013;162(4):793–798 e1.

51. Kapoor V, Malviya MN, Soll R. Lipid emulsions for parenterally fed term and late preterm infants. Cochrane Database Syst Rev 2019;6:CD013171.

52. Kapoor V, Malviya MN, Soll R. Lipid emulsions for parenterally fed preterm infants. Cochrane Database Syst Rev 2019;6:CD013163.

53. Hojsak I, Colomb V, Braegger C, et al. ESPGHAN committee on nutrition position paper. intravenous lipid emulsions and risk of hepatotoxicity in infants and

children: a systematic review and meta-analysis. J Pediatr Gastroenterol Nutr 2016;62(5):776–92.

54. Lonnerdal B. Bioactive proteins in human milk-potential benefits for preterm infants. Clin Perinatol 2017;44(1):179–91.

55. Andorsky DJ, Lund DP, Lillehei CW, et al. Nutritional and other postoperative management of neonates with short bowel syndrome correlates with clinical outcomes. J Pediatr 2001;139(1):27–33.

56. Channabasappa N, Girouard S, Nguyen V, et al. Enteral nutrition in pediatric short-bowel syndrome. Nutr Clin Pract 2020;35(5):848–54.

57. Bach AC, Babayan VK. Medium-chain triglycerides: an update. Am J Clin Nutr 1982;36(5):950–62.

58. Vanderhoof JA. Short bowel syndrome in children and small intestinal transplantation. Pediatr Clin North Am 1996;43(2):533–50.

59. Parker P, Stroop S, Greene H. A controlled comparison of continuous versus intermittent feeding in the treatment of infants with intestinal disease. J Pediatr 1981; 99(3):360–4.

60. Rogers SP, Hicks PD, Hamzo M, et al. Continuous feedings of fortified human milk lead to nutrient losses of fat, calcium and phosphorous. Nutrients 2010;2(3): 230–40.

61. Rayyan M, Rommel N, Allegaert K. The fate of fat: pre-exposure fat losses during nasogastric tube feeding in preterm newborns. Nutrients 2015;7(8):6213–23.

62. Aynsley-Green A, Adrian TE, Bloom SR. Feeding and the development of enteroinsular hormone secretion in the preterm infant: effects of continuous gastric infusions of human milk compared with intermittent boluses. Acta Paediatr Scand 1982;71(3):379–83.

63. Ichimaru S. Methods of enteral nutrition administration in critically ill patients: continuous, cyclic, intermittent, and bolus feeding. Nutr Clin Pract 2018;33(6): 790–5.

64. Hwang TL, Lue MC, Chen LL. Early use of cyclic TPN prevents further deterioration of liver functions for the TPN patients with impaired liver function. Hepatogastroenterology 2000;47(35):1347–50.

65. Richardson L, Banerjee S, Rabe H. What is the evidence on the practice of mucous fistula refeeding in neonates with short bowel syndrome? J Pediatr Gastroenterol Nutr 2006;43(2):267–70.

66. Wong KK, Lan LC, Lin SC, et al. Mucous fistula refeeding in premature neonates with enterostomies. J Pediatr Gastroenterol Nutr 2004;39(1):43–5.

67. Yabe K, Kouchi K, Takenouchi A, et al. Safety and efficacy of mucous fistula refeeding in low-birth-weight infants with enterostomies. Pediatr Surg Int 2019; 35(10):1101–7.

68. Koletzko B, Goulet O, Hunt J, et al. 1. Guidelines on paediatric parenteral nutrition of the European Society of paediatric gastroenterology, Hepatology and nutrition (ESPGHAN) and the European Society for clinical nutrition and metabolism (ESPEN), supported by the European Society of paediatric research (ESPR). J Pediatr Gastroenterol Nutr 2005;41(Suppl 2):S1–87.

69. Jensen AR, Goldin AB, Koopmeiners JS, et al. The association of cyclic parenteral nutrition and decreased incidence of cholestatic liver disease in patients with gastroschisis. J Pediatr Surg 2009;44(1):183–9.

70. Salvador A, Janeczko M, Porat R, et al. Randomized controlled trial of early parenteral nutrition cycling to prevent cholestasis in very low birth weight infants. J Pediatr 2012;161(2):229–233 e1.

71. Sigalet D, Boctor D, Brindle M, et al. Elements of successful intestinal rehabilitation. J Pediatr Surg 2011;46(1):150–6.
72. Ng E, Shah VS. Erythromycin for the prevention and treatment of feeding intolerance in preterm infants. Cochrane Database Syst Rev 2008;(3):CD001815.
73. Gomez R, Fernandez S, Aspirot A, et al. Effect of amoxicillin/clavulanate on gastrointestinal motility in children. J Pediatr Gastroenterol Nutr 2012;54(6): 780–4.
74. Tolia V, Calhoun J, Kuhns L, et al. Randomized, prospective double-blind trial of metoclopramide and placebo for gastroesophageal reflux in infants. J Pediatr 1989;115(1):141–5.
75. Beattie DT, Smith JA. Serotonin pharmacology in the gastrointestinal tract: a review. Naunyn Schmiedebergs Arch Pharmacol 2008;377(3):181–203.
76. Kubota A, Okada A, Imura K, et al. The effect of metronidazole on TPN-associated liver dysfunction in neonates. J Pediatr Surg 1990;25(6):618–21.
77. Tolga Muftuoglu MA, Civak T, Cetin S, et al. Effects of probiotics on experimental short-bowel syndrome. Am J Surg 2011;202(4):461–8.
78. Mogilner JG, Srugo I, Lurie M, et al. Effect of probiotics on intestinal regrowth and bacterial translocation after massive small bowel resection in a rat. J Pediatr Surg 2007;42(8):1365–71.
79. Kunz AN, Noel JM, Fairchok MP. Two cases of Lactobacillus bacteremia during probiotic treatment of short gut syndrome. J Pediatr Gastroenterol Nutr 2004; 38(4):457–8.
80. Hennequin C, Kauffmann-Lacroix C, Jobert A, et al. Possible role of catheters in Saccharomyces boulardii fungemia. Eur J Clin Microbiol Infect Dis 2000;19(1): 16–20.
81. Reddy VS, Patole SK, Rao S. Role of probiotics in short bowel syndrome in infants and children–a systematic review. Nutrients 2013;5(3):679–99.
82. Piper HG, Coughlin LA, Hussain S, et al. The impact of lactobacillus probiotics on the gut microbiota in children with short bowel syndrome. J Surg Res 2020;251: 112–8.
83. Premkumar MH, Calkins KL. A neonatologist's perspective: is the quest for an "ideal" lipid emulsion over? JPEN J Parenter Enteral Nutr 2018;42(1):12–3.
84. Carter BA, Cohran VC, Cole CR, et al. Outcomes from a 12-week, open-label, multicenter clinical trial of teduglutide in pediatric short bowel syndrome. J Pediatr 2017;181:102–111 e5.
85. Kocoshis SA, Merritt RJ, Hill S, et al. Safety and efficacy of teduglutide in pediatric patients with intestinal failure due to short bowel syndrome: a 24-week, phase III study. JPEN J Parenter Enteral Nutr 2020;44(4):621–31.

Moving?

Make sure your subscription moves with you!

To notify us of your new address, find your **Clinics Account Number** (located on your mailing label above your name), and contact customer service at:

Email: journalscustomerservice-usa@elsevier.com

800-654-2452 (subscribers in the U.S. & Canada)
314-447-8871 (subscribers outside of the U.S. & Canada)

Fax number: 314-447-8029

Elsevier Health Sciences Division
Subscription Customer Service
3251 Riverport Lane
Maryland Heights, MO 63043

*To ensure uninterrupted delivery of your subscription, please notify us at least 4 weeks in advance of move.

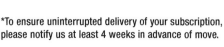

Printed and bound by CPI Group (UK) Ltd, Croydon, CR0 4YY

03/10/2024

01040469-0008